SKIN CANCER PREVENTION

SKIN CANCER PREVENTION

Edited by

Ulrik Ringborg
Karolinska Institute
Karolinska University Hospital Solna
Stockholm, Sweden

Yvonne Brandberg
Karolinska Institute
Karolinska University Hospital Solna
Stockholm, Sweden

Eckhard W. Breitbart
Center of Dermatology
Buxtehude, Germany

Rudiger Greinert
Center of Dermatology
Buxtehude, Germany

informa
healthcare

New York   London

Informa Healthcare USA, Inc.
270 Madison Avenue
New York, NY 10016

© 2007 by Informa Healthcare USA, Inc.
Informa Healthcare is an Informa business

No claim to original U.S. Government works
Printed in the United States of America on acid-free paper
10 9 8 7 6 5 4 3 2 1

International Standard Book Number-10: 0-8493-9889-4 (Hardcover)
International Standard Book Number-13: 978-0-8493-9889-6 (Hardcover)

Visit the Informa Web site at
www.informa.com

and the Informa Healthcare Web site at
www.informahealthcare.com

Preface

The increase in the cancer incidence has created a problem worldwide. Skin cancer is an important part of the problem. In countries with a white population there is an increasing incidence of cutaneous malignant melanoma as well as squamous cell and basal cell carcinoma. Skin cancer overall, including both malignant melanoma and nonmelanoma skin cancer, is the most frequent tumor type, resulting in decreased quality of life for patients and relatives as well as increasing health economy costs. In addition to the burden of skin cancer on morbidity, mortality is a consequence of cutaneous malignant melanoma including young individuals.

Prevention is an important strategy for reducing the cancer problem. For skin cancer, risk factors have been identified, making it possible to identify individuals at increased risk and behaviors that decrease both mortality and morbidity. Ultraviolet radiation, both from the sun and artificial ultraviolet sources, is the most important external risk factor for all three types of skin cancer. Over time more information about constitutional risk factors has been generated, among which the genetic background of the familial aggregation of skin cancer will significantly improve the identification of high-risk individuals. Early detection, no doubt, is a powerful tool for the improvement of prognosis for patients with cutaneous malignant melanoma. In this respect, understanding tumor progression and identification of precursor lesions most probably will improve prevention. Thus, both primary prevention and early detection are powerful strategies for decreasing mortality and morbidity as well as increasing the quality of life and cost-effectiveness in the skin cancer area.

The aim of this book is a comprehensive review of skin cancer prevention. Epidemiology gives us information about the extent of the problem and identifies the risk factors for skin cancer (external behavioral and constitutional). An expanding knowledge in the basic research area creates new possibilities for developing more effective prevention strategies. An important question is whether all ultraviolet radiation is harmful, or if lower doses are beneficial. Relationships between knowledge, attitudes and behavior are complex and we need more research in order to establish effective primary prevention aiming at behavioral change. Whether screening strategies are rational for early detection is another question yet to be answered. Communication strategies are crucial when conveying health messages and must be elaborated in different ways depending on the target population. The knowledge of the cost-effectiveness of skin cancer prevention programs is however limited, and must be studied in more detail.

A comprehensive view of skin cancer prevention shows the importance of developing translational research in order to establish evidence-based prevention. We hope this book will stimulate thinking to proceed in this direction.

The book editors are members of the European Society of Skin Cancer Prevention (EUROSKIN), an organization formed in 1999. An important mission for EUROSKIN is to harmonize skin cancer prevention in Europe. So far four international conferences have been arranged with the aim of improving communication among epidemiologists and basic researchers with researchers and actors in prevention programs to establish translational research in this area. The ultimate aim is to develop evidence-based and cost effective skin cancer prevention. We hope that this book will help us to move into this direction.

Ulrik Ringborg
Yvonne Brandberg
Eckhard W. Breitbart
Rudiger Greinert

Contents

v

Contributors

Honnavara N. Ananthaswamy   Department of Immunology, The University of Texas MD Anderson Cancer Center, Houston, Texas, U.S.A.

Philippe Autier   International Agency for Research on Cancer, Lyon, France

Chris D. Bajdik   Cancer Control Research Program, British Columbia Cancer Agency, Vancouver, and Department of Health Care and Epidemiology, University of British Columbia, Vancouver, British Columbia, Canada

Frederick C. Beddingfield   Department of Medicine, Division of Dermatology, David Geffen School of Medicine at UCLA, Los Angeles, California, U.S.A.

Cara L. Benjamin   Department of Immunology, The University of Texas MD Anderson Cancer Center, Houston, Texas, U.S.A.

Cecilia Boldemann   Center for Public Health, Stockholm County Council, Stockholm, Sweden

Mathieu Boniol   International Agency for Research on Cancer, Lyon, France

Peter Boyle   International Agency for Research on Cancer, Lyon, France

Richard Bränström   Department of Oncology-Pathology, Karolinska Institute, Stockholm, Sweden

Eckhard W. Breitbart   Center of Dermatology, Elbe Kliniken, Klinikum Buxtehude, Buxtehude, Germany

Jean-Pierre Césarini   Agence Française de Sécurité Sanitaire de l'Environnement et du Travail—Unité Agents Physiques, Maisons-Alfort, France

Marie-Christine Chignol   INSERM Unit 590, Centre Léon Bérard, Lyon, France

James E. Cleaver   Department of Dermatology and UCSF Cancer Center, University of California San Francisco, San Francisco, California, U.S.A.

Arne Dahlback   Department of Physics, University of Oslo, Oslo, Norway

Jean-François Doré   International Agency for Research on Cancer and INSERM Unit 590, Centre Léon Bérard, Lyon, France

David E. Elder   Department of Pathology and Laboratory Medicine, Hospital of the University of Pennsylvania, Philadelphia, Pennsylvania, U.S.A.

Richard P. Gallagher   Division of Dermatology and Cancer Control Research Program, British Columbia Cancer Agency, and Department of Health Care and Epidemiology, University of British Columbia, Vancouver, British Columbia, Canada

Alan C. Geller   Department of Dermatology, School of Medicine, School of Public Health, Boston University, Boston, Massachusetts, U.S.A.

Karen Glanz   Department of Behavioral Sciences and Health Education, Rollins School of Public Health, Emory University, Atlanta, Georgia, U.S.A.

Rudiger Greinert   Center of Dermatology, Elbe Kliniken, Klinikum Buxtehude, Buxtehude, Germany

Johan Hansson   Department of Oncology-Pathology, Karolinska Institute and Karolinska University Hospital Solna, Stockholm, Sweden

Meenhard Herlyn   Program in Molecular and Cellular Oncogenesis, The Wistar Institute, Philadelphia, Pennsylvania, U.S.A.

Michael F. Holick   Boston University Medical Center, Boston, Massachusetts, U.S.A.

Gunilla Jarlbro   Media and Communication Studies, Lund University, Lund, Sweden

Bengt Jönsson   Stockholm School of Economics, Center for Health Economics, Stockholm, Sweden

Steven Kazianis   Program in Molecular and Cellular Oncogenesis, The Wistar Institute, Philadelphia, Pennsylvania, U.S.A.

Nigel Kirkham   Department of Cellular Pathology, Royal Victoria Infirmary, Newcastle upon Tyne, U.K.

Rajiv Kumar   Division of Molecular Genetic Epidemiology, German Cancer Research Center, Heidelberg, Germany and Department of Bioscience, Karolinska Institute, Huddinge, Sweden

Tim K. Lee   Cancer Control Research Program, British Columbia Cancer Agency, Vancouver, and School of Computing Sciences, Simon Fraser University, Burnaby, British Columbia, Canada

David L. Mitchell   Department of Carcinogenesis, The University of Texas MD Anderson Cancer Center, Science Park—Research Division, Smithville, Texas, U.S.A.

Johan Moan   Department of Radiation Biology, Institute for Cancer Research, Montebello and Department of Physics, University of Oslo, Oslo, Norway

Alina Carmen Porojnicu   Department of Radiation Biology, Institute for Cancer Research, Montebello, Oslo, Norway and Department of Biophysics and Cell Biotechnology, Carol Davila University of Medicine and Pharmacy, Bucharest, Romania

Eva Rehfuess   Department of Public Health and Environment, World Health Organization, Geneva, Switzerland

Ulrik Ringborg   Department of Oncology-Pathology, Karolinska Institute and Karolinska University Hospital Solna, Stockholm, Sweden

Craig Sinclair   The Cancer Council Victoria, Carlton, Victoria, Australia

David H. Sliney   U.S. Army Center for Health Promotion and Preventive Medicine, Aberdeen Proving Ground, Maryland, U.S.A.

Michel Smans   International Agency for Research on Cancer, Lyon, France

Ulf Staginnus   European Health Economics, Madrid, Spain

B. Volkmer   Center of Dermatology, Elbe Kliniken, Klinikum Buxtehude, Buxtehude, Germany

S. Welz   Commentum Public Relations, Hamburg, Germany

Photobiology of Photocarcinogenesis

David L. Mitchell

Department of Carcinogenesis, The University of Texas MD Anderson Cancer Center, Science Park—Research Division, Smithville, Texas, U.S.A.

James E. Cleaver

Department of Dermatology and UCSF Cancer Center, University of California San Francisco, San Francisco, California, U.S.A.

INTRODUCTION—THE PROBLEM

Numerous studies have indicated an alarming increase in melanoma and non-melanoma skin cancer in Europe over the past two decades (1,2). Epidemiological and laboratory studies provide evidence for a direct causal role of sunlight exposure in the induction of skin cancer (3,4), and the high rate of skin carcinogenesis is a direct result of the high dose rate from the ultraviolet radiation (UVR) component. Both basal and squamous cell carcinomas (BCCs and SCCs, respectively) are found on sun-exposed parts of the body (e.g., the face and trunk in men, face and legs in women), and their incidence is correlated with cumulative sunlight exposure. Several lines of evidence support this conclusion: (*i*) tumor incidence and mortality increase with decreasing latitude, corresponding to exposure, (*ii*) skin cancers are less frequent in dark-skinned populations than in lighter-skinned peoples, owing to dose reduction and photoprotection afforded by skin pigmentation (i.e., melanin), and (*iii*) skin cancer increases with recreational (5) and occupational exposures, such as in ranchers and fishermen (6,7). Melanoma, although also associated with sunlight exposure, shows a weaker dependence on total exposure to sunlight and a distribution over the body that is not correlated to exposed areas but is more closely related to intermittent exposures and sunburn in childhood (8). There may be solar-dependent and -independent pathways for melanoma.

Exposure to direct sunlight in the mid-U.S. latitudes results in the accumulation of a mean lethal dose to unprotected human cells within approximately 30 minutes (9). The only other human carcinogen that even approaches these exposure levels would be cigarette smoke in very heavy smokers. Variations in individual susceptibility are also clearly observed in skin carcinogenesis. Human skin can be classified into types I–IV, ranging from individuals who always burn and never tan, to those who tan but never burn; skin cancer susceptibility varies accordingly (10). The most dramatic examples of variations in human susceptibility occur in certain human genetic disorders, especially xeroderma pigmentosum (XP), Cockayne syndrome (CS), trichothiodystrophy (TTD), basal cell nevus syndrome (BCNS), the porphyrias, and phenylketonuria (11). Sunlight exposure also has a major immunosuppressive effect leading to loss of antigen-presenting Langerhans cells and the appearance of dyskeratotic keratinocytes (apoptotic sunburn cells) in the upper epidermis, together with the erythemal sunburn response associated with vasodilation caused by a release of prostaglandin (12). Immunosuppression in organ transplant and HIV patients also increases skin cancer incidence (13).

UVR damage in cellular DNA can be resolved in several different ways (Fig. 1) depending on the type of lesion produced, the genomic location of the damage, the type of cell affected, and the developmental state of the cell. It is plausible that some lesions are not perceived as different from normal DNA by the cell. However, it is more probable that, unless the damage is repaired, it will disrupt the normal operation of vital cellular processes such as DNA replication or transcription. In this event, cell proliferation will cease or, if the lesion is situated in a gene required for an essential metabolic function, the cell will die.

Some types of photodamage are more effective than others at blocking the progression of DNA or RNA polymerases. Types of DNA damage that facilitate lesion bypass by the replication machinery may allow misincorporation of an incorrect complementary base, thus producing a mutation. A mutation may have several outcomes: (*i*) it may be benign, neither altering the genetic code nor affecting normal metabolism, (*ii*) it may create a truncated or partial RNA transcript and a dysfunctional protein; if the protein is essential, then the mutation is lethal, and (*iii*) finally, it may result in activation of an oncogene or inactivation of a tumor suppressor gene, resulting in the initiation of cell transformation and carcinogenesis. Although a direct role of DNA damage in replication and transcription is well-documented, other pathways in which DNA damage can affect cell fate and metabolism have been described and operate through various signal transduction pathways. For instance, DNA damage in the skin resulting from extended exposure to solar UVR is implicated in immunosuppression, erythema (sunburn), and photoaging.

The UVR component of sunlight is the major environmental agent that precipitates the clinical symptoms of skin carcinogenesis. This is well established for

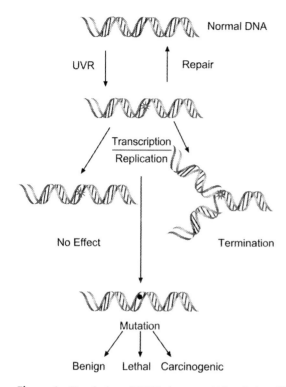

Figure 1 Resolution of DNA damage. *Abbreviation*: UVR, ultraviolet radiation.

SCC and BCC but still controversial for melanoma (14–16). Nonmelanoma skin cancers are by far the most common cancers (17,18), comprising 30% to 40% of all cancers and showing a significant increase over the past 100 years (19,20). As a consequence, there is a wealth of human epidemiological data on skin cancer risks that are associated with geographical locations, skin type, and various photosensitizing, enhancing, and protective applications (4,6,20–24). There is also a possibility of greater risk when the exposure is received during childhood and adolescence (4,25). Nonmelanoma skin cancer is therefore one of the few malignancies for which there is clear evidence for the identification of the initiating agent. The relationship of melanoma to sun exposure and the possible action spectrum are less clear (14), but may be related to acute burns rather than accumulated dose (4). Neonatal sunburn in mice can induce melanoma, but not exposures later in life (16). Over the past few years, the importance of ultraviolet-A (UVA) in skin cancer etiology has become an important question, particularly with the emergence of the artificial tanning industry that relies heavily on lamps emitting UVA wavelengths. Through the course of this introductory chapter, the molecular biology and biological effects of UVA and ultraviolet-B (UVB) will be compared with respect to their potential roles in the early stages of carcinoma and melanoma formation.

PHOTOCHEMISTRY OF DNA IN THE SKIN

The sun emits a broad array of energies at wavelengths ranging through 11 orders of magnitude from 1 nm to 100 m. Much of this energy is biologically irrelevant; long wavelength, low-energy emissions such as far infrared and microwaves are highly unlikely to impart sufficient energy to influence biochemical reactions. Likewise, visible and near infrared wavelengths, although very important for vision and photosynthesis, are not considered hazardous to living organisms. Finally, ionizing radiations such as high-energy particles, X rays, and gamma rays are expended by atomic collisions in the upper atmosphere. Hence, UVR emerges as the most biologically relevant component of the solar spectrum with respect to DNA damage.

UVR is divided into three spectral regions: ultraviolet-C (UVC) (240–290 nm), UVB (290–320 nm), and UVA (320–400 nm) (Fig. 2). Because of their high energies and availability, germicidal (UVC) lamps have historically been used for basic research studies in photobiology. However, as the earth's atmosphere absorbs UVR wavelengths below 295 to 300 nm, other components of the solar spectrum, such as UVB and UVA, are of much more concern. Although the UVA and UVB constitute a negligible portion of the sun's energy, they are primarily responsible for the pathological effects of solar radiation. For this reason, recent research has been directed more toward characterizing DNA damages produced by these biologically relevant solar wavelengths.

Photon absorption rapidly converts a pyrimidine base to an excited state (Fig. 3) (26). This event promotes an electron in a filled bonding π orbital in the singlet ground state into a higher-energy, empty π^* anti-bonding orbital, thus initiating photoproduct formation. Formation of an excited base occurs within 10^{-12} seconds after photon absorption. Various pathways are then available for resolution of this unstable electronic configuration. The major pathway involves rapid dissipation of the energy of the excited singlet base to the ground state (10^{-9} seconds) by non-radiative transition or by fluorescence, yielding heat or light in the process. Second, the excited base can react with other molecules to form unstable intermediates (i.e., free radicals) or stable photoproducts. Finally, there is a low probability that intersystem crossing, a non-radiative pathway, can transfer a base from the excited singlet state to the excited triplet state. The

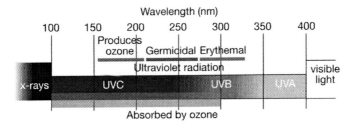

Figure 2 Ultraviolet spectrum.

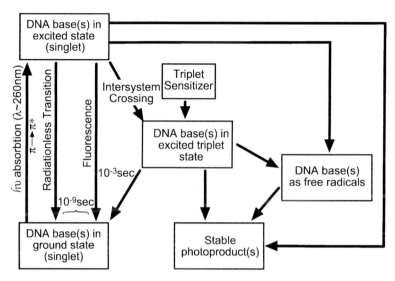

Figure 3 Photochemistry of DNA damage.

lifetime of the triplet state is several orders of magnitude longer than the excited singlet state (10^{-3} seconds), increasing the chance of photoproduct formation. Formation of the triplet state can be greatly enhanced in the presence of sensitizers such as acetone or acetophenone.

The most abundant photoproduct induced by UVR is the cyclobutane pyrimidine dimer (CPD) linked by a cyclobutyl ring between the five and six carbons of adjacent thymine (T) or cytosine (C) bases (Fig. 4 and Table 1). The CPD forms through the excited triplet state; other photoproducts form by other mechanisms. Of the four possible CPD combinations (T <> T, C <> T, T <> C, and C <> C), the T <> T dimer occurs with greatest frequency in 40% to 60% of the sum of cytosine-containing dimers. At wavelengths above 300 nm, photochemical alterations of cytosine, rather than thymine, may account for most biological effects. The pyrimidine (6–4)pyrimidone dimer [(6–4)PD] is the second most prevalent type of UV damage, occurring at a significant frequency compared to the CPD. In this photoproduct, the sixth carbon of a 3′ pyrimidine (either cytosine or thymine) is linked to the fourth carbon of a 5′ pyrimidine (primarily cytosine) by way of an unstable oxetane or azetidine intermediate. Unlike CPDs, the formation of (6–4)PDs does not proceed via an excited triplet state (Fig. 3), hence is less dependent on the photochemical behavior of thymine bases in DNA. Infrared spectroscopic and nuclear magnetic resonance analyses of the (6–4)PD indicate that the plane of the 3′ cytosine base is shifted 90° relative to the 5′ thymine. As shown in the reaction scheme for dimer formation (Fig. 4), absorption of UVB light by the (6–4)PD results in formation of a structurally related photoisomer, the Dewar pyrimidinone.

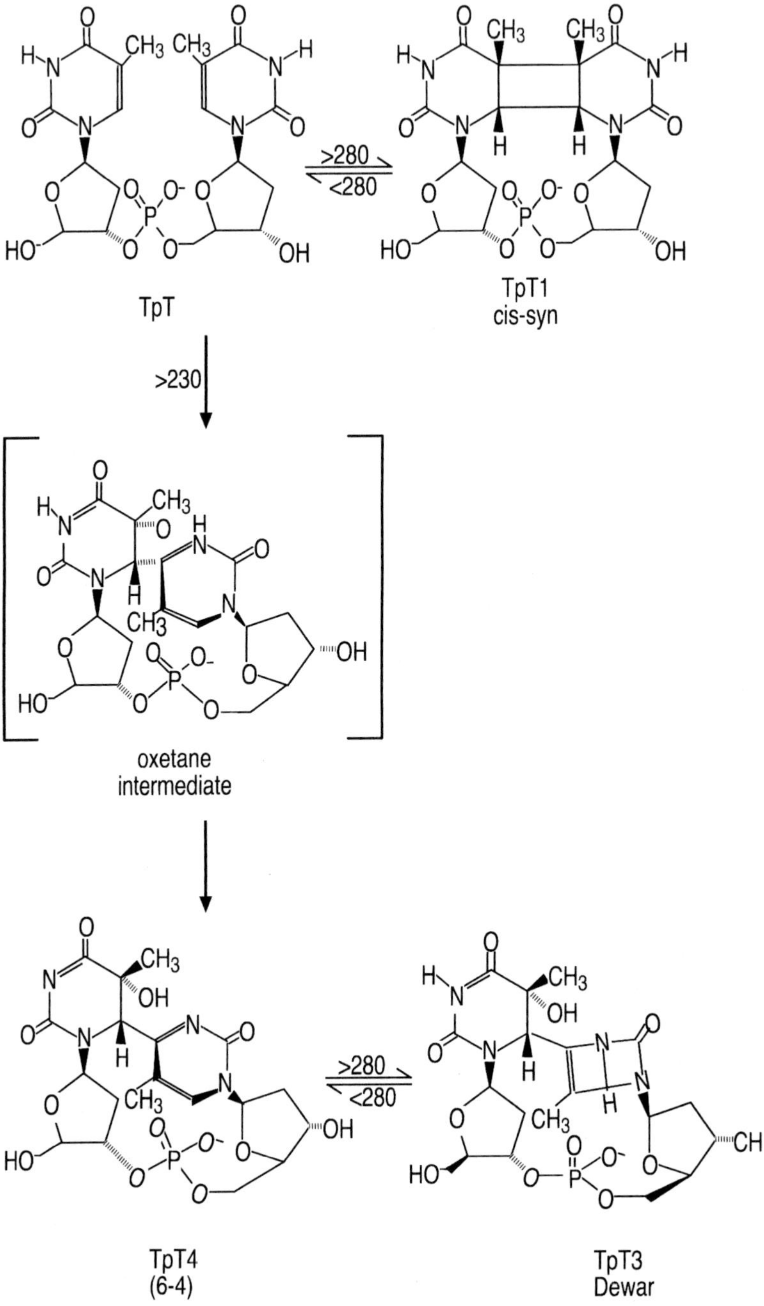

Figure 4   Reaction scheme for pyrimidine dimer formation.

Table 1 Distribution of Pyrimidine Dimers in CHO DNA Exposed to UVB, UVA and SSL Expressed as Lesions in 10^6 Bases DNA

	UVB (per J/m^2)	UVA (per kJ/m^2)	SSL (per kJ/m^2)
TT CPD	0.0175	0.0192	0.0159
TC CPD	0.0139	0.0012	0.0062
CC CPD	0.0012	0.0001	0.0006
TT (6–4)PD	0.0017	n.d.	0.0001
TC (6–4)PD	0.0143	n.d.	0.0021
TT Dewar	n.d.	n.d.	0.0009
TC Dewar	n.d.	n.d.	0.0037

Abbreviations: T, thymine; C, cytosine; CPD, cyclobutane pyrimidene dimer; PD, pyrimidine dimer; CHO, Chinese hamster ovary. *Source*: From Ref. 27.

Recently, a very thorough study comparing the relative induction rates of the major dimeric photoproducts in DNA has been published (27). In this work, high-performance liquid chromatography–tandem mass spectrometry was used to quantify CPDs, (6–4) PDs, and Dewar photoproducts in the same sample DNA extracted from Chinese hamster ovary (CHO) cells exposed to UVB, UVA, or solar-simulated sunlight (SSL). In Table 1, the frequencies are shown as lesions induced per joule (for UVB) or kilojoule (for UVA and SSL) in 10^6 bases of DNA. Several patterns are noteworthy. First, the predominant photoproducts produced by UVB at comparable levels are the TT CPD, TC CPD, and TC (6–4)PD, the latter two of which are considered the probable sources of the UVB signature mutations observed in skin tumors. Second, although the TT CPD and TC CPD are induced at considerably lower rates by UVA and SSL compared to UVB (note the 10^3-fold difference in dose), they do occur at sufficiently high frequencies to justify significant roles in the biological effects of these wavelengths, particularly considering the overwhelming proportion of UVA compared to UVB in the solar spectrum. Third, the Dewar pyrimidinone, although not observed after exposure to narrow-band UVA or UVB, is significantly induced by simulated (and presumably natural) sunlight.

Compared to photoproducts involving two pyrimidines, those involving a single base occur in DNA at very low frequencies (0.1–2.0% of dimers) after exposure to UVR. Because of its instability, the photobiology of the cytosine photohydrate has been difficult to study using the conventional analytical procedures for quantifying DNA damage. It should be kept in mind, however, that the half-life of the cytosine photohydrate is not trivial (i.e., 24 hours at room temperature), and this lesion may indeed pose a viable biological threat to a proliferating cell system. Recent data using sequencing analysis indicate that saturated thymine photoproducts, such as the thymine glycol, do not occur in UVC- or UVB-irradiated DNA at a significant rate, and hence, do not appear to contribute significantly to the biological effects of UVR. In contrast to the induction of DNA damage resulting from the direct absorption of UVC light, UVA and UVB may produce damage indirectly through highly reactive chemical intermediates. Similar to ionizing radiation, these wavelengths generate reactive oxygen species that can form, for example, singlet oxygen, hydroxyl and peroxyl radicals, and superoxide anions which in turn can react with DNA to form single base damage, such as 8-oxodeoxyguanosine, as well as strand breaks and DNA–protein crosslinks. Although the number of cytosine photohydrates compared to CPDs and (6–4)PDs remains constant throughout the UVR, the relative proportion of single-strand breaks and protein–DNA crosslinks increases significantly in DNA irradiated with UVB and UVA light. It should be kept in mind that the relationship between photoproduct frequency and biological effectiveness depends on the intrinsic capability of that lesion to kill cells or induce mutations. Hence, even though a photoproduct may occur at a very low frequency (e.g., the cytosine photohydrate or Dewar pyrimidinone), its structure and location may elicit a potent biological effect.

DNA DAMAGE AND SKIN CANCER

The idea that DNA damage is an essential component of photocarcinogenesis arose from the discovery that cells from patients suffering from XP are deficient in DNA repair (28). In this disease, a failure in one cellular protective mechanism, DNA repair, is associated with a major increase in the rate of onset of SCC, BCC, and melanoma (11). Median onset for skin cancer in the general U.S. population occurs at 50 to 60 years of age. In contrast, in XP patients, carcinogenesis is accelerated and median onset is within the first decade. This early onset is a direct consequence of sunlight-induced changes in DNA of skin cells and the inability to rectify these changes.

Nucleotide excision repair (NER) is the most important repair process concerned with UV damage in humans. Two major pathways of NER are known: transcription-coupled repair (TCR) and global genome repair (GGR) (Fig. 5). These NER pathways remove dimeric damage in DNA [e.g., CPDs and (6–4)PDs] caused by UVR as well as large chemically induced adducts and replace the damaged site with a newly synthesized polynucleotide patch approximately 29 bases in length (29,30). TCR removes damage more rapidly from the transcribed strands of transcriptionally-active genes, whereas GGR acts more slowly on non-transcribed regions (31) and is regulated by p53 through control of XPC and XPE (p48) expression (32).

NER requires a temporary relaxation of the nucleosomal structure such that the damaged regions are more accessible to exogenous nucleases. The continuous excision and re-synthesis of DNA is associated with a very low net frequency of DNA strand breaks, no more than about 1 in 3×10^5 DNA bases. Only about 1% of the CPDs produced in DNA are therefore being excised at any given time, but it takes only minutes to complete repair of an individual lesion. Excision, therefore, sets up a dynamic balance between strand breakage and rejoining, and is rate limited by the enzymes involved in the early steps of repair.

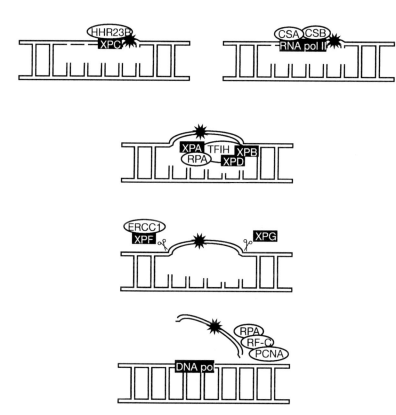

Figure 5 Nucleotide excision repair pathways.

Excision repair is a heterogeneous process both between species and within the genome. There is considerable difference between the rates of CPD and (6–4)PD excision from the overall genome of rodent and human fibroblasts and skin (33), even though the basic mechanisms and patch sizes are essentially the same (34). (6–4)PDs are more rapidly excised with 50% removed from human and rodent cells in two to six hours. CPDs are much more slowly repaired with 50% of the lesions removed from human cell DNA in 12 to 24 hours (35,36). The excision of CPDs may be partly delayed because the strong affinity of the excision system for (6–4)PDs initially sequesters available enzymes. There are also large variations in CPD excision between human subjects (36). The different rates of excision may reflect the fact that (6–4)PDs are considerably more distortive in DNA and are preferentially located in internucleosomal regions of DNA, which can lead to differences in binding between the damage recognition proteins and the lesion.

Additional variation in CPD repair occurs on an individual gene basis according to transcriptional activity (37). An increased excision rate in active genes (TCR) is also observed for (6–4)PDs (38), but this is less pronounced due to the greater overall rate of excision of these photoproducts in the genome as a whole. The differences in excision from active versus inactive genes occur because a basal transcription factor, TFIIH, and two gene products, CSA and CSB, regulate both basal transcription and the bypass of damage by RNA polymerase II (39,40). A detailed study of the promoter and first exons of the *PGK1* gene has indicated that excision is slow in regions of promoter binding but increases immediately after the transcription start site (41). Many of the genes that regulate TCR are associated with the human disorders XP, CS, TTD, and others. Two of the helicases in TFIIH correspond to the *XPB* and *XPD* genes. TCR also involves the CS genes *CSA* & *CSB*, *XPG* (42), and the mismatch repair (MMR) gene *MLH2* (43).

Evidence is accumulating suggesting that in addition to repairing replication errors, the MMR system may also be involved in other pathways affecting skin cancer etiology, including cell cycle arrest, apoptosis, and even NER. Double knockout mice for the *msh2* gene (the *Escherichia coli* mutS homolog that recognizes and binds G/T mismatches), coupled with either $XPC^{-/-}$ or $XPA^{-/-}$ deficiency, show an increased susceptibility to UVB-induced skin cancer, significantly greater than the single knockouts (44,45). In addition, cell lines derived from $XPA^{-/-}$ UVB-induced skin tumors show truncated cell cycle arrest with reduced apoptosis and MMR (45). It has been suggested that an MMR heterodimer containing msh2 may actually sense UV damage and influence the initiation of apoptosis (and NER) (46,47). Mouse embryonic fibroblasts derived from *msh2* knockouts show reduced apoptosis and higher skin cancer rates in response to UVB (48). It was intriguing that higher levels of residual DNA damage were observed in the knockout mice 24 hours after exposure, suggesting that msh2 plays a role in NER.

MECHANISMS OF SUNLIGHT MUTAGENESIS

Most types of photoproducts block the progression of replicative class B polymerases, including Pol A, D, and E. Depending on their structures, many photoproducts are, however, bypassed to different degrees during DNA replication by damage-specific class Y DNA polymerases including Pol H, I, and K that have low fidelities due to expanded active sites that facilitate read-through of non-informative sequence information (e.g., abasic sites). Pol H has the greatest capacity to replicate a large variety of DNA lesions and preferentially inserts adenine in the nascent strand opposite to the lesion (called the "A rule"). Pol I preferentially inserts guanine and is capable of replicating C-containing photoproducts. Pol H or I therefore can insert bases opposite to dipyrimidine photoproducts with the potential that the 3' complementary base may be mismatched either by an erroneous insertion or the distortion caused by the photoproduct. The absence of Pol H results in increased mutagenesis and has the most recognizable pathological consequence in the XP variant complementation group.

This mechanism has two important implications regarding the mutagenicity of different photoproducts. First, mutations will most often occur where cytosine is a component of the photoproduct since insertion of adenine opposite to thymine is a correct and non-mutagenic event. Hence, most CPDs, because they are formed between two thymine bases, are not mutagenic. Second, the more distortive a lesion is, the more likely it will block DNA synthesis and result in a lethal rather than mutagenic event. Since the $(6-4)$PD is considerably more distortive than the CPD (i.e., it causes a $47°$ as opposed to a $7°$ helical bend), it is more likely to be lethal rather than mutagenic. Because damage bypass and base insertion depend on a variety of conditions, both CPDs and $(6-4)$PDs contribute to tumorigenesis in a complex manner.

A comparison of photoproduct yields, rates of repair, and mutations in the *PGK1* and *p53* genes has shown that regions of high UV-induced mutation can be caused by high photoproduct yield and/or low repair. A combination of initial yields and rates of repair that leave a high net persistent load of photoproducts in a particular site appear to be directly related to the mutational yield. Using ligation-mediated polymerase chain reaction that allows precise location of damaged bases, the photoproduct distribution in exons 1 and 2 of three *ras* proto-oncogenes was mapped and no correlation between photoproduct frequency and mutation induction in codon 12 of H-*ras* and K-*ras* was found. DNA repair at individual nucleotides in the *p53* tumor-suppressor gene was highly variable and sequence dependent with slow repair observed at seven of eight of the positions associated with mutations. UV-induced mutations in the *p53* gene are a probable step in the formation of SCC and may arise at DNA repair "cold spots" rather than photoproduct "hot spots."

Additional work by Pfeifer and colleagues has shed considerable light on the fine structure and mechanisms of mutagenesis in human cells and the relative importance of UVA and UVB in affecting these DNA changes [for review, see (49)]. Of particular interest is the effect methylation has on mutagenesis. 5-Methylcytosine (5-^{m}Cyt) occurs almost exclusively at CpG sequences, which are known mutation hotspots in cancer-relevant genes (e.g., *p53*). As many as 30% of sunlight-induced mutations in the *p53* gene and lacI transgene are dipyrimidines that contain 5-^{m}Cyt. The increased mutability of CpG sequences is probably due to preferential targeting of CpG sequences by UVB for CPD and $(6-4)$PD formation and spontaneous deamination of 5-^{m}Cyt leading to thymine. Deamination is followed by either error-free replication by polη (i.e., the polH/XPV gene product) or direct lesion bypass by an error-prone polymerase (i.e., the "A rule").

Additional work for Pfeifer's group added additional insight into the differences in mutation spectra between UVA and UVB (50,51) (Fig. 6). As previously known, C → T transition mutations dominate the UVB spectrum accounting for nearly two-thirds of the total mutations detected. Coupled with the CC → TT double transition mutations, this type of "signature" mutation occurs at an extremely high frequency in response to UVB at sites where CPDs and $(6-4)$PDs

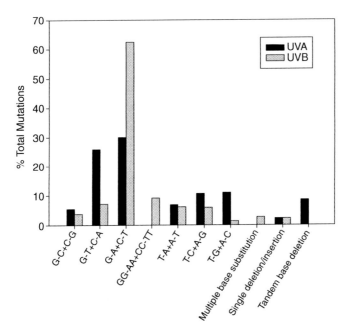

Figure 6 UVA and UVB mutation spectra.

also occur at high frequencies. In contrast, C → T transitions account for less than one-third of the total mutations induced by UVA with no double transition mutations detected. From these data, it appears that photoproducts occurring at T → C dipyrimidines are considerably less important in mutations induced by UVA compared to UVB. Not surprisingly, significantly greater levels of mutations form at sites containing thymine, including T → C transitions and T → A/G transversions, perhaps correlating with the prominent TT CPD induction recently shown for UVA exposure. In addition, G → T/A transversions take on a much more prominent role in UVA mutagenesis compared to UVB, perhaps reflecting the induction of photo-oxidative damage in DNA such as 8-oxodGuo.

BIOCHEMICAL PATHWAYS OF CARCINOGENESIS

Skin cancers include at least three categories of tumor type: SCC, BCC, and melanoma. These have distinct origins, molecular changes and etiology, and eventual outcomes, and each has characteristic genetic and solar components to their development. SCCs and BCCs appear to originate from different locations in the skin, and melanoma from the pigment cells. The initial damage produced by solar UV to the skin is eliminated either by repair or by proliferation and exfoliation from the skin's surface. Some cells in the skin are also removed by apoptosis, resulting in the elimination of these damaged "sunburn" cells. Epidermal stem cells are thought to reside in the bulge region of the hair follicles (52), but there are also secondary stem cells at the base of each column of epidermal transit amplifying cells in the epidermal proliferative units (53). Whether SCCs and BCCs come from different stem cells is currently a matter of investigation. A very low frequency of quiescent cells have been observed to retain DNA damage for long periods seemingly without repair or proliferation (54,55). The carcinogen-retaining cells may be stem cells or damaged cells with the potential to become mutants once stimulated to proliferate. Recent work by de Gruijl (personal communication) examined this phenomenon after UVB exposure in repair-proficient and -deficient mouse skin and found that while CPDs alone accumulated in repair-competent mice, both CPDs and (6–4)PDs persisted in $XPC^{-/-}$ knockout mice. In addition, the CPD-retaining cells co-localized with BrdU label–retaining cells and began to divide in response to treatment with the promoter 12-*o*-tetra decanoylphorbol 13-acetate (TPA). From these data, it is concluded that these cells are indeed stem cells that are not defective in NER, accumulating damage only in rarely dividing stem cells. It is very probable that these cells are the targets of sunlight-induced nonmelanoma skin cancer.

The progression of molecular changes involved in SCC appears to be initiated by inactivating mutations in p53 that result in expanding clones in the sun-exposed areas of the skin that are initially confined within the proliferating units (56). These clones can be very frequent and can escape the confines of the proliferative units after chronic UVB irradiation. Over 90% of SCCs are reported to have p53 mutations that are characteristic of UV exposure, being in dipyrimidine sequences with notable frequencies of CC → TT transitions (57–59). Loss of p53 function can result in multiple pleiotropic effects, ultimately increasing genomic instability especially during DNA replication and exposure to further UVR (Fig. 7). Several investigations have also identified activating mutations in the H-*ras* and N-*ras* oncogenes at codon 61, from solar UV exposure (60–62). However, although over 75% of UV-induced mutations are generally T → C at TC → CC transitions at CPD or (6–4)PD photoproduct sites, the H-*ras* and N-*ras* activation occurred in tumors at TT sites where transversions not previously identified in model culture systems were detected (63).

An understanding of BCCs is best illustrated in the hereditary disease BCNS. The defect in BCNS appears to be in the human homolog of the *Drosophila* gene *PATCHED* (*PTCH*). The gene is involved in embryonic patterning as well as determining the fate of multiple structures in the developing embryo. Both somatic mutations in sporadic BCCs and single-allele mutations in patients with BCNS (64,65) have provided strong evidence that this tumor suppressor is important in BCC tumorigenesis.

The patched protein (PTC) is a transmembrane receptor, and with the co-receptor membrane protein Smoothened (SMO), regulates signal transduction by the extracellular protein Hedgehog (hH) that binds to PTC (66) (Fig. 8). PTC represses the pathway by inhibiting signaling by SMO (67,68). SMO is released from PTC repression if (*i*) Hh binds to PTC, (*ii*) PTC is mutationally inactivated,

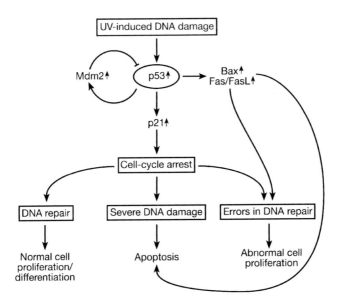

Figure 7 Pleiotropic effects of p53.

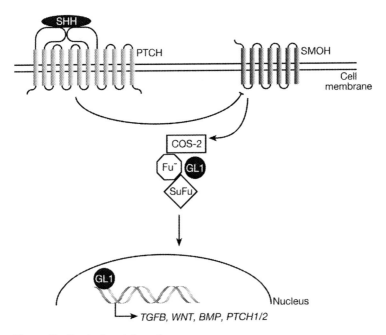

Figure 8 Patched protein pathway.

or (*iii*) SMO mutation impedes PTC–SMO protein interaction (69). Once released from PTC repression, SMO signaling activates transcription factor Gli that in turn upregulates expression of *PTC* itself and of a variety of other genes depending on tissue, organism, and stage of development. Mutations in *SMO* have been identified in BCCs and in these tumors, as in BCCs with *PTC* mutations, in situ studies detected increased *PTC* transcript in BCCs as compared to overlying epidermis and stroma (70). Thus, increased *PTC* message levels correlate with decreased PTC protein function.

More than 50% of BCCs and 90% of SCCs also contain mutations in p53 with a specific signature induced by ultraviolet light, and many other gene amplifications and deletions have been detected (71). However, studies on mutation frequencies in skin tumors from XP patients show significant differences in mutation frequencies in target genes in BCC and SCC (72). For instance, mutation frequencies are comparable in the *p53* gene of SCC but much greater in the *PTCH*, *SMO*, and *SHH* genes of BCC. In contrast, mutation frequencies are significantly greater in *ras* and *p16* in SCC compared to BCC.

Melanoma occurs in a hereditary form among approximately 5% to 12% of all patients (73). Although this is clinically and histologically indistinguishable from non-familial melanoma, there are differences in the age of diagnosis, lesion thickness, and frequency of multiple lesions (74–76). Significant differences occur in the genetic changes in melanomas according to whether the sites are exposed to chronic (face and hands) or intermittent (trunk and legs) sun damage or are not exposed at all (palms and soles) (77). Melanomas that are not driven by high levels of sun exposure involve a series of mutations, deletions, and amplifications (copy number changes) along the MAP kinase pathway (78–83). This pathway involves *N-ras*, *BRAF*, p16, the pair of *Cyclin D1* and *CDK4*, and *PTEN*. Copy number changes of *Cyclin D1* and *CDK4* are mutually exclusive, as are mutations in *ras* and *BRAF*. *PTEN*, being a negative regulator on a parallel *RAS*-activated pathway, can occur along with mutations in the *BRAF* arm, but is retained in melanomas on chronically sun-exposed skin. Although C → T transitions are commonly found in "sunlight-induced" melanomas, they are also found in other tumor types not associated with sunlight.

BRAF, a cytoplasmic serine/threonine kinase regulated by *RAS*, is mutated in a large fraction of melanoma on unexposed skin (84). BRAF has been successfully targeted by a small molecule inhibitor in clinical trials in combination with chemotherapy, and may become the first line of treatment for certain classes of melanoma (85). The role of sun damage in chronically exposed regions remains to be fully explored, but melanomas in these regions have fewer mutations and less copy number changes.

CONCLUSIONS

Significant advances in our understanding of the etiology of sunlight-induced skin cancer have been made in the recent past. The biochemical mechanism of

DNA repair has been extensively explored and its contribution to abrogating the initiation of skin cancer is now well understood. Indeed, the types of DNA damage, and by inference the wavelengths of UVR, responsible for initiating skin cancer are finally being recognized. Current thought suggests that the CPD is the major mutagenic lesion induced in mammalian cells by UVB due to its high induction levels, slow repair, and high bypass tolerance. Recently, researchers have used transgenic mice expressing inducible CPD or (6–4)PD photolyases in the skin to significantly advance our understanding of the biological effects of these two lesions with regard to skin cancer (86). From this work, it is evident that, at least in mice, most of the acute effects of UVB, including erythema, apoptosis, hyperplasia, and mutations are caused by CPDs and that CPDs are the principal cause of nonmelanoma skin cancer. Coupled with the recent finding that CPDs are induced at significant levels by UVA, this suggests that this lesion, the first to be identified in DNA by Beukers and Behrends in 1960, is probably the most important player in the etiology of skin cancer. Unfortunately, unlike nonmelanoma skin cancer, the etiology of melanoma is still far from clear.

REFERENCES

1. de Vries E, Louwman M, Bastiaens M, et al. Rapid and continuous increases in incidence rates of basal cell carcinoma in the southeast Netherlands since 1973. J Invest Dermatol 2004; 123:634–638.
2. Rosso S, Budroni M. Skin cancers: melanoma, non-melanoma cancers and Kaposi's sarcoma. Epidemiol Prev 2004; 28:57–63.
3. Fitzpatrick TB, Sober AJ. Sunlight and skin cancer [editorial]. N Engl J Med 1985; 313:818–820.
4. Armstrong BK, Kricker A. The epidemiology of UV induced skin cancer. J Photochem Photobiol B 2001; 63:8–18.
5. de Vries E, Schouten LJ, Visser O, et al. Rising trends in the incidence of and mortality from cutaneous melanoma in the Netherlands: a Northwest to Southeast gradient? Eur J Cancer 2003; 39:1439–1446.
6. Jablonski NG, Chaplin G. The evolution of human skin coloration. J Hum Evol 2000; 39:57–106.
7. Grossman L, Wei Q. DNA repair and epidemiology of basal cell carcinoma. Clin Chem 1995; 41:1854–1863.
8. Armstrong BK. Epidemiology of malignant melanoma: intermittent or total accumulated exposure to the sun? J Dermatol Surg Oncol 1988; 14:835–849.
9. Trosko JE, Krause D, Isoun M. Sunlight-induced pyrimidine dimers in human cells in vitro. Nature 1970; 228:358–359.
10. Vitaliano PP, Urbach F. The relative importance of risk factors in nonmelanoma carcinoma. Arch Dermatol 1980; 116:454–456.
11. Bootsma D, Kraemer KH, Cleaver JE. Nucleotide excision repair syndromes: xeroderma pigmentosum, Cockayne syndrome, and trichothiodystrophy. In: Vogel-stein V, Kinzler KW, eds. The genetic basis of human cancer. New York: McGraw-Hill, 1998:245–274.

12. Kripke ML. Immunological effects of ultraviolet radiation. J Dermatol 1991; 18:429–433.
13. London NJ, Farmery SM, Will EJ, et al. Risk of neoplasia in renal transplant patients. Lancet 1995; 346:403–406.
14. Kraemer KH, Lee MM, Andrews AD, et al. The role of sunlight and DNA repair in melanoma and nonmelanoma skin cancer. The xeroderma pigmentosum paradigm. Arch Dermatol 1994; 130:1018–1021.
15. De Fabo EC, Noonan FP, Fears T, et al. Ultraviolet B but not ultraviolet A radiation initiates melanoma. Cancer Res 2004; 64:6372–6376.
16. Noonan FP, Recio JA, Takayama H, et al. Neonatal sunburn and melanoma in mice. Nature 2001; 413:271–272.
17. Serrano H, Scotto J, Shornick G, et al. Incidence of nonmelanoma skin cancer in New Hampshire and Vermont. J Am Acad Dermatol 1991; 24:574–579.
18. Scotto J, Fraumeni JF Jr. Skin (other than melanoma). In: Schottenfeld D, Fraumeni JR Jr, eds. Cancer epidemiology and prevention. Philadelphia: Saunders, W. B., 1982:996–1011.
19. Boring CC, Squires TS, Tong T. Cancer statistics, 1993. CA Cancer J Clin 1993; 43:7–26.
20. Gallagher RP, Ma B, McLean DI, et al. Trends in basal cell carcinoma, squamous cell carcinoma, and melanoma of the skin from 1973 through 1987. J Am Acad Dermatol 1990; 23:413–421.
21. Davies RE, Forbes PD, Urbach F. Effects of chemicals on photobiologic reactions of skin. Basic Life Sci 1990; 53:127–135.
22. Robinson JK, Rademaker AW. Relative importance of prior basal cell carcinomas, continuing sun exposure, and circulating T lymphocytes on the development of basal cell carcinoma. J Invest Dermatol 1992; 99:227–231.
23. Marks R, Staples M, Giles GG. Trends in non-melanocytic skin cancer treated in Australia: the second national survey. Int J Cancer 1993; 53:585–590.
24. Thompson SC, Jolley D, Marks R. Reduction of solar keratoses by regular sunscreen use. N Engl J Med 1993; 329:1147–1151.
25. Marks R, Jolley D, Lectsas S, et al. The role of childhood exposure to sunlight in the development of solar keratoses and non-melanocytic skin cancer. Med J Aust 1990; 152:62–66.
26. Patrick MH. Physical and chemical properties of DNA. In: Wang SY, ed. Photochemistry and Photobiology of Nucleic Acids. Vol. II. New York: Academic Press, 1976:1–142.
27. Cadet J, Sage E, Douki T. Ultraviolet radiation-mediated damage to cellular DNA. Mutat Res 2005; 571:3–17.
28. Cleaver JE. Defective repair replication of DNA in xeroderma pigmentosum. Nature 1968; 218:652–656.
29. Sancar A, Sancar GB. DNA repair enzymes. Annu Rev Biochem 1988; 57:29–67.
30. Sancar A. Mechanisms of DNA excision repair. Science 1994; 266:1954–1956.
31. Hanawalt PC. Transcription-coupled repair and human disease. Science 1994; 266:1957–1958.
32. Ford JM, Hanawalt PC. Expression of wild-type p53 is required for efficient global genomic nucleotide excision repair in UV-irradiated human fibroblasts. J Biol Chem 1997; 272:28073–28080.
33. Mitchell DL, Nairn RS. The biology of the (6-4) photoproduct. Photochem Photobiol 1989; 49:805–819.

34. Cleaver JE, Jen J, Charles WC, et al. Cyclobutane dimers and (6-4) photoproducts in human cells are mended with the same patch sizes. Photochem Photobiol 1991; 54:393–402.
35. Cleaver JE, Kraemer KH. Xeroderma pigmentosum. In: Scriver CR, Beaudet AL, Sly WS, Valle D, eds. The Metabolic Basis of Inherited Disease. Vol. 2. New York: McGraw-Hill, 1989:2949–2971.
36. Freeman SE. Variations in excision repair of UVB-induced pyrimidine dimers in DNA of human skin in situ. J Invest Dermatol 1988; 90:814–817.
37. Mellon I, Bohr VA, Smith CA, et al. Preferential DNA repair of an active gene in human cells. Proc Natl Acad Sci USA 1986; 83:8878–8882.
38. Link CJ Jr, Mitchell DL, Nairn RS, et al. Preferential and strand-specific DNA repair of (6-4) photoproducts detected by a photochemical method in the hamster DHFR gene. Carcinogenesis 1992; 13:1975–1980.
39. Schaeffer L, Roy R, Humbert S, et al. DNA repair helicase: a component of BTF2 (TFIIH) basic transcription factor [see comments]. Science 1993; 260:58–63.
40. Licht CL, Stevnsner T, Bohr VA. Cockayne syndrome group B cellular and biochemical functions. Am J Hum Genet 2003; 73:1217–1239.
41. Gao S, Drouin R, Holmquist GP. DNA repair rates mapped along the human PGK1 gene at nucleotide resolution [see comments]. Science 1994; 263:1438–1440.
42. Cooper PK, Nouspikel T, Clarkson SG, et al. Defective transcription-coupled repair of oxidative base damage in Cockayne syndrome patients from XP group G. Science 1997; 275:990–993.
43. Leadon SA, Avrutskaya AV. Requirement for DNA mismatch repair proteins in the transcription-coupled repair of thymine glycols in Saccharomyces cerevisiae. Mutat Res 1998; 407:177–187.
44. Meira LB, Cheo DL, Reis AM, et al. Mice defective in the mismatch repair gene Msh2 show increased predisposition to UVB radiation-induced skin cancer. DNA Repair (Amst) 2002; 1:929–934.
45. Yoshino M, Nakatsu Y, te Riele H, et al. Additive roles of XPA and MSH2 genes in UVB-induced skin tumorigenesis in mice. DNA Repair (Amst) 2002; 1:935–940.
46. Peters AC, Young LC, Maeda T, et al. Mammalian DNA mismatch repair protects cells from UVB-induced DNA damage by facilitating apoptosis and p53 activation. DNA Repair (Amst) 2003; 2:427–435.
47. Young LC, Peters AC, Maeda T, et al. DNA mismatch repair protein Msh6 is required for optimal levels of ultraviolet-B-induced apoptosis in primary mouse fibroblasts. J Invest Dermatol 2003; 121:876–880.
48. Young LC, Thulien KJ, Campbell MR, et al. DNA mismatch repair proteins promote apoptosis and suppress tumorigenesis in response to UVB irradiation: an in vivo study. Carcinogenesis 2004; 25:1821–1827.
49. Pfeifer GP, You YH, Besaratinia A. Mutations induced by ultraviolet light. Mutat Res 2005; 571:19–31.
50. You YH, Pfeifer GP. Similarities in sunlight-induced mutational spectra of CpG-methylated transgenes and the p53 gene in skin cancer point to an important role of 5-methylcytosine residues in solar UV mutagenesis. J Mol Biol 2001; 305:389–399.
51. Besaratinia A, Pfeifer GP. Enhancement of the mutagenicity of benzo(a)pyrene diol epoxide by a nonmutagenic dose of ultraviolet A radiation. Cancer Res 2003; 63:8708–8716.

52. Rochat A, Kobayashi K, Barrandon Y. Location of stem cells of human hair follicles by clonal analysis. Cell 1994; 76:1063–1073.
53. Potten CS. The epidermal proliferative unit: the possible role of the central basal cell. Cell Tissue Kinet 1974; 7:77–88.
54. Morris RJ, Fischer SM, Slaga TJ. Evidence that a slowly cycling subpopulation of adult murine epidermal cells retains carcinogen. Cancer Res 1986; 46:3061–3066.
55. Mitchell DL, Volkmer B, Breitbart EW, et al. Identification of a non-dividing subpopulation of mouse and human epidermal cells exhibiting high levels of persistent UV photodamage. J Invest Dermatol 2001; 117:590–595.
56. Zhang W, Remenyik E, Zelterman D, et al. Escaping the stem cell compartment: sustained UVB exposure allows p53-mutant keratinocytes to colonize adjacent epidermal proliferating units without incurring additional mutations. Proc Natl Acad Sci USA 2001; 98:13948–13953.
57. Brash DE, Rudolph JA, Simon JA, et al. A role for sunlight in skin cancer: UV-induced p53 mutations in squamous cell carcinoma. Proc Natl Acad Sci USA 1991; 88:10124–10128.
58. Ziegler A, Jonason AS, Leffell DJ, et al. Sunburn and p53 in the onset of skin cancer. Nature 1994; 372:773–776.
59. Nataraj AJ, Trent JC 2nd, Ananthaswamy HN. p53 gene mutations and photocarcinogenesis. Photochem Photobiol 1995; 62:218–230.
60. Ananthaswamy HN, Price JE, Goldberg LH, et al. Detection and identification of activated oncogenes in human skin cancers occurring on sun-exposed body sites. Cancer Res 1988; 48:3341–3346.
61. Keijzer W, Mulder MP, Langeveld JC, et al. Establishment and characterization of a melanoma cell line from a xeroderma pigmentosum patient: activation of N-ras at a potential pyrimidine dimer site. Cancer Res 1989; 49:1229–1235.
62. Suarez HG, Daya-Grosjean L, Schlaifer D, et al. Activated oncogenes in human skin tumors from a repair-deficient syndrome, xeroderma pigmentosum. Cancer Res 1989; 49:1223–1228.
63. Bredberg A, Kraemer KH, Seidman MM. Restricted ultraviolet mutational spectrum in a shuttle vector propagated in xeroderma pigmentosum cells. Proc Natl Acad Sci USA 1986; 83:8273–8277.
64. Johnson RL, Rothman AL, Xie J, et al. Human homolog of patched, a candidate gene for the basal cell nevus syndrome. Science 1996; 272:1668–1671.
65. Hahn H, Wicking C, Zaphiropoulous PG, et al. Mutations of the human homolog of Drosophila patched in the nevoid basal cell carcinoma syndrome. Cell 1996; 85:841–851.
66. Toftgard R. Hedgehog signalling in cancer. Cell Mol Life Sci 2000; 57:1720–1731.
67. Marigo V, Davey RA, Zuo Y, et al. Biochemical evidence that patched is the Hedgehog receptor. Nature 1996; 384:176–179.
68. Stone DM, Hynes M, Armanini M, et al. The tumour-suppressor gene patched encodes a candidate receptor for Sonic hedgehog. Nature 1996; 384:129–134.
69. Xie J, Murone M, Luoh SM, et al. Activating smoothened mutations in sporadic basal-cell carcinoma. Nature 1998; 391:90–92.
70. Reifenberger J, Wolter M, Weber RG, et al. Missense mutations in SMOH in sporadic basal cell carcinomas of the skin and primitive neuroectodermal tumors of the central nervous system. Cancer Res 1998; 58:1798–1803.

71. Ashton KJ, Weinstein SR, Maguire DJ, et al. Molecular cytogenetic analysis of basal cell carcinoma DNA using comparative genomic hybridization. J Invest Dermatol 2001; 117:683–686.
72. Daya-Grosjean L, Sarasin A. The role of UV induced lesions in skin carcinogenesis: an overview of oncogene and tumor suppressor gene modifications in xeroderma pigmentosum skin tumors. Mutat Res 2005; 571:43–56.
73. Goldstein AM, Tucker MA. Genetic epidemiology of cutaneous melanoma: a global perspective. Arch Dermatol 2001; 137:1493–1496.
74. Barnhill RL, Roush GC, Titus-Ernstoff L, et al. Comparison of nonfamilial and familial melanoma. Dermatology 1992; 184:2–7.
75. Kopf AW, Hellman LJ, Rogers GS, et al. Familial malignant melanoma. Jama 1986; 256:1915–1919.
76. Aitken JF, Duffy DL, Green A, et al. Heterogeneity of melanoma risk in families of melanoma patients. Am J Epidemiol 1994; 140:961–973.
77. Whiteman DC, Watt P, Purdie DM, et al. Melanocytic nevi, solar keratoses, and divergent pathways to cutaneous melanoma. J Natl Cancer Inst 2003; 95:806–812.
78. Kamb A, Gruis NA, Weaver-Feldhaus J, et al. A cell cycle regulator potentially involved in genesis of many tumor types [see comments]. Science 1994; 264:436–440.
79. Nobori T, Miura K, Wu DJ, et al. Deletions of the cyclin-dependent kinase-4 inhibitor gene in multiple human cancers. Nature 1994; 368:753–756.
80. Bastian BC, LeBoit PE, Hamm H, et al. Chromosomal gains and losses in primary cutaneous melanomas detected by comparative genomic hybridization. Cancer Res 1998; 58:2170–2175.
81. Bastian BC, Wesselmann U, Pinkel D, et al. Molecular cytogenetic analysis of Spitz nevi shows clear differences to melanoma. J Invest Dermatol 1999; 113:1065–1069.
82. Bastian BC, LeBoit PE, Pinkel D. Mutations and copy number increase of HRAS in Spitz nevi with distinctive histopathological features. Am J Pathol 2000; 157:967–972.
83. Pollock PM, Trent JM. The genetics of cutaneous melanoma. Clin Lab Med 2000; 20:667–690.
84. Davies H, Bignell GR, Cox C, et al. Mutations of the BRAF gene in human cancer. Nature 2002; 417:949–954.
85. Flaherty LE, Gadgeel SM. Biochemotherapy of melanoma. Semin Oncol 2002; 29:446–455.
86. Jans J, Schul W, Sert YG, et al. Powerful skin cancer protection by a CPD-photolyase transgene. Curr Biol 2005; 15:105–115.

2

Etiology of Nonmelanocytic Skin Cancer

Cara L. Benjamin and Honnavara N. Ananthaswamy

Department of Immunology, The University of Texas MD Anderson Cancer Center, Houston, Texas, U.S.A.

INTRODUCTION

The incidence of skin cancer is rapidly rising with an occurrence of 1.2 million new cases each year in the United States alone (1) and 1% to 2% of the Australian population being affected by nonmelanoma skin cancer (NMSC) annually (2). NMSCs, including squamous cell carcinoma (SCC) and basal cell carcinoma (BCC), are the most frequently diagnosed neoplasm. Epidemiological evidence of chronic overexposure in sun-exposed areas of the body shows that people with outdoor occupations have a higher incidence of SCC than do people who work indoors (3). Additionally, the face, head, neck, back of the hands, and arms are predominant sites for development of NMSCs. It is becoming increasingly clear that solar ultraviolet (UV) radiation is a major causative factor in the development of NMSC and was the first identified human carcinogen. Sun exposure is currently the leading environmental risk factor for the development of NMSC in humans (4,5). There are several reviews that discuss evidence showing that solar radiation is strongly implicated in the induction of human skin cancer (6–9).

Lifestyle changes have occurred over the years that have led to increased UV exposure. Examples include increased outdoor recreational activities, changes in clothing styles, and longevity. UV radiation (UVR) from sunlight is divided into three major categories separated by wavelength: UVC (200–280 nm), UVB (280–320 nm), and UVA (320–400 nm). Shorter wavelengths have higher energy and are therefore more biologically damaging. The earth's ozone filters out wavelengths below 280 nm, preventing UVC from reaching the earth's surface and becoming a factor in UV carcinogenesis, leaving UVB and UVA. UVB may have the potential to be the most damaging due to its higher energy, but UVA accounts for greater than 90% of the solar radiation that reaches the earth's surface. Although UVA is the predominant component of solar UVR to which we are exposed, it was believed to be non-carcinogenic or weakly carcinogenic. However, a few studies have demonstrated that wavelengths in the UVA region not only cause aging and wrinkling of the skin, but they have also been shown to cause skin cancer in animals when given in high doses over a long period of time (10–12). More recently, Agar et al. (13) demonstrated that human SCCs harbored UVB-type mutations in the upper part of the lesions and UVA-type mutations in the lower part of the tumor tissue, suggesting a role for UVA in the pathogenesis of human SCC. Interestingly, UVA radiation has been shown to be involved in the development of melanoma in fish (14,15). In contrast, wavelengths in the UVC region are not present in natural sunlight because they are filtered out by the ozone in the atmosphere. Thus, UVC radiation, though more effective in inducing DNA damage, mutation, and cell lethality in vitro, is not relevant to the problem of skin cancer in humans.

Additionally, there is growing concern over the depletion of the ozone layer that will increase the amount of UVB that reaches the earth's surface, and therefore increase the incidence of skin cancer. Data show a decrease in the ozone over the Antarctic, and ground level measurements in Argentina at the southern tip of South America have shown a 45% increase of UVB radiation (16). The major effect of a decrease in ozone layer would be an increase in the amount of UVR present in natural sunlight. Wavelengths in the UVB region are particularly sensitive to changes in ozone concentration. Although UVA radiation would also be expected to increase if the ozone concentration decreases, the increase would be very small in relation to the amount of UVA already present in sunlight. Even a small increase in the amount of UVB radiation present in sunlight is likely to have important consequences for plant and animal life on earth and will almost certainly affect human health adversely. As the incidence of skin cancer increases with age, it is implied that the lifetime cumulative exposure to UVR is responsible for the induction of skin cancer (17). The relatively recent decrease seen in the ozone would therefore not be entirely responsible for the increasing incidence of NMSCs. Additionally, it has been shown that the action spectra for induction of pyrimidine dimers, cell death, mutation, and transformation is similar to the DNA absorption spectrum (18–20).

UV Effects

It has been well documented that UVR causes DNA damage (21), inflammation (22), photoaging (23,24), erythema, sunburn (25), eye damage (26), immunosuppression (27–29), and skin cancer (30–32). A person's susceptibility to NMSC is dependent on several factors, including sun exposure habits, occupation, degree of skin pigmentation, and general health status. The incidence of skin cancer in light-skinned individuals increases closer to the equator, and Caucasians in Australia have the highest incidence of NMSC in the world (33). An individual's health status is also important. Interaction between papilloma viruses and sunlight exposure has been shown to increase the risk for SCC in sun-exposed body sites (34,35). Chronic immunosuppression, such as in renal transplant patients, causes a four- to seven-fold increase in low sun exposure areas and greater than 20-fold increase in sun-exposed sites of developing NMSC (36). In fact, patients with genetic irregularities, such as Xeroderma pigmentosum (XP), have an extreme sensitivity to the sun and develop multiple skin cancers on sun-exposed parts of the body.

These factors, among others, suggest that UVR in sunlight is a significant contributor to NMSC (37). Data obtained in laboratory models such as mice, rats, guinea pigs, and opossums confirm these observations, but it should be noted that the tumor type can vary depending on the species, and as seen in mice, the tumor development can also be strain dependent. Skin cancer development is a multi-step process that involves initiation, promotion, and progression. Initiation is the irreversible genetic alteration, followed by promotion, which is typically a signal for clonal expansion, which gives rise to pre-malignant or malignant lesions. Finally, progression is the transformation of the lesion into an invasive tumor that may have metastatic potential.

UV DAMAGE TO DNA

Pyrimidine Dimers

UVR produces very specific mutations, primarily from cyclobutane-type pyrimidine dimers (CPD) and pyrimidine (6–4)pyrimidone or (6–4) photoproducts (38,39). Both lesions are formed exclusively in runs of tandemly-located pyrimidine residues, which are often "hot spots" for UV-induced DNA damage and mutation (40–42). These unique lesions in the DNA give rise to unique mutations. UVR predominantly induces C → T and CC → TT transitions at dipyrimidine sequences, which have become the "signature" of UV-induced mutagenesis (40). Both the dimers and photoproducts in the DNA cause a distortion of the double helix due to the reduction in the angle between the bases. This alteration leads to mutation by misincorporation of A residues at the unreadable region during semi-conservative replication (43). Hallmark UV-induced mutations are recognizable by C → T and CC → TT transitions at the dipyrimidine sequences (40).

Reactive Oxygen Species

Skin is a very unique and complex organ. As a perimeter between the body and the outside environment, it suffers the direct insult of UVR. UVR results in the increased generation of reactive oxygen species (ROS) (44), which can lead to oxidative stress, depending on the dose, time of exposure, or wavelength (45). Although the keratinocytes within the epidermis are rich in antioxidants such as superoxide dismutase, catalase, thioredoxin reductase, glutathione peroxidase, tocopherol, glutathione, and ascorbic acid, ROS may still interact with protein, lipids, and DNA (46). These highly reactive molecules can produce single-strand break, DNA–protein cross-linking, and altered nucleic bases (46). UVA and visible light can produce more 7,8-dihydro-8-oxoguanine (8-hydroxyguanine) altered bases than single-strand breaks or DNA–protein cross-linking (47,48). Additionally, UV-mediated oxidative stress has been shown to activate redox-sensitive transcription factors, such as nuclear factor kappa B (49,50), activator protein-1 complex, c-Fos, and c-Jun (51,52).

EPIDEMIOLOGICAL EVIDENCE

Xeroderma Pigmentosa

Pigmentation, which protects against sunburning, also protects against skin cancer. A striking example of this is seen in the high incidence and early onset of SCC in African albinos, compared with their pigmented counterparts (53). In addition to albinism, there are other genetic diseases that demonstrate that DNA is the direct target of UV damage resulting in cell death. It has been noted that individuals with xeroderma pigmentosa (XP) have an increased propensity for sun sensitivity. XP is a genetically inherited disease in which the patients are extremely sensitive to solar irradiation and frequently develop skin cancer as a result of exposure (54). XP individuals develop numerous skin cancers and ocular abnormalities at a very early age, with the average age of onset being eight years, while the general population median is 60 years of age. This leaves the XP individual with a 1000- to 2000-fold greater chance than a normal individual of developing skin cancer. It is unclear if the transmission of the disease is autosomal recessive or by some complex mode of genetic mechanisms, but the increased sensitivity to sunlight is due to a defect in the somatic cell's ability to repair UV-induced DNA damage (55,56).

There are eight XP genetic complementation groups (A through G and a variant) that have been identified with defective DNA repair (57). It was first discovered that skin cells from XP patients are defective in the repair of UV-induced DNA damage by Cleaver, who found that UV irradiation in vitro left skin cells with diminished rates of unscheduled DNA synthesis (55). Later, the same defect in unscheduled DNA repair synthesis was demonstrated in vivo in XP individual's skin (58). Subsequent studies revealed that skin cells from XP patients were defective in the repair of UV-induced pyrimidine dimers; the defect, in particular, was the absence of a functional UV-specific endonuclease that is involved in the initial steps of the excision repair mechanism (59). Following the identification of (6–4) photoproducts, it is discovered that XP cells are also defective in the repair of this lesion (60). Studies utilizing skin fibroblasts from excision repair–deficient XP patients have shown that they exhibit a higher frequency of UV-induced mutation and transformation than normal human skin fibroblasts (61,62). Taken together, these results suggest that defects in DNA repair predispose XP cells to UV-induced skin cancer because UVR induces a much higher frequency of mutation in XP cells than in normal cells, and some of these mutations may be involved in cancer induction.

Immunosuppressed Individuals

One factor that has been clearly associated with an increased risk of NMSCs is chronic immunosuppression. This observation came from studies of malignancies arising in renal transplant patients, which demonstrated that the risk of developing skin cancer was increased four- to seven-fold in areas of low sun exposure and more than 20-fold in areas of high sun exposure (36). These tumors appear predominantly on sun-exposed body sites and generally occur within a few years of transplantation. Careful examination of the skin of such patients revealed a high incidence of warts as well as carcinoma in situ and SCC (63). Human papillomavirus (HPV) has been associated with the skin cancers as well as with benign warts, suggesting that immune suppression, papillomaviruses, and UVR may all interact to produce skin cancer in these individuals. These observations imply that a person's immune status is an important component in the risk of developing skin cancer.

Exposure to certain chemicals may enhance the induction of skin cancers by UVR. Studies in animal models have demonstrated that there are many possible types of interactions between chemicals and UVR that can increase or even decrease tumor formation. For example, repeated application of a chemical tumor-promoting agent such as croton oil to murine skin initiated with UVR results in a high incidence of skin cancers, even though treatment with either agent alone produces few or no tumors (64). In humans, however, such interactions have been documented only in the case of psoralens, which are photosensitizing compounds. The long-term use of 8-methoxypsoralen plus UVA radiation (PUVA) for therapy of psoriasis has been associated with an increased incidence of SCC in some studies (65). However, these skin cancers do not occur preferentially on parts of the body that receive the highest solar UVR, suggesting that they are related to the therapy alone rather than to an interaction between solar UVR and PUVA therapy. Recent molecular studies support the view that PUVA is carcinogenic for humans by itself.

There is sufficient data that demonstrate the relationship of UV irradiation and suppression of the immune system (66,67). UVR induces both a local and systemic immune suppression that include depletion of Langerhans cells (antigen presenting cells) from the skin, infiltration of inflammatory macrophages, disruption of cytokine production, and isomerization of urocanic acid from the *trans* to the *cis* form (68). UV-induced murine skin cancers are antigenic and can only be propagated in immunodeficient hosts (69). Studies also showed that UVR produces a systemic effect by the inability to reject tumors when injected intravenously or at unexposed sites in UV-irradiated mice (69). Additionally, these experiments demonstrated that UV-induced suppressor T cells play a role in tumor induction by shortening the latent period (70). The immune response is very complex and not completely understood. UVR stimulates the production of several immunosuppressive molecules such as interleukin-1, tumor necrosis factor-alpha (TNF-α), interleukin-10, and prostaglandin E_2 (PGE$_2$) in keratinocytes, which also has systemic effects (71).

The initial molecule that interacts with UVR to cause immunosuppression is debated. Candidates include DNA and urocanic acid, among other molecules within the cell membrane. DNA is proposed as a target due to the evidence that UV-induced immunosuppression can be reversed by treatment with DNA repair enzymes (72,73). Urocanic acid is a deamination product of histidine. High levels of *trans*-urocanic acid are produced by sweat glands within the stratum corneum of skin, and a photochemical isomerization converts the compound from *trans*- to the *cis*-urocanic acid. In animal models, the *cis* presentation can suppress delayed-type hypersensitivity (74) and contact hypersensitivity (75). It appears that *cis*-urocanic acid interferes with the antigen presenting cells (76) and acts as a stimulus for TNF-α to act as an immunosuppressant (75). UVR damages cell membranes either directly or indirectly by the release of ROS. One result is the increased production of PGE$_2$ (77,78), which is known to serve as an immunosuppressive agent (79,80).

Maryland Watermen

Persons who spend the most time outdoors, such as those with outdoor occupations, generally have a higher incidence of SCC than those who work indoors, suggesting that there is a dose–response relationship between sunlight exposure and skin cancer incidence. An interesting illustration of this point comes from a case study of a stable and homogeneous group of Caucasians who make their living fishing on the Chesapeake Bay. In this group of Maryland watermen, the incidence of SCC, but not BCC, correlated directly with the individual's personal exposure to sunlight. The higher the UVB radiation received, the higher the probability of developing SCC (3).

EXPERIMENTAL EVIDENCE

UV Carcinogenesis in Mice

Early evidence of the carcinogenic effects on mouse skin showed that a single dose of UV light at a carcinogenic wavelength caused necrosis and ulceration, followed by scarring, but failed to produce tumors, but in the case of repeated small doses, the neoplastic response was predominantly epithelial, resulting in formation of papillomas and SCCs (81). The results emphasize the significance of dose and wavelength in evaluating effects of UV light skin carcinogenesis. Further experiments on the UV effects on DNA were studied in skin from animal models, but great advances were made with the advent of transgenics. Mouse models with varying genetics were generated to assess the role of numerous cellular components in the neoplastic transformation of normal tissue in response to UVR. Some of the more recent and exciting data come from studies on the mouse models for XP.

Patients with the autosomal recessive DNA repair disorder XP suffer high incidence of skin cancer after sunlight exposure. XP-mutant mice are attractive models to study this syndrome, as they, too, develop UVR-induced skin tumors, mimicking the human phenotype. Of the seven classic XP complementation groups (A through G), XPA and XPC are only involved in nucleotide excision repair (NER). Recombinant adenovirus carrying the human *XPA* gene was used for in vivo gene therapy in UVB-irradiated skin of XP-mutant mice. Virus subcutaneous injection led to the expression of the XPA protein in basal keratinocytes and prevented deleterious effects in the skin, including the delayed development of SCC (82).

The XPC protein complex plays a key role in recognizing DNA damage throughout the genome for mammalian NER. It has been shown that XPC undergoes reversible ubiquitylation upon UV irradiation of cells (83). UVR radiation-induced skin cancer is significantly enhanced in XPC mice when they also carry a mutation in one copy of the *Trp53* gene ($Xpc^{-/-}$ $Trp53^{+/-}$). Skin tumors in these mice often contain inactivating mutations in the remaining Trp53 allele, and there is a novel mutational hot spot at a non-dipyrimidine site (ACG) in codon 122 of the *Trp53* gene in the tumors. The mutation in codon T122 can be identified in mouse skin DNA from ($Xpc^{-/-}$ $Trp53^{+/-}$) mice as early as two weeks after exposure to UVB radiation, well before histological evidence of dysplastic or neoplastic changes. As this mutational hot spot is not at a dipyrimidine site and is apparently Xpc-specific, it is suggested that some form of non-dipyrimidine base damage is normally repaired in a manner that is distinct from conventional NER, but that requires XPC protein (84).

Photoreactivation Experiments in Opossum

Another line of experimental evidence is provided by the gray, short-tailed opossum from South America, *Monodelphis domestica*, which has the unique ability to photoreactivate UV-induced pyrimidine dimers. The process requires the presence of photoreactivating enzyme, photolyase, and photoreactivating light. Post-UV treatment of the opossum with photoactivating light (320–400 nm) decreased the appearance of erythema, and the minimal erythema dose is significantly higher in animals that have been treated with photoactivating light post-UV (85). Post-UV treatment also suppressed the induction of histopathological alterations in the skin. This study identifies DNA as a primary chromophore involved in the induction of various photobiological responses of the skin such as hyperplasia and sunburn cell (SBC) formation, and also identified pyrimidine dimers as the one responsible DNA lesion (86). Further investigation of the opossum showed induction of SBCs and hyperplasia of the epidermis by UVR. A dose of 500 J/m^2 (approximately one minimal erythemal dose) from an FS-40 sunlamp induced measurable numbers of SBCs with a peak at 32 to 48 hours, while post-UVR exposure of skin to photoreactivating light suppressed the induction of SBCs by approximately 75%. Pre-UVR exposure to photoreactivating light had no effect on the induction of SBCs. Hyperplasia was also suppressed to a similar extent by post-UVR photoreactivation treatment (87). These studies demonstrate that pyrimidine dimers in DNA are the major photoproduct involved in the induction of SBCs and hyperplasia in *M. domestica* by UVR.

Photoreactivation Experiments in Fish

UV-induced pyrimidine dimers can also be enzymatically repaired to reduce the incidence of tumors in the Amazon molly, *Poecilia formosa* (88). Cells taken from the thyroid and surrounding area were UV irradiated and injected into the abdomen of isogenic recipients, which resulted in development of thyroid tumors. If the UV irradiation is followed by photoreactivating light the incidence of thyroid tumors is significantly reduced (88). Subsequent studies with an animal model from crosses and backcrosses of platyfish (*Xiphophorus maculatus*) and swordtails (*Xiphophorus helleri*) revealed that these two strains of fish are susceptible to invasive melanoma induction by exposure to filtered radiation from sunlamps. Post-UV exposure to photoreactivating light reduced the incidence to background (14). The presence of photolyase in humans has been debated until Li et al. (89) used a very specific and sensitive assay to compare photoreactivation activity in human, rattlesnake, yeast, and *Escherichia coli* cells. Photolyase was easily detected in *E. coli*, yeast, and rattlesnake cell-free extracts but none was detected in cell-free extracts from HeLa cells or human white blood cells with an assay capable of detecting 10 molecules/cell. It was therefore concluded that humans most likely do not have DNA photolyase.

MOLECULAR EVIDENCE

Role of *p53* Tumor Suppressor Gene in Nonmelanoma Skin Cancer

The *p53* tumor suppressor gene is involved in the cell cycle arrest and activation of programmed cell death (90,91). Individuals with Li-Fraumeni syndrome inherit a mutation in one allele of the *p53* gene (92). These individuals have a high incidence of malignancies including NMSC. These data, along with observations that many cancers have a mutated or lost *p53* gene, suggest that alterations in either pathway contributes to neoplastic transformation. Inactivation of the p53 plays an important role in the induction of skin cancer by UVR.

Mutations in the *p53* gene have been detected in 50% of all human cancers and in almost all skin carcinomas (93). *p53* codes for a 53-kDa phosphoprotein involved in gene transcription and control of the cell cycle by coordinating transcriptional control of regulatory genes (94–96). Human *p53* is a highly conserved 11-exon gene that is located on the short arm of chromosome 17 (97).

Analysis of mutations in *p53* gene has established an unequivocal connection between UV exposure, DNA damage, and skin carcinogenesis. UVB and UVC radiations induce unique types of DNA damage, producing CPD and pyrimidine (6–4)pyrimidone or (6–4) photoproducts (38,39,98), and it has been shown that p53 plays an important role in the protection of cells from DNA-damage from UVB exposure (99,100). UV-induced DNA damage activates mechanisms for removal of DNA damage, delay in cell cycle progression, DNA repair, or apoptosis by transcriptional activation of p53-related genes, such as *p21* (101), Murine double minute 2 (*MDM2*) (102), and *Bax*. Normally, there is little p53 protein in the cell, but in response to UV damage, high levels of p53 are induced (103,104). With high levels of p53 protein, there is a G1 arrest, allowing the cellular repair pathway to remove DNA lesions before DNA synthesis and mitosis (100,105) and an increase in apoptosis (106,107). Therefore, p53 aids in the DNA repair or the elimination of cells that have excessive DNA damage (91,108).

An important finding about p53 was the fact that upon UV irradiation, there is an increased half-life of the p53 protein in murine 3T3 fibroblasts (109). Typically, wild-type p53 has a relatively short half-life, but stabilization and elevation of p53 protein levels may signify early events in tumorigenesis. This information is important when considering that M1 leukemia cells arrest at the G1-S and G2-M phases of the cell cycle when irradiated (100,110,111). Additionally, the levels of p53 induction in human skin is proportional to the level of UVB exposure, although there is no correlation between UVB-induced p53 levels and erythema (104). Several DNA damaging agents have been shown to induce p53 and growth arrest (111,112), but only by those agents that induce strand breaks. Pyrimidine dimers alone do not trigger p53 induction, unless accompanied by excision repair-associated DNA strand breaks (113).

In UV-induced skin cancer, the frequency of C to T transitions is especially frequent at the trinucleotide sequence 5′-PyCG in the *p53* gene (38). There are several "hot spot" mutation sites within the *p53* gene. Data collected from Pfeifer et al. show that of the most commonly mutated sites in *p53*, five are mutated dipyrimidine in the sequence context 5′-CCG or 5′-TCG (codons 196, 213, 245, 248, and 282). Additionally, they found only 19 5′-CCG or 5′-TCG transitions in the target sequence occurring between codons 120 and 290 (114). Mouse tumors induced by irradiation with UVB lamps or solar simulators have identified a hot spot mutation at codon 270 of the *p53* gene, which correlates to a sequence change from 5′-TCGT to 5′-TTGT (115). Codon 270 of the mouse *p53* gene is equivalent to codon 273 of the human *p53* gene, but there is no dipyrimidine sequence at this location. Codon 270 is methylated at the CpG site and UVB produced the strongest CPD at the 5′-TCG. Time course experiments have shown that the CPD at this sequence persists longer than average, which suggests that the CPD is responsible for the induction of this mutational hot spot in UV-induced skin tumors (116). In fact, CPDs are responsible for majority of mutations induced by UVB irradiation in mammalian cells. Using mammalian cells containing the mutational reporter genes *lacI* and *cII*, You et al. (117) concluded that CPDs are responsible for at least 80% of the UVB-induced mutations in this model.

p53 Mutations in Human Precancerous Skin Lesions

The mutations in *p53* gene appear to be an early genetic change in the development of UV-induced skin cancers. Thousands of *p53*-mutant cell clones are found in normal-appearing sun-exposed skin (118–120). There is a high frequency of *p53* mutations reported in pre-malignant actinic keratosis (AK) lesions, which are considered to be pre-SCCs. In an AK study by Ziegler et al. (121), *p53* mutations were found at a 66% frequency and a high proportion of them (23/35) were C → T transitions. Nelson et al. (122) showed that 8 of 15 (53%) AKs had C → T transition in *p53* gene. A study by Campbell et al. (123) showed that 40% (8 out of 20) of individuals with Bowen's disease carried *p53* mutations as well. These early findings suggested that *p53* mutations may be involved in the malignant conversion of pre-cancerous lesions to SCCs and that mutations in *p53* and/or *p53* over-expression may be used as biomarkers for skin cancer susceptibility. Since then, the presence of UV-signature C → T and CC → TT mutations in the *p53* gene in human and experimental mouse skin cancers has been well documented (124–134).

p53 Mutations in Squamous and Basal Cell Carcinoma of the Skin

A number of investigators have detected *p53* gene mutations in a large proportion of human SCCs and BCCs (121,124–132,135,136). Initial studies by Brash and co-workers (43) revealed *p53* mutation in 58% of human SCC. Later studies by Ziegler et al. (121) and Rady et al. (125) have demonstrated *p53* mutations in human BCCs at 56% and 50% frequencies, respectively. Interestingly, Ziegler et al. (121) found that 45% of human BCCs contained a second point mutation on the other *p53* allele. More recently, Bolshakov et al. (131) analyzed 342 tissues from patients with aggressive and non-aggressive BCCs and SCCs for *p53* mutations. *p53* mutations were detected in 66% BCCs, 38% of non-aggressive BCCs, 35% of aggressive SCCs, 50% of non-aggressive SCCs, and 10% of samples of sun-exposed skin. About 71% of the *p53* mutations detected in aggressive and non-aggressive BCCs and SCCs were UV-signature mutations (131).

Most recently, Agar et al. have examined eight primary SCCs and eight pre-malignant solar keratosis lesions for *p53* mutations separately, in basal and supra-basal layers of keratinocytes using laser capture microdissection (13). They were able to detect UVA-type mutations (A:T → C:G transversions) both in SCCs and squamous cell lesions mostly in the basal germinative layer, which contrasted with a predominantly suprabasal localization of UVB-signature mutations in these lesions (13). This epidermal layer bias was confirmed by immunohistochemical analyses with a superficial localization of UVB-induced CPD contrasting with the localization of UVA-induced 8-hydroxy-2′-deoxyguanine adducts to the basal epithelial layer. The basal location of UVA- rather than UVB-induced DNA damage and mutation suggests that the UVA component of solar radiation is an important carcinogen in the stem cell compartment of the skin.

Analyses of mouse skin cancers induced by UVR have provided strong evidence for the involvement of *p53* mutation in the pathogenesis of UV-induced murine skin cancer. Analogous to human skin cancers, UV-induced mouse skin cancers also display *p53* mutations (133,134,137,138), although the frequency of mutations and the exons in which they occur differ among mouse strains, for reasons that are not yet clear. For example, in our study, *p53* mutations were detected at 70% to 100% frequency in UV-induced SKH-hr1 and C3H mouse skin tumors (134,138). In contrast, 20% of SCC from SKH-1/hr hairless mice and 50% of SCC from BALB/c mice exhibited *p53* mutations in another study (133). Nonetheless, most of the mutations detected in UV-induced mouse skin tumors were C → T and CC → TT transitions at dipyrimidine sites, like those found in human skin cancers, and most were located on the non-transcribed DNA strand.

Further evidence for the involvement of mutations in *p53* on the development of cancer is supplied by studies on p53 knockout mice. Heterozygous (+/−) and homozygous (−/−) p53 mice have been shown to develop spontaneous tumors of both primary lymphoid malignancies and various sarcomas (139,140). Ionizing radiation can enhance the frequency of these tumors even with a single dose (141). Interestingly, these mice failed to develop skin tumors. Chemical induction of skin cancer on these mice did not yield an increase in the frequency of papillomas, but there was a enhanced progression from papillomas to carcinomas compared with wild-type mice (142). As there is a strong association between UV-induced skin cancers and *p53* mutations, studies using congenic *p53* mutant mice and UV irradiation revealed that heterozygous mice had increased susceptibility to skin cancer induction, and p53$^{-/-}$ mice were at an even greater risk of developing skin cancer. Tumors in the heterozygous (+/−) mice were predominantly sarcomas, while the tumors from homozygous (−/−) mice were mostly SCCs associated with pre-malignant lesions resembling AKs (143). Point mutations in the *p53* gene affect the tumor susceptibility differently than allelic loss. Point mutations are generally associated with early stages of skin tumors, while allelic loss enhances tumor development at high levels of UVB exposure and increases progression of skin tumors to a higher malignancy (144).

p53 Mutations in Nonmelanoma Skin Cancer of Patients with Xeroderma Pigmentosa and Recipients of Renal Allografts

p53 mutations have also been found at high frequencies in skin cancers from patients with the genetic disorder XP (128,129). Studies by Sato et al. (129)

revealed that five of eight XP skin cancers had *p53* mutations, and of the six mutations seen, two were C → T transitions and two were CC → TT double-base substitutions. Dumaz et al. (128) showed that *p53* mutations were present in 17 of 43 (40%) skin cancers from XP patients and 61% of these mutations were tandem CC → TT base substitutions.

Immunosuppressed recipients of renal allografts (RAR) are also at much higher risk for skin cancer development. Over-expression of p53 protein and *p53* mutations has been detected in a large proportion of SCCs and pre-malignant lesions in RAR patients. In one study, accumulated p53 was present in 41% of pre-malignant keratoses, 65% of intraepidermal carcinomas, and 56% of SCCs from RAR patients (145). McGregor et al. (146) have shown similarly high incidence of *p53* mutations in nonmelanoma skin tumors from RAR patients and sporadic NMSC from immune-competent patients of 48% and 63%, respectively. Seventy-five percent of all mutations in transplant patients and 100% of mutations in non-transplant tumors were UV-signature mutations. Some evidence suggests that arginine/arginine genotype at a common polymorphism site at *p53* codon 72 may confer a susceptibility to the development of NMSC in RAR patients (147). Finally, some evidence suggest a role for HPV and its p53 protein-inhibitory activity in skin carcinogenesis within the immunosuppressed population (148).

p53 Mutations Are an Early Event in UV Carcinogenesis in Human and Mouse Skin

Mutations in *p53* arise early in UV-induced skin cancer (120,121,123,149) and have been identified in normal sun-exposed skin (118,120) as well as UV-irradiated mouse skin (150). This differs from other cancers such as colon cancer in that *p53* mutations are a late event marking the progression from a late adenoma to a carcinoma (151) as well as with melanoma marking the progression to a higher-grade malignancy (152). Non-cancerous skin adjacent to cancerous tumors has been shown to harbor *p53* mutations that are different from those contained within the tumor (119,153). AKs carry *p53* mutations at about 60%, with 89% of them being UV signature-type mutations. This can suggest that AKs are a clonal expansion of the cells that already contain the 53 mutation. Recent data investigating the role of clonal expansion suggest that it is more involved than hyperproliferation. Brash et al. has shown that UV not only can induce mutations, but that it drives clonal expansion of these cells by inducing apoptosis in surrounding normal cells and creating a micro-environment in need of repopulating. Thus, the repopulation is an enrichment for the death-resistant mutant cells. Using a mouse model that over-expresses Survivin, a molecule that functions in suppressing apoptosis, clonal expansion of mutated cells was suppressed due to the reduced apoptotic death of the surrounding normal cells within the micro-environment (154).

Mechanisms of Clonal Expansion

Murine model of UV-induced carcinogenesis allowed a unique opportunity for investigating the fate of *p53*-mutant keratinocytes during various stages of skin cancer development. In the skin of hairless mice, *p53* mutations induced by chronic UV exposure could be detected by allele-specific PCR as early as one week after initiation of the experiment, with 100% of the animals incurring *p53* mutations after eight weeks of UV treatment (155). Two to three weeks after beginning the UV treatment, clones of keratinocytes carrying mutant *p53* could already be visualized using immunohistochemical assays (149,156,157). As a tumor promoter, UV induces cell proliferation by stimulating the production of various growth factors and cytokines, as well as activation of their receptors (158–165). Repeated exposure of skin to UVR therefore results in clonal expansion of initiated *p53*-mutant cells (149,156,157). Brash and colleagues have shown that every successive UVB exposure allows *p53*-mutant keratinocytes to colonize adjacent epidermal stem-cell compartments without incurring additional mutations (156). Two mechanisms are believed to contribute to selective expansion of *p53*-mutant cells: their resistance to UV-induced apoptosis and their proliferative advantage over normal keratinocytes in response to stimulation with UV. Indeed, single UV exposure was shown to stimulate the proliferation of *p53*-mutant cells while inducing apoptosis in normal keratinocytes in culture and in artificial skin models (121,166,167). However, chronic UV irradiation of skin quickly induces apoptosis resistance and stimulates hyperproliferation throughout the epidermis as an adaptive response (155). The mechanism of selective proliferative advantage of *p53*-mutant cells is yet unclear, but it may be a critical factor promoting clonal expansion of initiated cells.

One mechanism that may contribute to expansion of initiated keratinocytes is the deregulation of UV-induced Fas/Fas-ligand-mediated apoptosis in skin. Hill et al. (168) showed that accumulation of p53 mutations in the epidermis of FasL-deficient mice occurred at much higher frequency compared with wild-type mice after chronic UV irradiation. Authors concluded that FasL-mediated apoptosis is important for skin homeostasis, and that the dysregulation of Fas–FasL interactions may be central to the development of skin cancer. Ouhtit et al. (155) further found that in skin of chronically irradiated SKH-hr1 mice, the progressive decrease of FasL expression was paralleled by accumulation of *p53* mutations and decrease in the number of apoptotic cells. These findings suggest that chronic UV exposure would induce a loss of FasL expression and a gain in *p53* mutations, leading to dysregulation of apoptosis, expansion of mutated keratinocytes, and initiation of skin cancer.

While patches of *p53*-mutant keratinocytes grow in density and size when UV treatment continues, they decline rapidly once the UV exposures are ceased (149,157,169). Remenyik et al. (169) showed that regression of pre-cancerous p53-positive clones occurs due to mechanisms other than antigen-specific immunity, proceeding with similar kinetics in the skin of $Rag1^{-/-}$ antigen-specific immunity incompetent mice and their wild-type counterparts. Our preliminary results suggest that elimination of *p53*-mutated keratinocytes occurs due to normal skin turnover.

Both continued and discontinued regiments of chronic UV treatment ultimately result in skin tumor development with 100% incidence, although the kinetics of tumor occurrence is delayed in the latter case (170). De Gruijl and coworkers have used a mathematical model that relates tumor occurrence to the daily dose of UV and the time needed to contract tumors. This model also offers prediction of skin cancer susceptibility depending on the load of *p53*-mutated keratinocyte clones in skin (157). Thus, these studies suggest that skin cancer development can be delayed but not abrogated upon further avoidance of exposure to UV.

Inhibition of UV-Induced *p53* Mutations Protects Against Skin Cancer in Mice

Our studies have shown that *p53* mutations can be detected in UV-irradiated mouse skin months before the gross appearance of skin tumors, suggesting that *p53* mutations can serve as a surrogate early biological endpoint in skin cancer prevention studies (150,171). To determine whether there is an association between reduction of UV-induced *p53* mutations and protection against skin cancer, sunscreen (SPF-15 to 22) was applied onto the shaved dorsal skin of C3H mice 30 minutes before each exposure to 4.54 kJ/m^2 of UVB (290–400 nm) radiation. Control mice were treated five days/wk with UV only or vehicle + UV. *p53* mutation analysis indicated that mice exposed to UV only or vehicle + UV for 16 weeks (cumulative exposure to 359 kJ/m^2 of UVB) developed *p53* mutations at a frequency of 56% to 69%, but less than 5% of mice treated with sunscreens + UV showed evidence of *p53* mutations. More importantly, 100% of mice that received a cumulative dose of 1000 kJ/m^2 of UVB only, or vehicle + UVB developed skin tumors, whereas, the probability of tumor development in all the mice treated with the sunscreens + 1000 kJ/m^2 of UVB was 2% and mice treated with sunscreens + 1500 kJ/m^2 of UVB was 15%. These results demonstrate that the sunscreens used in this study not only protect mice against UV-induced *p53* mutations, but also against skin cancer. Because of this association, it was concluded that inhibition of *p53* mutations is a useful early biological endpoint of photoprotection against an important initiating event in UV carcinogenesis.

CELLULAR AND MOLECULAR MECHANISMS

Downstream Effectors

More recent data investigating the role of p53 in UV-induced skin carcinogenesis have revealed other factors that are important to mention, such as the molecular downstream targets of p53: MDM2, growth arrest and DNA damage-inducible gene 45 (GADD45), and p21CIP/WAF1. MDM2 protein is a transcriptional target of p53, which binds to the *N*-terminus of p53 to promote degradation through the ubiquitin–proteasome pathway (172–175). Under normal cellular circumstances, in the presence of DNA damaging agents, p53 protein is stabilized by inhibition of the Mdm2-mediated p53 ubiquination (176). GADD45 is a member of a group of genes induced in response to growth–arrest signals and it is a p53-regulated gene that can suppress cell growth. Loss of GADD45 results in reduced NER activity (177). p21CIP/WAF1 is a moderator of p53-mediated cell-cycle arrest, by directly interfering with DNA synthesis by binding to PCNA. Its role is largely unknown, but there are two observations to support its importance. First, the p21CIP/WAF1 promoter has a p53 protein-binding site. Second, there is a significant increase in p21CIP/WAF1 mRNA following UVR in cells with intact *p53*, but not in cells with mutant *p53* (178).

Calpains are calcium-dependent cytoplasmic proteases that are involved in various cellular functions, including exocytosis, cell fusion, apoptosis, and the differentiation and proliferation of keratinocytes. Inhibition of calpains has been correlated with the enhanced stability of the p53 protein, suggesting that the calpain system can also cleave the p53 protein (179). Several studies have shown that calpains cleave the p53 protein to generate an *N*-terminally truncated protein (179,180). In vitro addition of calpastatin, a calpain inhibitor, to reconstructed human epidermis resulted in the total inhibition of proteolysis of p53 and an increase in Mdm2 expression, binding, and ultimate stabilization of p53 in response to UV irradiation (181).

Model of UV-Induced Initiation and Progression of Squamous Cell Carcinomas

The best-characterized model of carcinogenesis is that of the UV-induced development of skin carcinomas. Figure 1 depicts the stages of initiation and progression of SCC, in which mutation-associated inactivation of *p53* tumor-suppressor gene plays a critical role (43,99,121,150,182,183). Analysis of data on gene mutations in human pre-malignant AK lesions, as well as data from the UV-induced carcinogenesis experiments in mice, has suggested that the first step involves acquisition of UV-induced mutations in the *p53* by epidermal keratinocytes (121,182,183). This defect diminishes SBC formation and enhances cell survival allowing retention of initiated, pre-cancerous keratinocytes (121). Second, chronic exposures to solar UV results in the accumulation of *p53* mutations in skin, which confer a selective growth advantage to initiated keratinocytes and allow their clonal expansion, leading to formation of pre-malignant AK (121). The expanded cell death–defective clones represent a larger target for additional UV-induced *p53* mutations or mutations in other genes, thus enabling progression to carcinomas.

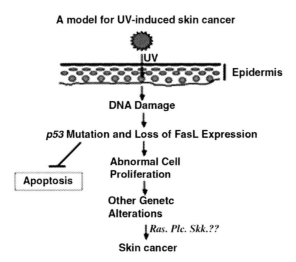

Figure 1   Pathway involved in skin cancer development.

DIFFERENT MECHANISMS FOR DIFFERENT TUMOR TYPES

Despite similarly high frequencies of UV-induced *p53* mutations in BCCs and SCCs of the skin, some differences exist in the mechanisms of their UV induction. The originating cells may arise from interfollicular basal cells, hair follicles, or sebaceous glands, thus from a deeper zone than the SCC ones, which probably means exposure to different doses or wavelengths of UV. Some of the genetic alterations in BCC pathway include those in the sonic hedgehog pathway of oncogenic transformation. Patched gene (*PTCH*) is a tumor-suppressor gene that encodes for a regulatory protein. Under normal conditions, PTCH conveys extracellular growth regulatory signals to the nucleus. Reifenberger et al. has shown that 67% of BCC carry a mutation in the *PTCH* gene (184). *PTCH* mutations are more frequent in BCC and are typically UV-specific C:T transitions and represent earlier events than *p53* mutations (185). Additionally, XP patients have more *PTCH* mutations than sporadic mutations, which may be associated with allelic loss at chromosome region 9q22.3 (186,187). Nonsense, missense, and silent *PTCH* mutations were found in SCCs from individuals with Gorlin's syndrome or a history of sporadic BCC (188). Besides mutations in the *p53* and *PTCH* genes, a small subset of SCC and BCC of the skin also carries mutations in INK4a/ARF tumor suppressor gene products and *ras* oncogene (189).

TNF-related apoptosis-inducing ligand (TRAIL), is an ubiquitously-expressed member of the TNF family that has been found to preferentially induce apoptosis in tumor cells, but not in normal cells (190). SCC and BCC do not express TRAIL while AKs and Bowen's disease show reduced levels of

TRAIL (191). Additionally, acute UVB does not alter the levels of TRAIL, but chronic UV as seen in elderly individuals shows a reduction of TRAIL (190).

NMSCs are derived from the keratinocytes that lie within the basal and squamous layers of the epidermis, while melanoma originates from the pigmented melanocytes. There are three lines of evidence that show how different *p53* mutations are in NMSC and melanomas. *p53* mutations occur more frequently in NMSC with 10% to 90% versus 1% to 20% in melanoma (192). Second, mutations in *p53* of NMSC are generally C → T and CC → TT transitions at dipyrimidine sites and melanomas display C:G → T:A, suggesting an absence of UV mutational influence (126). Lastly, *p53* mutations are early events in NMSC and late events in melanoma (121). *Ras* mutations also differ in NMSC and melanoma. While data have shown that H-ras is more commonly mutated in NMSC, a mutationally-activated N-ras contributes to melanogenesis (193,194).

SUMMARY

It is well known that UVR present in sunlight is a potent human carcinogen. Epidemiological evidence suggested the role of sunlight in skin cancer, and both experimental and molecular evidences have shown that UVR is a significant contributor to its pathology. The mutagenic and carcinogenic effects of UV light can be attributed to the induction of DNA damage and errors in repair and replication. Approximately, 80,000 pyrimidine dimers/cell are induced in human epidermis in one hour of sunlight exposure (195). Fortunately, cells are equipped with a variety of mechanisms that constantly monitor and repair most of the damage inflicted by UV light. However, occasional mistakes in DNA repair and replication can introduce mutations in the genome. Accumulation of several mutations in key genes due to chronic exposure to sunlight can lead to the development of skin cancer. Mutations in *ras* oncogenes do not appear to be as important as mutations in the *p53* tumor suppressor gene in skin cancer development. As skin cancers do not arise immediately after exposure to UV light, mutated *ras* or *p53* genes must remain latent for long periods of time. Tumor growth and progression into the more malignant stages may require additional events involving alterations of other oncogenes or growth suppressor genes. Identification of these genes should provide new insights into the mechanisms by which UV light induces skin cancer.

REFERENCES

1. Parker SL, Tong T, Bolden S, et al. Cancer statistics. CA Cancer J Clin 1997; 47:5–27.
2. Diepgen TL, Mahler V. The epidemiology of skin cancer. Br J Dermatol 2002; 61:1–6.
3. Vitasa BC, Taylor HR, Strickland PT, et al. Association of nonmelanoma skin cancer and actinic keratosis with cumulative solar ultraviolet exposure in Maryland watermen. Cancer 1990; 65:2811–2817.

4. Rosso S, Zanetti R, Martinez C, et al. The mulicentre south European study "Helios." II: Different sun exposure patterns in the aetiology of basal cell and squamous cell carcinomas of the skin. Br J Cancer 1996; 73:1447–1454.
5. Armstrong BK, Kricker A. The epidemiology of UV induced skin cancer. J Photochem Photobiol 2001; 63:8–18.
6. de Gruijl FR. UVA vs. UVB. Methods Enzymol 2000; 319:359–366.
7. van der Leun JC, de Gruijl FR. Climate change and skin cancer. Photochem Photobiol Sci 2002; 1:324–326.
8. Matsumura Y, Ananthaswamy HN. Toxic effects of ultraviolet radiation on skin. Toxicol Appl Pharmacol 2004; 195:298–308.
9. Kraemer KH. Sunlight and skin cancer: another link revealed. Proc Natl Acad Sci USA 1997; 94:11–14.
10. Zigman S, Fowler J, Kraus AL. Black light induction of skin tumors in mice. J Invest Dermatol 1976; 67:723–725.
11. Strickland P. Photocarcinogenesis by near ultraviolet (UVA) radiation in Sencar mice. J Invest Dermatol 1986; 87:272–275.
12. de Gruijl FR. p53 mutations as a marker of skin cancer risk: comparison of UVA and UVB effects. Exp Dermatol 2002; 11:37–39.
13. Agar NS, Halliday GM, Barnetson RS, et al. The basal layer in human squamous tumors harbors more UVA than UVB fingerprint mutations: a role for UVA in human skin carcinogenesis. Proc Natl Acad Sci USA 2004; 101:4954–4959.
14. Setlow RB, Woodhead AD, Grist E. Animal model for ultraviolet radiation-induced melanoma: platyfish-swortail hybrid. Proc Natl Acad Sci USA 1989; 86:8922–8926.
15. Setlow RB, Grist E, Thompson K, et al. Wavelengths effective in induction of malignant melanoma. Proc Natl Acad Sci USA 1993; 90:6666–6670.
16. Frederick JE, Soulen PF, Diaz SB, et al. Solar ultraviolet irradiance observed from southern Argentina—September 1990 to March 1991. J Geophys Res 1993; 98:8891–8897.
17. Fears TR, Scotto J, Schneiderman MA. Mathematical models of age and ultraviolet effects on the incidence of skin cancer among whites in the United States. Am J Epidemiol 1977; 105:420–427.
18. Doniger J, Jacobson ED, Krell K, et al. Ultraviolet light spectra for neoplastic transformation and lethality of Syrian hamster embryo cells correlate with spectrum for pyrimidine dimer formation in cellular DNA. Proc Natl Acad Sci USA 1981; 78:2378–2382.
19. Sutherland BM, Delihas NC, Oliver RP, et al. Action spectra for ultraviolet light-induced transformation of human cells to anchorage-independent growth. Cancer Res 1981; 41:2211–2214.
20. Rosenstein BS, Mitchell DL. Action spectra for the induction of pyrimidine (6-4) pyrimidone photoproducts and cyclobutane pyrimidine dimers in normal human skin fibroblasts. Photochem Photobiol 1987; 45:775–780.
21. Wikonkal NM, Brash DE. Ultraviolet radiation induced signature mutations in photocarcinogenesis. J Invest Dermatol Symp Proc 1999; 4:6–10.
22. Eaglestein WH, Ginsberg LD, Mertz PM. Ultraviolet irradiation-induced inflammation: effects of steroid and nonsteroid anti-inflammatory agents. Arch Dermatol 1979; 115:1421–1423.

23. Yaar M, Gilcrest BA. Aging and photoaging: postulated mechanisms and effectors. J Invest Dermatol Symp Proc 1998; 3:47–51.
24. Godar DE, Swicord ML, Kligman LH. Photoaging. In: Schopka HJ, Steinmetz M, eds. Environmental UV Radiation and Health Effects. Munich-Neuherberg: BfS-ISH-Berichte, 1995:123–131.
25. Daniels F Jr, van der Leun JC, Johnson BE. Sunburn. Sci Am 1968; 219:38–46.
26. Sliney DH. Epidemiological studies of sunlight and cataract: the critical factor of ultraviolet exposure geometry. Ophthalmic Epidemiol 1994; 1:107–119.
27. Vink AA, Yarosh DB, Kripke ML. Chromophore for UV-induced immunosuppression: DNA. Photochem Photobiol 1996; 63:383–386.
28. Nishigori C, Yarosh DB, Donawho C, et al. The immune system in ultraviolet carcinogenesis. J Invest Dermatol Symp Proc 1996; 1:143–146.
29. Kripke ML. Immunology and photocarcinogenesis: new light on an old problem. J Am Acad Dermatol 1986; 14:149–155.
30. Urbach F. Incidence of nonmelanoma skin cancer. Dermatol Clin 1991; 9:751–755.
31. Elwood JM, Jopson J. Melanoma and sun exposure: an overview of published studies. Int J Cancer 1997; 73:198–203.
32. Ley RD, Reeves VE. Chemoprevention of ultraviolet radiation-induced skin cancer. Environ Health Perspect 1998; 105:981–984.
33. McCarthy WH. The Australian experience in sun protection and screening for melanoma. J Surg Oncol 2004; 86:236–245.
34. Jablonska S, Dabrowski J, Jakubowicz K. Epidermodysplasia verruciformis as a model in studies on the role of papovaviruses in oncogenesis. Cancer Res 1972; 32:583–589.
35. Schaper ID, Marcuzzi GP, Weissenborn SJ, et al. Development of skin tumors in mice transgenic for early genes of human papillomavirus type 8. Cancer Res 2005; 65:1394–1400.
36. Penn I. Tumors of the immunocompromised patient. Annu Rev Med 1988; 39:63–73.
37. Ananthaswamy HN, Pierceall WE. Molecular mechanisms of ultraviolet radiation carcinogenesis. Photochem Photobiol 1990; 52:1119–1136.
38. Setlow RB, Carrier WL. Pyrimidine dimers in ultraviolet-irradiated DNA's. J Mol Biol 1966; 17:237–254.
39. Mitchell DL, Nairn RS. The biology of the 6-4 photoproducts and cyclobutane dimers in mammalian cells. Photochem Photobiol 1989; 49:805–819.
40. Brash DE. UV mutagenic photoproducts in *Escherichia coli* and human cells: a molecular genetics perspective on human skin cancer. Photochem Photobiol 1988; 49:59–66.
41. Mitchell DL, Jen J, Cleaver JE. Sequence specificity of cyclobutane pyrimidine dimers in DNA treated with solar (ultraviolet B) radiation. Nucleic Acid Res 1992; 20:225–229.
42. Sage E, Brash D. Distribution and repair of photolesions in DNA: genetic consequences and the role of sequence context. Photochem Photobiol 1993; 57:163–174.
43. Brash DE, Rudolph JA, Simon JA, et al. A role for sunlight in skin cancer: UV-induced p53 mutations in squamous cell carcinoma. Proc Natl Acad Sci USA 1991; 88:10124–12128.
44. Afaq F, Mukhtar H. Effects of solar radiation on cutaneous detoxification pathways. J Photochem Photobiol 2001; 63:61–69.

45. Katiyar SK, Afaq F, Azizuddin K, et al. Inhibition of UVB-induced oxidative stress-mediated phosphorylation of mitogen-activated protein kinase signalling pathways in cultured human epidermal keratinocytes by green tea polyphenol(−)-epigallocatechin-3-gallate. Toxicol Appl Pharmacol 2001; 176:110–117.
46. Berton TR, Mitchell DL, Fischer SM, et al. Epidermal proliferation but not the quantity of DNA photodamage is correlated with UV-induced mouse skin carcinogenesis. J Invest Dermatol 1997; 109:340–347.
47. Tchou J, Kasai H, Shibutoni S, et al. 8-Oxoguanine (8-hydroxyguanine) DNA glycosylase and it substrate specificity. Proc Natl Acad Sci USA 1991; 88:4690–4694.
48. Boiteux S, Gajewski E, Laval J, et al. Substrate specificity of the *Escherichia coli* Fpg protein (formamidopyrimidine-DNA glycosylase): excision of purine lesions in DNA produced by ionizing radiation or photosensitization. Biochemistry 1992; 31:106–110.
49. Afaq F, Ahmad N, Mukhtar H. Suppression of UVB-induced phosphorylation of mitogen-activated protein kinases and nuclear factor-kappa B by green tea polyphenol in SKH-1 hairless mice. Oncogene 2003; 22:9254–9264.
50. Afaq F, Adhami VM, Ahmad N, et al. Inhibition of ultraviolet B-mediated activation of nuclear factor-kappa B in normal human epidermal keratinocytes by green tea constituent (−)-epigallocatechin-3-gallate. Oncogene 2003; 22:1035–1044.
51. Isoherranen K, Westermarck J, Kahari VM, et al. Differential regulation of the AP-1 family members by UV irradiation in vitro and in vivo. Cell Signal 1998; 10:191–195.
52. Kramer-Strickland K, Edmonds A, Bair WB, et al. Inhibitory effects of deferoxamine on UVB-induced AP-1 transactivation. Carcinogenesis 1999; 20:2137–2142.
53. Kricker A, Armstrong BK, English DR. Sun exposure and non-melanocytic skin cancer. Cancer Causes Control 1994; 5:367–392.
54. Kraemer KH, Lee MM, Scotto J. Xeroderma pigmentosum. Cutaneous, ocular, and neurologic abnormalities in 830 published cases. Arch Dermatol 1987; 123:241–250.
55. Cleaver JE. Defective repair replication of DNA in xeroderma pigmentosum. Nature 1968; 218:652–656.
56. Cleaver JE, Bootsma D. Xeroderma pigmentosum: biochemical and genetic characteristics. Annu Rev Genet 1975; 9:19–38.
57. Hoeijmakers JH, Bootsma D. Molecular genetics of eukaryotic DNA excision repair. Cancer Cells 1990; 2:311–320.
58. Epstein JH, Fukuyama K, Reed WB, et al. Defect in DNA synthesis in skin of patients with xeroderma pigmentosum demonstrated in vivo. Science 1970; 168:1477–1478.
59. Setlow RB, Regan JD, German J, et al. Evidence that xeroderma pigmentosum cells do not perform the first step in the repair of ultraviolet damage to their DNA. Proc Natl Acad Sci USA 1969; 64:1035–1041.
60. Cleaver JE. DNA damage and repair in normal, xeroderma pigmentosum and XP revertant cells analyzed by gel electrophoresis: excision of cyclobutane dimers from the whole genome is not necessary for cell survival. Carcinogenesis 1989; 10:1691–1696.
61. Maher VM, Ouellette LM, Curren RD, et al. Frequency of ultraviolet light-induced mutation is higher in xeroderma pigmentosum variant cells than in normal human cells. Nature 1976; 261:593–595.

62. Maher VM, Rowan LA, Silinskas KC, et al. Frequency of UV-induced neoplastic transformation of diploid human fibroblasts is higher in xeroderma pigmentosum cells than in normal cells. Proc Natl Acad Sci USA 1982; 79:2613–2617.
63. Bouwes Bavinck JN. Epidemiological aspects of immunosuppression: role of exposure to sunlight and human papillomavirus on the development of skin cancer. Hum Exp Toxicol 1995; 14:98.
64. Epstein JH, Roth HL. Experimental ultraviolet light carcinogenesis: a study of croton oil promoting effects. J Invest Dermatol 1968; 50:387–389.
65. Stern RS, Thibadeau LA, Kleinerman RA, et al. Risk of cutaneous carcinoma in patients treated with oral methoxsalen photochemotherapy for psoriasis. N Engl J Med 1979; 300:809–813.
66. Kripke ML. Effects of UV radiation on tumor immunity. J Natl Cancer Inst 1982; 82:1392–1396.
67. Ullrich SE, Kim T-H, Ananthaswamy HN, et al. Sunscreen effects on UV-induced immune suppression. J Invest Dermatol 1999; 4:65–69.
68. Vainio H, Bianchini F. IARC Handbooks of Cancer Prevention, Sunscreens. Lyon, France: International Agency for Research on Cancer, 2001.
69. Kripke ML. Immunological mechanisms in UV radiation carcinogenesis. Adv Cancer Res 1981; 34:69–106.
70. Fischer SM, Kripke ML. Suppressor T lymphocytes control the development of primary skin cancers in ultraviolet-irradiated mice. Science 1982; 216:1133–1134.
71. Ullrich SE. The role of epidermal cytokines in the generation of cutaneous immune reactions and ultraviolet radiation-induced immune suppression. Photochem Photobiol 1995; 62:389–401.
72. Applegate LA, Ley RD, Alcalay J, et al. Identification of the molecular target for the suppression of contact hypersensitivity by ultraviolet radiation. J Exp Med 1989; 170:1117–1131.
73. Kripke ML, Cox PA, Alas LG, et al. Pyrimidine dimers in DNA initiate systemic immunosuppression in UV-irradiated mice. Proc Natl Acad Sci USA 1992; 89:7516–7520.
74. Ross JA, Howie SE, Norval M, et al. Ultraviolet-irradiated urocanic acid suppressed delayed-type hypersensitivity to herpes simplex virus in mice. J Invest Dermatol 1986; 87:630–633.
75. Kurimoto I, Streilein JW. *cis*-Urocanic acid contact hypersensitivity induction is mediated via tumor necrosis factor-α. J Immunol 1992; 148:3072–3078.
76. Noonan FP, DeFabo EC, Morrison H. Cis-urocanic acid, a product formed by ultraviolet B irradiation of the skin, initiates an antigen presentation defect in splenic dendritic cells. J Invest Dermatol 1988; 90:92–99.
77. Pentland AP, Mahoney M, Jacobs SC, et al. Enhanced prostaglandin synthesis after ultraviolet injury is mediated by endogenous histamine stimulation. J Clin Invest 1990; 86:566–574.
78. Chen X, Gresham A, Pentland A. Oxidative stress mediates synthesis and phosphorylation of cytosolic phospholipase A_2 after UVB injury. Biochim Biophys Acta 1996; 1299:23–33.
79. Chung HT, Burnham DK, Robertson B, et al. Involvement of prostaglandins in the immune alterations caused by the exposure of mice to ultraviolet radiation. J Immunol 1986; 137:2478–2484.

80. Jun BD, Roberts LK, Cho BH, et al. Parallel recovery of epidermal antigen-presenting cell activity and contact hypersensitivity responses in mice exposed to ultraviolet irradiation: the role of a prostaglandin-dependent mechanism. J Invest Dermatol 1988; 90:311–316.
81. Stenback F. Cellular injury and cell proliferation in skin carcinogenesis by UV light. Oncology 1975; 31:61–75.
82. Marchetto MC, Muotri AR, Burns DK, et al. Gene transduction in skin cells: preventing cancer in xeroderma pigmentosum mice. Proc Natl Acad Sci USA 2004; 101:17759–17764.
83. Sugasawa K, Okuda Y, Saijo M, et al. UV-induced ubiquitylation of XPC protein mediated by UV-DDB-ubiquitin ligase complex. Cell 2005; 121:387–400.
84. Nahari D, McDaniel LD, Task LB, et al. Mutations in the *Trp53* gene of UV-irradiated *Xpc* mutant mice suggest a novel *Xpc*-dependent DNA repair process. DNA Repair 2004; 3:379–386.
85. Ley RD. Photoreactivation of UV-induced pyrimidine dimers and erythemia in the marsupial Monodelphis domestica. Proc Natl Acad Sci USA 1985; 82: 2409–2411.
86. Applegate LA, Stuart TD, Ley RD. Ultraviolet radiation-induced histopatholgical changes in the skin of the marsupial Monodelphis domestica. I. The effects of acute and chronic exposures and of photoreactivation treatment. Br J Dermatol 1985; 113:219–227.
87. Ley RD, Applegate LA. Ultraviolet radiation-induced histopathologic changes in the skin of the marsupial Monodelphis domestica. II. Quantitative studies of the photoreactivation of induced hyperplasia and sunburn cell formation. J Invest Dermatol 1985; 85:365–367.
88. Hart RW, Setlow RB, Woodhead AD. Evidence that pyrimidine dimers in DNA can give rise to tumors. Proc Natl Acad Sci USA 1977; 75:5574–5578.
89. Li YF, Kim ST, Sancar A. Evidence for lack of DNA photoreactivating enzyme in human. Proc Natl Acad Sci USA 1993; 90:4389–4393.
90. Hartwell LH, Weinert TA. Checkpoints: controls that ensure the order of cell cycle events. Science 1989; 246:629–634.
91. Lane D. p53, guardian of the genome. Nature 1992; 358:15–16.
92. Malkin D, Li FP, Strong LC, et al. Germ line p53 mutations in a familial syndrome of breast cancer, sarcomas, and other neoplasms. Science 1990; 250:1233–1238.
93. Basset-Seguin N, Moles JP, Mils V, et al. TP53 tumor suppressor gene and skin carcinogenesis. J Invest Dermatol 1994; 103:102S–106S.
94. Levine AJ, Momand J, Finlay CA. The *p53* tumor suppressor gene. Nature 1991; 351:453–456.
95. Vogelstein B, Kinzler KW. p53 function and dysfunction. Cell 1992; 70: 523–526.
96. Harris CC. Structure and function of the p53 tumor suppressor gene: clues for rational cancer therapeutic strategies. J Natl Cancer Inst 1996; 88:1442–1455.
97. Lamb P, Crawford L. Characterization of the human p53 gene. Mol Cell Biol 1986; 6:1379–1385.
98. Mitchell DL. The relative cytotoxicity of (6-4) photoproducts and cyclobutane dimers in mammalian cells. Photochem Photobiol 1988; 48:51–57.
99. Smith ML, Fornace AJ Jr. p53-mediated protective responses to UV irradiation. Proc Natl Acad Sci USA 1997; 94:12255–12257.

100. Kuerbitz SJ, Plunkett BS, Walsh WV, et al. Wild-type p53 is a cell cycle checkpoint determinant following irradiation. Proc Natl Acad Sci USA 1992; 89:7491–7495.
101. Brugarolas J, Chandrasekaran C, Gordon JI, et al: Radiation-induced cell cycle arrest compromised by p21 deficiency. Nature 1995; 377:552–557.
102. Kamijo T, Weber JD, Zambetti G, et al. Functional and physical interactions of the ARF tumorsuppressor with p53 and Mdm2. Proc Natl Acad Sci USA 1998; 95:8292–8297.
103. Hall PA, McKee PH, Menage HP, et al. High levels of p53 protein in UV-irradiated normal human skin. Oncogene 1993; 8:203–207.
104. Healy E, Reynolds NJ, Smith MD, et al. Dissociation of erythemia and p53 expression in human skin following UVB irradiation, and induction of p53 protein and mRNA following application of skin irritants. J Invest Dermatol 1994; 103:493–499.
105. Zahn Q, Carrier F, Fornace AJ Jr. Induction of cellular p53 activity by DNA-damaging agents and growth arrest. Mol Cell Biol 1993; 13:4242–4250.
106. White E. Life, death, and the pursuit of apoptosis. Genes Dev 1996; 10:1–15.
107. Yonish-Rouach E, Reznitzky D, Lotem J, et al. Wild type p53 induces apoptosis of myeloid leukemic cells that is inhibited by IL-6. Nature 1991; 352:345–347.
108. Levine AJ. p53, the cellular gatekeeper for growth and division. Cell 1997; 88: 323–331.
109. Maltzman W, Czyzyk L. UV irradiation stimulates levels of p53 cellular tumor antigen in nontransformed mouse cells. Mol Cell Biol 1984; 4:1689–1694.
110. Kastan MB, Onyekwere O, Sidransky D, et al. Participation of p53 protein in the cellular response to DNA damage. Mol Cell Biol 1991; 51:6304–6311.
111. Kastan MB, Zhan Q, El-Deiry S, et al. A mammalian cell cycle checkpoint pathway utilizing p53 and Gadd45 is defective in ataxia-telangiectasia. Cell 1992; 71:587–597.
112. Fritsche M, Haessler C, Brandner G. Induction of the nuclear accumulation of the tumor suppressor gene p53 by DNA damaging agents. Oncogene 1993; 8:307–318.
113. Nelson WG, Kastan MB. DNA strand breaks: the DNA template alterations that trigger p53-dependent DNA damage response. Mol Cell Biol 1994; 14:1815–1823.
114. Pfeifer GP, You Y-H, Besaratinia A. Mutations induced by ultraviolet light. Mut Res 2005; 571:19–31.
115. Tommasi S, Denissenko MF, Pfeifer GP. Sunlight induces pyrimidine dimers preferentially at 5-methylcytosine bases. Cancer Res 1997; 57:4727–4730.
116. You Y-H, Szabo PE, Pfeifer GP. Cyclobutane pyrimidine dimers form preferentially at the major p53 mutational hotspot in UVB-induced mouse skin tumors. Carcinogenesis 2000; 21:2113–2117.
117. You Y-H, Lee DH, Yoon JH, et al. Cyclobutane pyrimidine dimers are responsible for the vast majority of mutations induced by UVB irradiation in mammalian cells. J Biol Chem 2001; 276:44688–44694.
118. Nakazawa H, English D, Randell PL, et al. UV and skin cancer: specific p53 gene mutation in normal skin as a biologically relevant exposure measurement. Proc Natl Acad Sci USA 1994; 91:360–364.
119. Ren ZP, Hedrum A, Ponten F, et al. Human epidermal cancer and accompanying precursors have identical p53 mutations different from p53 mutations in adjacent areas of clonally expanded non-neoplastic keratinocytes. Oncogene 1996; 12:765–773.
120. Jonason AS, Kunala S, Price GL, et al. Frequent clones of p53-mutated keratinocytes in normal human skin. Proc Natl Acad Sci USA 1996; 93:14025–14029.

121. Ziegler A, Jonason AS, Leffell DJ, et al. Sunburn and p53 in the onset of skin cancer. Nature 1994; 372:730–731.
122. Nelson MA, Einspahr JG, Alberts DS, et al. Analysis of the p53 gene in human precancerous actinic keratosis lesions and squamous cell cancers. Cancer Lett 1994; 85:23–29.
123. Campbell C, Quinn AG, Ro YS, et al. p53 mutations are common and early events that precede tumor invasion in squamous cell neoplasia of the skin. J Invest Dermatol 1993; 100:746–748.
124. Greenblatt MS, Bennett WP, Hollstein M, et al. Mutations in the p53 tumor suppressor gene: clues to cancer etiology and molecular pathogenesis. Cancer Res 1994; 54:4855–4878.
125. Rady P, Scinicariello F, Wagner RF Jr, et al. p53 mutations in basal cell carcinomas. Cancer Res 1992; 52:3804–3806.
126. Ziegler A, Leffell DJ, Kunala S, et al. Mutation hotspots due to sunlight in the p53 gene of nonmelanoma skin cancers. Proc Natl Acad Sci USA 1993; 90:4216–4220.
127. Pierceall WE, Mukhopadhyay T, Goldberg LH, et al. Mutations in the p53 tumor suppressor gene in human cutaneous squamous cell carcinomas. Mol Carcinog 1991; 4:445–449.
128. Dumaz N, Drougard C, Sarasin A, et al. Specific UV-induced mutation spectrum in the p53 gene of skin tumors from DNA-repair-deficient xeroderma pigmentosum patients. Proc Natl Acad Sci USA 1993; 90:10529–10533.
129. Sato M, Nishigori C, Zghal M, et al. Ultraviolet-specific mutations in the p53 gene in skin tumors in xeroderma pigmentosum patients. Cancer Res 1993; 53:2944–2946.
130. van der Riet P, Karp D, Farmer E, et al. Progression of basal cell carcinoma through loss of chromosome 9q and inactivation of a single p53 allele. Cancer Res 1994; 54:25–27.
131. Bolshakov S, Walker CM, Strom SS, et al. p53 mutations in human aggressive and nonaggressive basal and squamous cell carcinoma. Clin Cancer Res 2003; 9:228–234.
132. Stern RS, Bolshakov S, Nataraj AJ, et al. p53 mutation in nonmelanoma skin cancers occurring in psoralen ultraviolet a-treated patients: evidence for heterogeneity and field cancerization. J Invest Dermatol 2002; 119:522–526.
133. Kress S, Sutter C, Strickland PT, et al. Carcinogen-specific mutational pattern in the p53 gene in ultraviolet B radiation-induced squamous cell carcinomas of mouse skin. Cancer Res 1992; 52:6400–6403.
134. Kanjilal S, Pierceall WE, Cummings KK, et al. High frequency of p53 mutations in ultraviolet radiation-induced muring skin tumors: evidence for strand bias and tumor heterogeneity. Cancer Res 1993; 53:2961–2964.
135. Pierceall WE, Goldberg LH, Tainsky MA, et al. Ras gene mutation and amplification in human nonmelanoma skin cancers. Mol Carcinog 1991; 4:196–202.
136. Moles JP, Moyret C, Guillot B, et al. p53 gene mutations in human epithelial skin cancers. Oncogene 1993; 8:583–588.
137. Dumaz N, van Kranen HJ, de Vries A, et al. The role of UV-B light in skin carcinogenesis through the analysis of p53 mutations in squamous cell carcinomas of hairless mice. Carcinogenesis 1997; 18:897–904.
138. Ananthaswamy HN, Fourtanier A, Evans RL, et al. p53 mutations in hairless SKH-1 mouse skin tumors induced by a solar simulator. Photochem Photobiol 1998; 67:227–232.

139. Donehower LA, Harvey M, Slagle BL, et al. Mice deficient for p53 are developmentally normal but susceptible to spontaneous tumours. Nature 1992; 356:212–215.
140. Jacks T, Remington L, Williams BO, et al. Tumor spectrum analysis in p53-mutant mice. Curr Biol 1994; 4:1–7.
141. Kemp CJ, Wheldon T, Balmain A. p53-deficient mice are extremely susceptible to radiation-induced tumorigenesis. Nat Genet 1994; 8:66–69.
142. Kemp CJ, Donehower LA, Bradley A, et al. Reduction of p53 gene dosage does not increase initiation or promotion but enhances malignant progression of chemically induced skin tumors. Cell 1993; 74:813–822.
143. Jiang W, Ananthaswamy HN, Muller HK, et al. p53 protects against skin cancer induction by UV-B radiation. Oncogene 1999; 18:4247–4253.
144. van Kranen HJ, Westerman A, Berg RJW, et al. Dose-dependent effects of UVB-induced skin carcinogenesis in hairless p53 knockout mice. Mut Res 2005; 571:81–90.
145. Stark LA, Arends MJ, McLaren KM, et al. Accumulation of p53 is associated with tumour progression in cutaneous lesions of renal allograft recipients. Br J Cancer 1994; 70:662–667.
146. McGregor JM, Berkhout RJ, Rozycka M, et al. p53 mutations implicate sunlight in post-transplant skin cancer irrespective of human papillomavirus status. Oncogene 1997; 15:1737–1740.
147. McGregor JM, Harwood CA, Brooks L, et al. Relationship between p53 codon 72 polymorphism and susceptibility to sunburn and skin cancer. J Invest Dermatol 2002; 119:84–90.
148. Purdie KJ, Pennington J, Proby CM, et al. The promoter of a novel human papillomavirus (HPV77) associated with skin cancer displays a UV responsiveness, which is mediated through a consensus p53 binding sequence. EMBO J 1999; 18: 5359–5369.
149. Berg RJW, van Kranen HJ, Rebel HG, et al. Early p53 alterations in mouse skin carcinogenesis by UVB radiation: immunohistochemical detection of mutant p53 protein in clusters of preneoplastic epidermal cells. Proc Natl Acad Sci USA 1996; 93:274–278.
150. Ananthaswamy HN, Loughlin SM, Cox P, et al. Sunlight and skin cancer: inhibition of p53 mutation in UV-irradiated mouse skin by sunscreens. Nature Med 1997; 3:510–514.
151. Fearon ER, Vogelstein B. A genetic model for colorectal tumorigenesis. Cell 1990; 61:759–767.
152. Hussein MR, Haemel AK, Wood GS. Apoptosis and melanoma: molecular mechanisms. J Pathol 2003; 199:275.
153. Kanjilal S, Strom SS, Clayman GL, et al. p53 mutations in nonmelanoma skin cancer of the head and neck: molecular evidence for field cancerization. Cancer Res 1995; 55:3604–3609.
154. Brash DE, Zhang W, Grossman D, et al. Colonization of adjacent stem cell compartments by mutant keratinocytes. Seminars in Cancer Biology 2005; 15:97–102.
155. Ouhtit A, Gorny A, Muller HK, et al. Loss of Fas-ligand expression in mouse keratinocytes during UV carcinogenesis. Am J Pathol 2000; 157:1975–1981.
156. Zhang W, Remenyik E, Zelterman D, et al. Escaping the stem cell compartment: sustained UVB exposure allows p53-mutant keratinocytes to colonize adjacent epidermal proliferating units without incurring additional mutations. Proc Natl Acad Sci USA 2001; 98:13948–13953.

157. Rebel H, Mosnier LO, Berg RJ, et al. Early p53-positive foci as indicators of tumor risk in ultraviolet-exposed hairless mice: kinetics of induction, effects of DNA repair deficiency, and p53 heterozygosity. Cancer Res 2001; 61:977–983.
158. De Meyts P, Urso B, Christoffersen CT, et al. Mechanism of insulin and IGF-I receptor activation and signal transduction specificity. Receptor dimer cross-linking, bell-shaped curves, and sustained versus transient signaling. Ann N Y Acad Sci 1995; 766:388–401.
159. Rosette C, Karin M. Ultraviolet light and osmotic stress: activation of the JNK cascade through multiple growth factor and cytokine receptors. Science 1996; 274:1194–1197.
160. Bender K, Blattner C, Knebel A, et al. UV-induced signal transduction. J Photochem Photobiol B 1997; 37:1–17.
161. Kuhn C, Hurwitz SA, Kumar MG, et al. Activation of the insulin-like growth factor-1 receptor promotes the survival of human keratinocytes following ultraviolet B irradiation. Int J Cancer 1999; 80:431–438.
162. Jost M, Kari C, Rodeck U. The EGF receptor—and essential regulator of multiple epidermal functions. Eur J Dermatol 10:505-510, 2000
163. Peus D, Vasa RA, Meves A, et al. UVB-induced epidermal growth factor receptor phosphorylation is critical for downstream signaling and keratinocyte survival. Photochem Photobiol 2000; 72:135–140.
164. Walterscheid JP, Ullrich SE, Nghiem DX. Platelet-activating factor, a molecular sensor for cellular damage, activates systemic immune suppression. J Exp Med 2002; 195:171–179.
165. Coffer PJ, Burgering BM, Peppelenbosch MP, et al. UV activation of receptor tyrosine kinase activity. Oncogene 1995; 11:561–569.
166. Oda K, Arakawa H, Tanaka T, et al. p53AIP1, a potential mediator of p53-dependent apoptosis, and its regulation by Ser-46-phosphorylated p53. Cell 2000; 102:849–862.
167. Mudgil AV, Segal N, Andriani F, et al. Ultraviolet B irradiation induces expansion of intraepithelial tumor cells in a tissue model of early cancer progression. J Invest Dermatol 2003; 121:191–197.
168. Hill LL, Ouhtit A, Loughlin SM, et al. Fas ligand: a sensor for DNA damage critical in skin cancer etiology. Science 1999; 285:898–900.
169. Remenyik E, Wikonkal NM, Zhang W, et al. Antigen-specific immunity does not mediate acute regression of UVB-induced p53-mutant clones. Oncogene 2003; 22:6369–6376.
170. de Gruijl FR, van der Leun JC. Development of skin tumors in hairless mice after discontinuation of ultraviolet irradiation. Cancer Res 1991; 51:979–984.
171. Ananthaswamy HN, Ullrich SE, Mascotto RE, et al. Inhibition of solar simulator-induced p53 mutations and protection against skin cancer development in mice by sunscreens. J Invest Dermatol 1999; 112:763–768.
172. Oliner JD, Pietenpol JA, Thiallingam S, et al. Oncoprotein MDM2 conceals the activation domain of tumour suppressor p53. Nature 1993; 362:857–860.
173. Kubbutat MH, Jones SN, Vousden KH. Regulation of p53 stability by Mdm2. Nature; 387:299–303.
174. Haupt Y, Maya R, Kazaz A, et al. 1997. Mdm2 promotes the rapid degradation of p53. Nature 1997; 387:296–299.
175. Giaccia AJ, Kastan MB. The complexity of p53 modulation emerging patterns from divergent signals. Genes Dev 1998; 12:2973–2983.

176. Weissman AM. Regulating protein degradation by ubiquination. Immunol Today 1997; 18:189–198.
177. Korabiowska M, Brinck U, Betke H, et al. Growth arrest DNA damage gene expression in naevi. In vivo. 1999; 13:247–250.
178. Hussein MR. Ultraviolet radiation and skin cancer: molecular mechanisms. J Cutan Pathol 2005; 32:191–205.
179. Kubbutat MH, Vousden KH. Proteolytic cleavage of human p53 by calpain: a potent regulator of protein stability. Mol Cell Biol 1997; 17:460–468.
180. Pariat M, Carillo S, Molinari M, et al. Proteolysis by calpains: a possible contribution to degradation of p53. Mol Cell Biol 1997; 17:2806–2815.
181. Gelis C, Mavon A, Vicendo P. The contribution of calpains in the downregulation of Mdm2 and p53 proteolysis in reconstituted human epidermis in response to solar irradiation. Photochem Photobiol 2005; 81:975–982.
182. Brash DE, Ziegler A, Jonason AS, et al. Sunlight and sunburn in human skin cancer: p53, apoptosis, and tumor promotion. J Invest Dermatol Symp Proc 1996; 1:136–142.
183. Leffell DJ, Brash DE. Sunlight and skin cancer. Sci Am 1996; 275:52–59.
184. Reifenberger J, Wolter M, Knobbe CB, et al. Somatic mutations in the PTCH, SMOH, SUFUH and TP53 genes in sporadic basal cell carcinomas. Br J Dermatol 2005; 152:43–51.
185. D'Errico M, Calcagnile A, Canzona F, et al. UV mutation signature in tumor suppressor genes involved in skin carcinogenesis in xeroderma pigmentosum patients. Oncogene 2000; 19:463–467.
186. Daya-Grosjean L, Sarasin A. UV-specific mutation of the human patched gene in basal cell carcinomas from normal individuals and xeroderma pigmentosum patients. Mut Res 2000; 450:193.
187. de Gruijl FR, van Kranen HJ, Mullenders LH. UV-induced DNA damage, repair, mutations and oncogenic pathways in skin cancer. J Photochem Photobiol 2001; 63:19.
188. Ping XL, Ratner D, Zhang H, et al. PTCH mutations in squamous cell carcinoma of the skin. J Invest Dermatol 2001; 116:614–616.
189. Matsumura Y, Ananthaswamy HN. Molecular mechanisms of photocarcinogenesis. Front Biosci 2002; 7:d765–d783.
190. Wiley SR, Schooley K, Smolak PJ, et al. Identification and characterization of a new member of the TNF family that induces apoptosis. Immunity 1995; 3:673–682.
191. Stander S, Schwarz T. Tumor necrosis factor-related apoptosis-inducing ligand (TRAIL) is expressed in normal skin and cutaneous inflammatory disease, but not in chronically UV-exposed skin and non-melanoma skin cancer. Am J Dermatopathol 2005; 27:116–121.
192. Rees JL. Genetic alterations in non-melanoma skin cancer. J Invest Dermatol 1994; 103:747.
193. Kreimer-Erlacher H, Seidl H, Back B, et al. High mutation frequency at Ha-ras exons 1-4 in squamous cell carcinomas from PUVA-treated psoriasis patients. Photochem Photobiol 2001; 74:323–330.
194. Chan J, Robinson ES, Yeh IT, et al. Absence of ras gene mutations in UV-induced malignant melanoma correlates with a dermal origin of melanocytes in Monodelphis domestica. Cancer Lett 2002; 184:73–80.
195. Setlow RB. DNA repair, ageing, and cancer. Natl Cancer Inst Monogr 1982; 60:249–255.

3

Etiology and Modeling of Human Melanoma

Illuminating the Dark Pathways of a Deadly Disease

Steven Kazianis and Meenhard Herlyn

Program in Molecular and Cellular Oncogenesis, The Wistar Institute, Philadelphia, Pennsylvania, U.S.A.

INTRODUCTION

Clinical Characteristics of Melanoma

Melanoma is a neoplastic disease, which resembles other malignancies in that normal cells are progressively transformed into a cell type that can be defined as showing proliferative, invasive, and metastatic properties. Melanoma is a difficult disease to treat when metastasis has occurred, although most primary melanomas are readily treated by simple or moderately complex surgical excision. Several subtypes of melanoma are described with distinct characteristics. Cutaneous lesions are predominantly broken down into superficial spreading, nodular, lentigo maligna, and acral lentiginous melanomas (1,2), however, several other rarer types exist, such as desmoplastic melanomas (3). Non-cutaneous melanomas such as ocular and mucosal lesions (4,5) comprise a lower overall percentage (6). However, these forms also contribute to a high mortality rate; uveal melanomas, for example, which comprise the majority of ocular melanomas, can be highly metastatic to the liver (6).

Although fair-skinned individuals generally show higher incidence of cutaneous melanoma, all humans, regardless of their skin type and geographic setting, can develop the disease in its various forms (7). In contrast to other cancers, the incidence has risen and is projected to continue to rise in older fair-skinned individuals (8,9). A recent study suggests that melanoma is more common in people of higher socioeconomic status than in lower status populations (10). However, the lower socioeconomic status group typically presents with more advanced stages at time of diagnosis, and in turn, experience worse survival rates from melanoma (10).

Metastatic melanoma is notoriously resistant to chemotherapy approaches (11,12), and one study has even suggested that chemotherapeutic agents can further mutate already aggressive melanoma cells (13). Patients can rapidly prognostically regress and also succumb to metastatic disease with melanoma cells located in liver, lung, spleen, brain, and other critical organs (14,15).

Cutaneous melanomas, regardless of subtype, typically develop in a stepwise manner (Fig. 1), progressing through radial, vertical, and the metastatic steps. In numerous cases, primary cutaneous melanomas are derived from nevi that can be congenital or acquired later in life. Primary lesions typically can be grossly identified by established warning signs, which include *A*symmetry, *B*order irregularity, *C*olor, and *D*iameter ("ABCD"). Currently, this mnemonic guide has been altered to include "*E*nlargement," "*E*levation," or "*E*volutionary change" (ABCDE) (16–18). When excised by dermatologists or surgeons, primary melanomas are typically collected for histological staging, and are analyzed using established criteria for "Breslow" thickness (19,20), and defined criteria regarding cell atypia in the local skin microenvironment (21). Stages vary from Stage 0, which describes radial growth phase (RGP) disease that is restricted to the epidermis, and Stage IV, which is characterized by distant metastases. A recent study has also examined long-term prognosis of patients with thin lesions that are less than 1.0 mm in "Breslow" thickness. This study established that growth phase, mitotic rate, and sex are important prognostic factors for patients with such melanomas, and the study identified subgroups at substantially greater risk for metastasis (22). In the near future, it is possible that melanomas could be primarily defined according to their RNA expression signatures, as it has begun for a few other cancer types (23–25).

Understanding the Melanocyte

In order to understand melanoma in its advanced form, one has to understand the normal developmental progression of the malignant cell precursors and try to elucidate how environmental factors interact with underlying genetic factors. All melanomas, regardless of which vertebrate species afflicted, are by definition derived from the melanocyte cell lineage (Fig. 1), which includes progenitor cells that have embryologically migrated from the neural crest (26,27). Such progenitor cells, currently referred to as "stem" cells (Fig. 1), subsequently

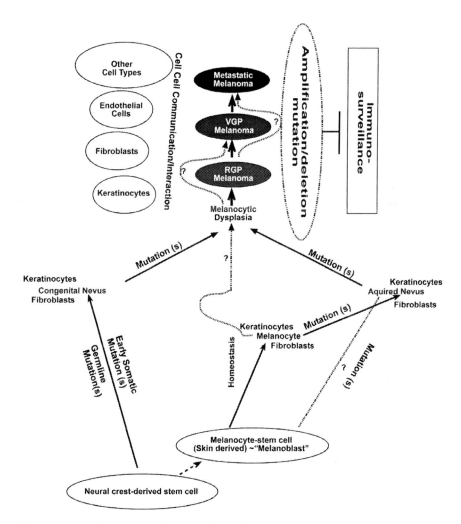

Figure 1 Developmental pathway depicting differentiation of melanocyte precursors, as well as indicating the areas where congenital or acquired mutations can contribute toward the development of malignant melanomas. *Abbreviations*: RGP, radial growth phase melanoma; VGP, vertical growth phase melanoma.

differentiate to become melanocytes (27). The term "melanoblast" (26,27), a term delineating an intermediate cell type between embryonally derived neural crest cells and melanocytes, is currently becoming less utilized and replaced with "melanocyte stem cell" (27,28). In certain vertebrates, including fishes, amphibians, and reptiles, melanocytes can also further differentiate and become melanophores, which are thought to be terminally differentiated (26,29).

Under normal physiological conditions, melanocytes are in a resting state forming the "epidermal melanin unit" with keratinocytes in the epidermis. It is in this unit where melanocytes and keratinocytes are aligned along the basement membrane zone (30). Each melanocyte, when surrounded by basal layer keratinocytes and attached to the basement membrane, transports pigment-containing melanosomes through its dendrites to approximately 35 surrounding keratinocytes. Melanocytes and keratinocytes maintain a life-long balance, which is only disturbed during transformation into a nevus or melanoma (30). During childhood, that is, during expansion of the total skin surface, there is a continuous need for melanocyte proliferation to maintain a stable ratio with the basal layer keratinocytes. Melanocytes decouple from keratinocytes prior to cell division and which growth factors induce them to divide. Our lab has demonstrated that dermis-derived growth factors, such as hepatocyte growth factor (HGF), downregulate E-cadherin and desmoglein 1 for decoupling from keratinocytes (31). ET-1 (endothelin-1) produced by keratinocytes can also downregulate E-cadherin (32). Similar functions are attributed to ET-3, produced by bFGF-stimulated fibroblasts (30,33) can exert the same functions. The growth factors bFGF, SCF, and ET-3/ET-1, alone or in combination, can initiate cell division (30,33). In summary, an imbalance in the expression of cadherins or production of growth factors leads to an imbalance in the ratio between keratinocytes and melanocytes as the first indication for a change toward transformation.

The melanocyte predominantly occupies a microenvironmental niche within the basal epidermal layer of the human epidermis (34–37), although it is also found in other parts of the body such as the inner ear, eye, peritoneal lining, and so on. It is a unique cell in that it produces and exports a class of related compounds named melanins (38) that are of variable biochemical makeup, depending upon a variety of factors, including the underlying genetics of an individual person (39,40). These melanins are hypothetically and experimentally shown to be photoprotective (41–43). This is of particular importance, because the neighboring keratinocytes respond to environmental stimuli such as UV irradiation by producing growth factors (Fig. 2) (44–51) that induce melanocytes to proliferate, produce, and export melanins (52).

Within the integument, melanocytes interact in a milieu that includes contact with matrix proteins, neighboring keratinocytes, and other cell types. All cells of the skin, to varying degrees, are subjected to environmental variables that can include physical agents, such as UV, as well as chemical agents. The skin has to retain a dynamic plasticity to enable quick wound healing, and also respond to DNA damage. In mammals, a major role of the skin is also the production of pigmented hairs, which are rejuvenated and replenished by a complex and co-ordinate symphony that includes progenitor cells, keratinocytes of different stages of differentiation, melanocytes, and other cell types (26,27). It is thought that the melanocyte is a long-lived cell that is induced to proliferate only after appropriate local stimuli (34–37). At present, it has been shown in mice that a pluripotent stem cell exists within the hair bulge, which, under

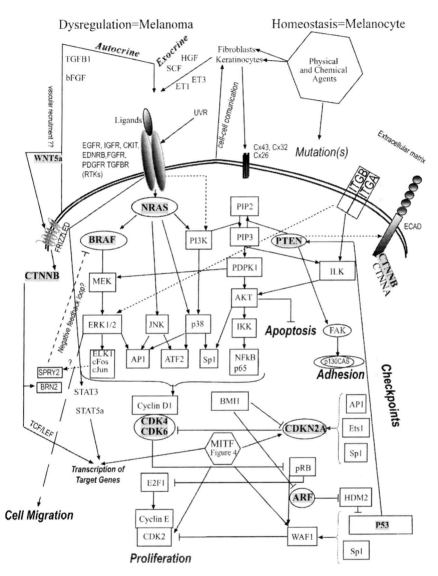

Figure 2 Simplified schematic of critical genes and pathways implicated in distinguishing melanoma from normal melanocytes. Genes depicted in bold letters and highlighted are implicated in being involved especially in melanoma signal transduction, as they are mutated (somatically or in the germline) or aberrantly expressed. Dotted lines represent indirect interactions. Pathway intermediate proteins are not shown due to space constraints. Numerous areas of crosstalk between pathways exist.

appropriate stimuli, periodically produces cells such as melanocytes. Some of these melanocytes clearly migrate to the neighboring hair bulb, and at the base of the hair shaft aggregate, produce, and export melanins. Melanocytes within hair bulbs consequently provide the distinct pigments for hair in mammals. Graying hair, typically a hallmark of aging, has recently been shown to be indicative of defective self-maintenance of melanocyte stem cells (27).

MODELING MELANOMA

In order to elucidate genetic and environmental mechanisms of melanocytic transformation, invasion, and metastasis, and to discover potential therapeutic approaches, numerous models of melanoma have been developed. Nearly a century ago, hybrid fishes between species of the genus *Xiphophorus* were created (53,54) that developed melanoma in the absence of environmental stimuli (Fig. 3A). The etiology of these spontaneous melanomas, which are typically extremely invasive but not highly metastatic, are relatively well understood and attributed to lack of gene regulation. Within the last two decades, a number of studies have shown that these fish melanomas occur due to the inheritance of a mutant, ligand-independent tyrosine kinase receptor, referred to as Xiphophorus melanoma receptor kinase (Xmrk) (29,55,56). The *Xmrk* gene is homologous but not orthologous to the mammalian *EGFR* locus (57). Hybrid fishes between different species of *Xiphophorus* overexpress this protein, which induces cellular proliferation within cells of the melanocytic lineage (29,55,56). Activation of several downstream protein targets, including members of the mitogen-activated protein kinase (MAPK) pathway, has been shown using the fish model as a consequence of the constitutively active Xmrk oncoprotein as well as by using chimaeric Xmrk/Egfr constructs in mammalian cell lines (58). In backcross *Xiphophorus* hybrids, differential susceptibility of malignant melanoma is associated with a locus that harbors a tumor suppressor gene currently referred to as *CDKNAB* (59). Evolutionary studies have shown that this locus is related to mammalian *CDKN2A* (59,60), which is clearly implicated in a large number of human melanoma cases. This model has been among the first to yield valuable data regarding the contribution of environmental factors in the development of melanoma and many other neoplastic diseases. These fishes are still exploited today and numerous submodels are utilized, including ones where melanomas occur only in aging fish derived from natural populations (61,62).

Most recently, in addition to *Xiphophorus*, another fish genus is also being utilized in melanoma research. In an exciting new model (63), zebrafish are utilized, which develop integumentary pigment cell aggregates referred to as fish nevi ("F-nevi") (Fig. 3). These fish were bred homozygously for a mutation in the zebrafish *TP53* locus and for a transgenic copy of human BRAFV600E mutant driven by an endogenously derived *MITF* promoter. Albeit with a relatively long latency, vertical growth phase (VGP) and nodular melanomas occur within three genetic backgrounds, with striping patterning of these strains

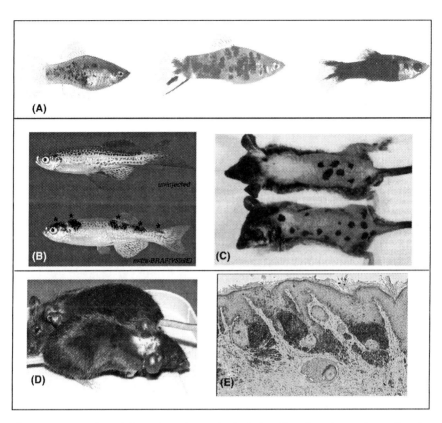

Figure 3 Depiction of five selected models depicting diversity of experimental mela-noma models: (**A**) *Xiphophorus* fish (*Left*): non-hybrid *X. maculatus* with the Sp pigment pattern. (*Right*): hybrid fishes (F₁ and backcross hybrids, respectively) progress-ively show greater phenotypic enhancement of the same pigment pattern. (**B**) The two zeb-rafish graphically illustrate the development of "F-nevi" derived only from a transgenic background of mutant (V600E) versus ectopically expressed wild-type human *BRAF*. (**C**) Two *Monodelphis domestica* that were UVB irradiated as neonates and developed nodular melanoma. (**D**) Two mice with nodular melanomas, resulting from overexpression of the metabotropic GRM1. (**E**) Histological section of neonatal human skin that has been grafted on severe combined immunodeficiency mouse. Melanocytes show transformed phenotype due to dermal injection of adenoviruses carrying human *FGF2, EDN3*, and *KITLG (SCF)* genes, in addition to UVB irradiation of the epidermis. *Abbreviations*: UVB, ultraviolet B; GRM1, glutamate receptor 1. *Source*: Figure 3B adapted from Ref. 202; Figure 3C adapted from Ref. 203; Figure 3D adapted from Ref. 204.

playing a role in the positioning of nevi and melanomas (63). The significance of using human oncogenes in a fish somewhat counterbalances the argument that fish are evolutionarily distant and not relevant for human melanoma research. On the other hand, fishes have an integumentary architecture that differs from human, and they are naturally exposed to much different environmental stimuli.

Marsupials such as *Monodelphis domestica*, the South American opossum, represent a model utilizing females with young that stay attached ex utero. Studies have shown that melanomas can occur after UV irradiation of the pups; UVB wavelengths have been statistically inductive, while UVA was not (64–66). While gene homologues such as *CDKN2A*, *NRAS*, and *KRAS* have been cloned and partially characterized (67–70), the marsupial genome–sequencing project has only recently been initiated (71). In addition, lack of inbred lines and additional strains such as immuno-compromised animals for research have somewhat impeded progress in this promising model where animals develop truly metastatic disease much akin to the human affliction.

Another relatively under utilized model traces melanoma development in miniature sinclair swine. In this model, regression of lesions is studied as individuals develop a mature immune system. This relatively under utilized model has shown immune recognition of early lesions and the possibility that loss of telomerase expression may be implicated in regression of lesions (72,73).

Rodents indisputably have been invaluable for the study of melanoma. Researchers have exploited the mouse *Mus musculus*, as well as the great number of tools associated with it. Genomic tools include completion of mouse genome mapping and sequencing, delineation of its transcriptome, and the powerful genetic approaches, which include "knockout," "knock-in," and now RNAi-mediated technologies (74–76). Additionally, great control could be utilized regarding tissue-specific expression of transgenes and inducability of genetic elements that can be difficult to carry into adulthood (75,76). A complete listing of all mouse melanoma models is beyond the scope of this chapter, and has not been extensively reviewed. However, the contributions of these in what we understand about melanoma development is profound, and some of these models will be specifically mentioned subsequently.

Melanoma biology can also be eloquently studied by using hybrid models, such as by studying the behavior of human melanocytes or human melanoma cells injected or transplanted into immune-deficient mice. In a now well-established model, human skin derived from adult or neonates is obtained from surgical procedures, including abdominoplasties and the routine circumcision of male infants. This skin represents a wide range of natural human genetic heterogeneity, indicative of the population it is derived from. Samples are subsequently surgically grafted onto the dorsum of immune-compromised mouse strains such as severe combined immunodeficiency (SCID) or nude varieties. The graft is incorporated in a mouse wound bed and becomes vascularized. Experimental manipulations can be carried out once the grafts are well healed and incorporated. This model has the advantage of studying melanocytes in a context of being surrounded by keratinocytes, matrix proteins, and fibroblasts as they are normally present in human skin. Using this grafting technique, our laboratory was able to progressively establish that several growth factors, injected into the human dermis using adenoviral vectors, could induce melanocytic proliferation (30,77,78). When a combination of FGF^{FGF2}, ET3^{EDN3}, and SCF^{KITLG} transgenes were used, and

UVB was added, primary cutaneous melanomas were induced that showed neoplasia, radial, and limited vertical growth characteristics (33,79). In a recently completed study, non-UV–irradiated skin samples, subjected to the above-mentioned mixture of transgenes, were analyzed for genomic instability and *TP53* pathway activation. A DNA damage response was strongly activated in these human skin xenografts, and derived lesions showed allelic imbalance at loci prone to DNA double-strand break formation when DNA replication is compromised (80). Gorgoulis et al. and Bartkova et al. (80,81) suggest that cancer development is associated with DNA replication stress, which leads to DNA double-strand breaks, genomic instability, and selective pressure for p53 mutations.

Grafting human skin onto rodents has the disadvantage of introducing genetic heterogeneity, as evidenced by the fact that melanomas do not develop in *all* skin samples due to the growth factor induction/UV irradiation regimen (33). Undoubtedly, skin type and genetic heterogeneity play a factor in such experimentation. Therefore, several laboratories, including ours, have developed a means to study melanocytes in a more controlled microenvironment that includes fibroblasts and keratinocytes (77,82–85). Although there are several permutations of this model, it generally involves embedding fibroblasts, such as in collagen(s), and then overlaying with keratinocytes, at which time melanocytes or melanoma cells can be incorporated into the mixture. Within this in-vitro microenviroment, melanocytes readily localize to the junction between the fibroblast and the keratinocyte layer, mimicking the in-vivo situation in human skin. Keratinocytes naturally form stratified layers forming an epidermis in vitro, and this is punctuated by exposing part of the reconstruct to air, at which point keratinocytes form the uppermost stratified layers. Models such as this undoubtedly will be further exploited because one can use a single source of cells. Additionally, one can overexpress or repress expression of selected genes using vectors, and utilize the rapidly expanding repertoire of RNA-interference methodologies.

ETIOLOGY

Physical Agents

Perhaps the most universal physical agent that most persons are variably exposed to is wavelengths that belong to the UV spectrum (200–400 nm). This is broken down into arbitrary segments referred to as UVA (320–400 nm), UVB (290–320 nm), and UVC (200–290 nm). UV irradiation causes DNA damage including cyclobutane pyrimidine dimers and (6–4) photoproducts; and these are usually repaired by endogenous nucleotide excision repair enzymes. Sun exposure in humans, especially in childhood and in individuals with a history of erythema (or "sunburn") is statistically linked with the development of melanoma (86,87). Fair-skinned individuals and particularly those with red or blond hair are at highest risk, and numerous research reports have closely examined the complex genetics that contribute to the production of such phenotypes

(88–90). Darker-skinned individuals, typically with higher levels of exported eumelanin derived from their melanocytes, are less prone to the development of most forms of cutaneous melanoma and show less UV-induced damage, expression of *IL-10*, and the recruitment of neutrophils (91). In addition, there is no significant correlation of melanoma development with geographical latitude in such darker-skinned individuals (7), although this is somewhat contrasted by another study (92). In light-skinned individuals, however, there exist a large number of independent studies, in different continents, positively correlating latitude, UV exposure, and melanoma formation (7,87,93,94).

For the study of UV-inducibility of melanoma, Setlow et al. (95–97) established using *Xiphophorus* fishes that UVB irradiation was statistically inductive toward the development of melanoma. These studies and others also eloquently pointed out that photolyase, an enzyme lost in the eutherian mammalian lineage which includes humans, could reverse DNA damage if fish were exposed to ambient light after irradiation (95–99). Within mammalian models, UVB has also been indisputably inductive toward the formation of melanoma. UVB wavelengths were effective at inducing melanoma formation in the marsupial *Monodelphis domestica*, in the absence of chemical agents, introduction of transgenes, or the use of gene knockout strategies (100,101). The animals are exposed as neonates, and develop the melanomas as they mature into adulthood (Fig. 3). In a genetically engineered mouse model carrying an *HRAS* transgene, and being null for *ARF*, it has been shown that UVB targets the Rb pathway and specifically *CDK6* or *CDKN2A*, resulting in an increased incidence of melanomagenesis (102). In another highly pertinent mouse model, animals transgenic for *HGF* develop primary and metastatic melanomas after a single erythemal dose of neonatal UVB radiation (103,104).

In xenografts models using human adult- and neonate-derived skin, UVB has also been shown to play a key role in melanoma formation (33,79,105). Melanocytic hyperplasia was seen when ectopic expression of bFGF was induced and in the presence of UVB (79). Later experiments using UVB and a combination of growth factors, as mentioned above, in neonatal foreskin xenografts led to the development of primary cutaneous melanomas (33,105).

The involvement of UVA in melanomagenesis is controversial and not proven. Setlow et al. (95,96) showed significant evidence and reason for alarm that UVA could also lead to melanoma induction in models using *Xiphophorus* fish (95,96). As UVA is ever-present in our outdoor environment and may be increasing due to ozone depletion, their landmark studies led to more studies using UVA and perhaps influenced sunscreen manufacturers to reformulate their compounds to block the UVA spectrum as well (95–97). UVA is even present within our indoor environments, as these wavelengths are found in a large variety of fluorescent, quartz halogen, and tungsten bulbs (106).

In contrast to the studies using *Xiphophorus*, experimentation in *Monodelphis* (64,65), *Mus* (107), and using human xenografts (33,79,105) has failed to clearly implicate UVA in the formation of melanoma. However, numerous studies have suggested that UVA can produce DNA damage through oxidative stress, including within melanocytes by the production of reactive oxygen species (108,109). In transgenic mutA mice and within epidermis, UVA induces C to T transitions at methylated CpG-associated dipyrimidine sites more frequently than UVB (110). Other studies have also suggested that compounds produced in the process of producing eumelanins and phaemelanins themselves could become genotoxic to melanocytes upon exposure to oxidative stress and contribute to microsatellite instability (43,111). In addition, it is well established that UV (in both UVB and UVA ranges) irradiation of skin suppresses the immune system (109,112).

Chemical Agents

Virtually nothing is known about the role that exogenous chemical compounds and topically applied compounds play in the formation of melanoma. Experimentally, however, numerous chemical carcinogens have been shown to be inductive for the development of melanoma in fishes as well as mammals. In hybrid fish that genetically show lack of gene regulation at two loci, methyl-N-nitrosourea is strongly inductive (61,113,114). In three of four tested mouse strains, a chronic (25-week) protocol of 7,12-dimethylbenz[a]anthracene as initiator and croton oil as promoter led to the development of melanomas with invasive properties (115). Hypothetically, it is possible that even compounds thought of as inert by majority of the human population, when applied to skin, could be melanomagenic. The use of antibacterial soaps, for example, are said to contain photosensitizing compounds, and in combination with sun exposure, may lead to free radical production in the skin and may contribute to the development of melanoma (116,117). Recently, the U.S. Food and Drug Administration (alert 3/2005) has issued a "black box" warning for the drug tacrolimus (marketed as Protopic® and used primarily to treat atopic dermatitis), and is investigating if the drug is linked to a few reported cancer cases, including melanoma, within human patients (118). Other chemicals are also raising an interest, including a class of parabens compounds, which have apparently been used extensively in cosmetics and sunscreens (119–121). A few studies have linked this class of chemicals to estrogenic activity (119–121), and one study established that these compounds could be detected in breast carcinomas of human patients (122). To date, no data seem to have been published regarding these compounds and melanoma, although the fact that they have been included in sunscreen compositions (119) may merit further study.

Genetic Etiology and Susceptibility

BRAF

Several loci have been implicated in melanoma formation in humans and modeled in vitro and in vivo. At the present time, *BRAF* is indisputably the most commonly implicated gene. In a simple but laborious screen of hundreds of patient melanoma and matched control samples, researchers were able to sequence several genes in the MAPK pathway (123). They discovered that these patients prominently showed somatic mutations in the *BRAF* gene within their tumors (123). The *BRAF* locus, comprising ~200 kb of genomic sequence is composed of 18 exons, and codes for a serine–threonine kinase of 767 amino acids. *BRAF* is most often mutated from a T to an A at nucleotide position 1799 [cDNA sequence position after the start codon, resulting in a V to E amino acid substitution at the 600th amino acid position (V600E); previously identified as V599E]. The mutant protein has been shown to have a ~100X higher kinase activity than the wild-type protein, and in certain in-vitro systems the ability to transform cells, including melanocytes (123,124).

The BRAF V600E position, as well as other somatic mutations predominantly in exons 15 and 11, has now been shown to be commonly mutated in melanoma. Of note, with the exception of one possible case (125), no account of a germline V600E BRAF mutation has been discovered, although it could have been easily detected by an appreciable number of studies (125–128). Intriguingly, at least one report suggests that there may be complex underlying genetics that may have familial predisposition implications (129).

It has been discovered that *BRAF* mutations, especially including V600E, are found in both congenital and acquired nevi that can exist in the body for decades with relative homeostasis (Table 1A) (130–134). It is possible, and perhaps likely, that BRAF mutation may represent a primary event in the progression toward melanoma formation. However, at least two studies suggest that *BRAF* mutations are found at a higher incidence in metastatic melanomas rather than primary melanomas, and so may be indicative of disease progression (135,136). Compiling published data (130,131,133,137–140) presented in Table 1A, one can see that indeed many different subtypes of nevi also display BRAF V600E somatic mutations (137/282; 49% total). However, when one more closely examines the subtypes of cutaneous nevi, it is obvious that spitz nevi (0/70) and possibly blue nevi (3/25) differ from other cutaneous aggregations, in showing a low incidence of BRAF somatic mutations (3/95 = 3.2%) compared with the corrected, combined value for other cutaneous nevi (134/ 187 = 72%; Table 1A).

When one examines primary melanomas of the skin (Table 1B), a high percentage shows BRAF somatic mutations (224/498; 45%) although this percentage is lower than that of nevi. This paradoxical situation has been the topic of considerable mention in the literature (132,135,141–144) and is still very much unresolved. Within metastatic melanomas (Table 1C), the percentage (56%) is somewhat higher than primary melanomas, although still not as high as the 72% of nevi.

Screens of other melanoma subtypes such as mucosal melanomas (4), desmoplastic melanomas (3), uveal melanomas (5,141,145–147), and so on, reveal much lower percentages of V600E BRAF mutations (Table 1D). Curiously, these other melanomas typically occur in less sun-exposed anatomical regions. However, the T1799A mutation is currently not considered to be a canonical "UV-signature" mutation (4). The fact that somatic *BRAF* mutations are frequent

Table 1A Detected *BRAF* Mutations in Nevi

Study	Type	N	N (%) w/*BRAF* mutations
Pollock et al. (130)	Congenital	7	6 (86)
Pollock et al. (130)	Intradermal	42	37 (88)
Pollock et al. (130)	Compound	23	16 (70)
Pollock et al. (130)	Dysplastic	5	4 (80)
Uribe et al. (131)	Common	22	16 (73)
Uribe et al. (131)	Atypical	25	13 (52)
Kumar et al. (133)	Intradermal	8	7 (88)
Kumar et al. (133)	Compound	11	8 (73)
Kumar et al. (133)	Junctional	6	2 (33)
Miller et al. (139,192)	Atypical	9	4 (44)
Mihic-Probst et al. (137)	Spitz	20	0 (0)
Turner et al. (138)	Spitz	24	0 (0)
Saldanha et al. 2005?	Spitz	26	0 (0)
Saldanha et al. 2005	Blue	25	3 (12)
Turner et al. (138)	Common	7	4 (58)
Turner et al. (138)	Dysplastic	6	3 (50)
Saldanha et al. 2005	Common acquired	16	14 (88)
Total		282	137 (49%)
Total (excluding spitz and blue nevi)		187	134 (72%)

in melanoma could imply a role of an etiologic agent, such as UV in inducing mutations such as V600E. The fewer percentage of *BRAF* V600E mutations in melanomas from non-sun-exposed sites suggests that UV irradiation may be causative, as others have noted (4), although the molecular mechanism has currently eluded discovery.

A particularly high incidence of V600E BRAF somatic mutations have been discovered in papillary carcinomas of the thyroid as well (148). In patients exposed to high levels of radiation resulting from the Chernobyl radioactive release accident, the *BRAF* locus has been found to be somatically recombined with the neighboring *AKAP9* locus, resulting in the formation of a fusion protein with the kinase domain of BRAF. This fusion protein exhibited kinase activity (123). Whether this mutation contributes to thyroid carcinoma or to melanoma has not currently been shown experimentally. Other mutations have also been discovered in *BRAF* within melanomas and other neoplasms (149). Some of these mutations have also been shown to be activating, although none are found at the incidence of the V600E mutation (123).

NRAS

The human Ras family of GTPases is encoded for by four loci: *HRAS*, *HRAS2* (*ERAS*), *NRAS*, and *KRAS*. Mutant forms of these genes have been discovered

Table 1B   Detected *BRAF* Mutations in Primary Cutaneous Melanomas[a]

Study	N	N (%) w/*BRAF* mutations
Davies et al. (123)	9	6 (67)
Pollock et al. (130)	5	4 (80)
Dong et al. (135)	28	7 (25)
Uribe et al. (131)	25	13 (52)
Yazdi et al. (132)	97	28 (29)
Cruz et al. (141)	44	16 (36)
Omholt et al. (142)	70	40 (57)
Miller et al. (139,192)	34	20 (59)
Reifenberger et al. (143)	15	8 (53)
Thomas et al. (144)	37	17 (46)
Sasaki et al. (158)	23	9 (39)
Turner et al. (138)	6	4 (67)
Goydos et al. 2005	36	20 (56)
Davison et al. (3)	57	23 (40)
Saldanha et al. 2005	12	9 (75)
	498	224 (45%)

[a]For brevity, studies with less than five total examined samples are not included.

in a large number of neoplasms, and studies have repeatedly documented that active forms of these proteins are oncogenic, in a large variety of cell types (150). Although *HRAS* has been shown to be inductive in classic melanoma models employing mice (151,152), and *KRAS* has been shown to be mutated in a small number of melanoma cases (143,153), *NRAS* seems to be involved in many more melanoma lesions (142,143,154–156). As NRAS activates the MAPK pathway and acts "upstream" of BRAF (Fig. 2), one would predict a mutually exclusive nature to mutations of these two genes. Several studies

Table 1C   Detected *BRAF* Mutations in Melanoma Metastases

Study	N	N (%) w/*BRAF* mutations
Pollock et al. (130)	60	41 (68)
Omholt et al. (142)	88	43 (49)
Miller et al. (139,192)	24	19 (79)
Reifenberger et al. (143)	22	6 (27)
Goydos et al. 2005	79	43 (54)
	273	152 (56%)

Table 1D   Detected *BRAF* Mutations in Other Melanomas

Study	Melanoma type	Patients	N (%) w/*BRAF* mutations
Cruz et al. (141)	Uveal	62	0 (0)
Edmunds et al. (146)	Uveal	48	0 (0)
Cohen et al. (147,148)	Uveal	29	0 (0)
Rimoldi et al. (5)	Uveal	10	0 (0)
Weber et al. (153)	Uveal	42	0 (0)
Klc et al. 2004	Uveal	33	0 (0)
Edwards (4)	Mucosal	12	0 (0)
Helmke et al. 2004	Anorectal	19	2 (11)[a]
Panagopoulos et al. 2005	MMSP	8	0 (0)
Davison et al. (3)	Desmoplastic	12	0 (0)
Total		275	2 (0.007%)

[a]Both cases were not V600E mutations.
Abbreviation: MMSP, malignant melanoma of soft parts.

have presented data to support this notion (108,123,142,154,157,158). However, it is distinctly possible that mutated *NRAS* can be more potently oncogenic than mutant forms of *BRAF*, because *NRAS* can also be involved in signaling with the PI3K pathway (Fig. 2) (2,159). In addition, several studies have indicated that within melanoma, NRAS and BRAF mutations may be mutually exclusive events potentially indicating the sufficiency of NRAS and BRAF at activating the same MAPK pathway (123,142,143,149,154,157). Eskandarpour et al. (156) also indicate a high percentage (95%) mutation rate of *NRAS* locus in a Swedish cohort of melanoma patients that have *CDKN2A* germline mutations. The same study found NRAS mutated in only 10% of sporadic melanomas. Furthermore, the authors discovered multiple activating *NRAS* mutations in tumor cells from the same patients. Based on this study (156), it may be possible that patients with *CDKN2A* germline mutations may predispose to high genomic instability and high frequencies of *NRAS* mutations.

CDKN2A

Several other loci have clearly been shown to be associated with melanoma formation in humans and implied in both familial and sporadic forms of the disease. Numerous families showing high to moderate risk of developing this disease have been studied, and the melanoma tumor suppressor gene candidate, *CDKN2A*, has been implicated (160–162). In addition, numerous publications have shown that within some families with atypical mole syndrome, there is an association with *CDKN2A* germline mutations (163–165). Although a small locus, it is quite a complex one, coding for two distinct transcripts/proteins derived from two promoters. The two proteins, which are structurally distinct, are named p14[ARF] and p16^{CDKN2A}. While p14^{ARF} has been shown to destabilize the hdm2 protein (Fig. 2), which in turn destabilizes p53, p16^{CDKN2A} is implicated in regulating G1 checkpoint through its interactions with CDK4 or CDKN6/cyclin D complexes, blocking phosphorylation of the Rb tumor suppressor protein by cyclin D proteins. In sum, *CDKN2A* locus codes for two proteins, each critically involved in distinct tumor suppression pathways.

In the sporadic version of cutaneous melanoma, it is thought that *CDKN2A* is sometimes mutated (166,167), deleted in a heterozygous or homozygous state (168–171), or RNA expression is dramatically reduced due to promoter hypermethylation (172–174). Although the mechanism of somatic deletion is not fully understood, it is thought that mutations that occur often show "UV signatures" that include nucleotide base changes such as C–T or CC–TT transitions (166,167). Although the majority of mutations exist in exon 2, the region transcribed to produce both p14arf and p16, some mutations only affect one of the two proteins (168–171).

Important and confirmatory experiments regarding the role of both mouse homologous proteins (p19arf and p16) have been completed (102,151,175,176). Using a transgenic mouse with a tyrosinase-driven mutant (v12G) *HRAS* and combination of a germline deleted *CDKN2A* locus that either abrogated p19^{ARF} (in the mouse this locus produces a 19 kD protein), p16^{CDKN2A}, or both proteins. Researchers were able to induce melanomagenesis in a variety of backgrounds with or without physical or chemical agents (102,151,175,176).

TP53

Somatic and germline mutations have been reported for *TP53* in virtually every human cancer and it has been demonstrated that ~50% of human tumors harbor *TP53* mutations (177). In melanoma, it has been noted that earlier studies using immuno-histochemistry to visualize p53 protein may have been flawed, because it has been reported that wild-type p53 can be robustly expressed in melanoma, and the technique may not exclusively indicate mutated protein (178–181). Due to this limitation in melanoma, a systematic sequencing study of the entire coding region of the *TP53* locus would have to be performed within tumors, in addition to examining control tissues. Additionally, one would have to address the status of the entire pathway, which includes the number of key proteins involved in the regulation of p53 as well as the mediation of DNA damage checkpoint control. To date, such approaches have not been performed. However, it is clear that p53 itself is mutated, at least in a low percentage of melanomas (178,179,181). In addition, these discovered mutations show UV signatures and overlap with mutations found in other skin cancers such as squamous cell carcinomas (178,179,181). It is even more obvious that inactivation of the p53 pathway, either through deletion of the *CDKN2A/ARF* locus or other means, is a common occurrence in melanoma. Additionally, within experimental animal models, *TP53* mutations can co-operate with mutant *BRAF* (63) or *HRAS* (175,176) to induce melanoma.

PTEN

Deletions of the *PTEN* tumor suppressor locus have been reported in melanoma cell lines as well as in both primary and metastatic melanomas (182–186). PTEN is a multifunctional protein that is involved in mediating signals of integrins, and also is involved in mediating signals from receptor tyrosine kinases (Fig. 2). In one study, substantial overlap of *NRAS* or *BRAF* somatic mutations existed with *PTEN* somatic alterations (154). These findings suggest the existence of possible cooperation between *NRAS* or *BRAF* activation and *PTEN* loss in melanoma development. In addition, restoration of *PTEN* in metastatic melanoma cells led to increased apoptosis, less invasion, vascularization, and metastasis (187). These data and others cumulatively and strongly implicate *PTEN* as a tumor suppressor locus in melanoma and also provide additional avenues for the treatment of metastatic melanoma.

MITF

The microphthalmia gene was first discovered in mouse, and encodes a basic helix–loop–helix zipper transcription factor that usually partners with other transcription factors. Mutations in this locus led to loss of pigmentation in numerous parts of the body where melanocytes normally occur, also resulting in reduced eye size (thus the original name "microphthalmia") and early onset deafness. The human homolog is also implicated in pigmentary abnormalities and deafness disorders (188). MITF plays a profound role in the commitment and homeostasis of melanocytes and their precursor cells (Fig. 4) (50,51,189–194). Genes such as tyrosinase, which confer melanocytes with unique properties, are strictly regulated by MITF. MITF is produced in several isoforms, and in melanocytes the MITF-M isoform predominates, enabling use of this transcript as a prognostic marker (195). MITF is truly a master regulator of melanocytes in that it not only turns on genes important for the synthesis of melanins, but also regulates genes involved in cell cycle regulation such as *CDKN2A* (51) and *CDKN1A* (Fig. 4) (50). It also transcriptionally regulates *BCL2*, which confers anti-apopotosis properties to cells (194). As MITF and its various transcriptional binding partners are implicated in both lineage commitment and differentiation and anti-apoptosis, it is a very complex but important locus to understand. Clearly, fully delineating the role of this locus in neural crest-derived cells would greatly serve toward the understanding of melanocyte biology and ultimately melanoma.

Other Loci

Despite a tremendous advancement of molecular genetics, there undoubtedly remain other loci that contribute to melanoma biology. As the genome sequence is complete, this implies that the correct genes have to be discovered as being implicated in melanoma formation. The advent and infiltration of microarray technologies, to assess RNA expression, but also to define regions of deletions

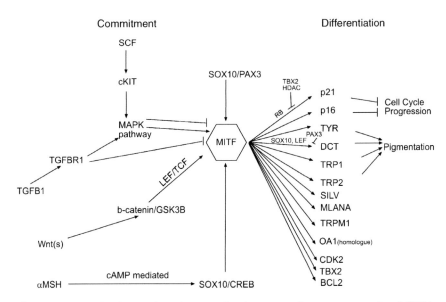

Figure 4 The role of MITF in melanocyte development and cancer progression. MITF is involved in melanocyte lineage commitment, differentiation, and in regulating the cell cycle. *Abbreviation*: MITF, microphthalmia-associated transcription factor.

and duplications will greatly assist our study of melanoma toward finding cures. As an example, consider a study using mice where a genomic screening technique for adipocyte-related phenotypes relying on random integration yielded unexpected results (196). The authors discovered a gene that was transcriptionally overexpressed as a result of a specific DNA integration event. Afflicted mice showed hyperpigmentation of the earlobes within 10–12 days of age, and developed metastatic melanoma by three months (Fig. 2). Chromosomal walking and cloning revealed that ectopic expression of the metabotropic glutamate receptor 1 (*GRM1*) was implicated (196–199). This G protein–coupled receptor was previously unstudied, and is the current focus of research by numerous investigators.

CONCLUSIONS AND FUTURE DIRECTIONS

The genetics of melanoma susceptibility in humans has long been studied and has been greatly assisted by the availability of samples from melanoma-prone kindreds. Availability of tumor material for genetic analysis and corresponding control tissue from patients has always been a particular issue when it comes to genetic testing, because material from small RGP or VGP melanomas are often prioritized for histologic examination. Luckily, newer technological advances in preservation enable a coordinated team to conduct research on the removed material as well as not compromise the pathology, which is typically prioritized for diagnostic purposes. In addition, techniques such as laser capture microdissection enable pathologists to extract ever more precise areas of tumors and surrounding tissue that can be used for DNA and, in some cases, RNA analyses as well.

At the current time, the advent of polymerase chain reaction (PCR), microarray printing, and advanced DNA sequencing methologies have advanced the field of melanoma research tremendously. It is currently possible to simultaneously collect information regarding sex, age, tumor topology, skin and hair color, sun exposure history, and melanoma biopsy, and then be able to correlate these data with pathological melanoma staging. A research team can theoretically also have information regarding mutation status of critical gene targets, expression for virtually every gene in the human genome, and resolute data regarding amplified or deleted regions. With control tissue, one can tell if changes in the melanoma genome arose somatically or from the germline.

The above-mentioned idealized scheme maximizes the information that can be gained from a patient for research purposes. Ultimately, this will not only enable an understanding of the disease but provide for better treatment options for each patient. The delineation of UV as a clear etiologic agent has greatly assisted in educating us all, in not overdoing our exposure to the sun and understanding that some of us are in especially higher risk groups. Fundamentally, the understanding of melanocyte biology will ultimately lead to cures that will be targeted and specific for melanoma. In addition, the discovery of somatic mutation of genes such as *BRAF* in large percentages of melanoma patients offers tremendous promise that targeting the mutant protein in melanoma cells, specifically, could have immediate benefit to patient survival. Some of these approaches have already been taken to the clinic with some degree of success (200,201). Undoubtedly, the next generation of treatments will work better, and these approaches will benefit many groups of patients. This is the goal that both basic researchers and clinicians have in common.

ACKNOWLEDGMENTS

We would like to thank all members of our laboratory for assisting with numerous aspects of this manuscript. Drs. Suzie Chen, Edward Robinson, and Leonard Zon are sincerely thanked for generously providing images of mice, South American opossum, and zebrafish, respectively. The *Xiphophorus* Genetic Stock Center is acknowledged for the assistance and service to the entire community of fish–melanoma researchers and for the studies conducted by Dr Steven Kazianis and colleagues. Funding for our laboratory is derived from the National Institutes of Health grants CA93372, CA098101, CA25874, CA47159, CA80999, CA76674, and RR017336-01A1, in addition to the Commonwealth Universal Research Enhancement Program, Pennsylvania Department of Health. We would also like to thank the donations from private organizations including the Sullivan Foundation and the Bill Walter III Melanoma Research Fund.

REFERENCES

1. Satyamoorthy K, Herlyn M. Cellular and molecular biology of human melanoma. Cancer Biol Ther 2002; 1:14–17.
2. Chudnovsky Y, Khavari PA, Adams AE. Melanoma genetics and the development of rational therapeutics. J Clin Invest 2005; 115:813–824.
3. Davison JM, Rosenbaum E, Barrett TL, et al. Absence of V599E BRAF mutations in desmoplastic melanomas. Cancer 2005; 103:788–792.
4. Edwards RH, Ward MR, Wu H, et al. Absence of BRAF mutations in UV-protected mucosal melanomas. J Med Genet 2004; 41:270–272.
5. Rimoldi D, Salvi S, Lienard D, et al. Lack of BRAF mutations in uveal melanoma. Cancer Res 2003; 63:5712–5715.
6. Singh AD, Bergman L, Seregard S. Uveal melanoma: epidemiologic aspects. Ophthalmol Clin North Am 2005; 18:75–84, viii.
7. Eide MJ, Weinstock MA. Association of UV index, latitude, and melanoma incidence in nonwhite populations—US Surveillance, Epidemiology, and End Results (SEER) Program, 1992 to 2001. Arch Dermatol 2005; 141:477–481.
8. Bevona C, Sober AJ. Melanoma incidence trends. Dermatol Clin 2002; 20: 589–595, vii.
9. Geller AC, Miller DR, Annas GD, et al. Melanoma incidence and mortality among US whites, 1969–1999. JAMA 2002; 288:1719–1720.
10. Reyes Ortiz CA, Goodwin JS, Freeman JL. The effect of socioeconomic factors on incidence, stage at diagnosis and survival of cutaneous melanoma. Med Sci Monit 2005; 11:RA163–RA172.
11. Serrone L, Hersey P. The chemoresistance of human malignant melanoma: an update. Melanoma Res 1999; 9:51–58.
12. Soengas MS, Lowe SW. Apoptosis and melanoma chemoresistance. Oncogene 2003; 22:3138–3151.
13. Lev DC, Onn A, Melinkova VO, et al. Exposure of melanoma cells to dacarbazine results in enhanced tumor growth and metastasis in vivo. J Clin Oncol 2004; 22:2092–2100.
14. Rodolfo M, Daniotti M, Vallacchi V. Genetic progression of metastatic melanoma. Cancer Lett 2004; 214:133–147.
15. Chang DZ, Panageas KS, Osman I, et al. Clinical significance of BRAF mutations in metastatic melanoma. J Transl Med 2004; 2:46.
16. Thomas L, Tranchand P, Berard F, et al. Semiological value of ABCDE criteria in the diagnosis of cutaneous pigmented tumors. Dermatology 1998; 197:11–17.
17. Hazen BP, Bhatia AC, Zaim T, et al. The clinical diagnosis of early malignant melanoma: expansion of the ABCD criteria to improve diagnostic sensitivity. Dermatol Online J 1999; 5:3.
18. Strumia R, Montanari A. Low positive predictive value of ABCD-E rule for dermatoscopy of small melanocytic naevi. Melanoma Res 2003; 13:631–632.
19. Breslow A. Prognosis in cutaneous melanoma: tumor thickness as a guide to treatment. Pathol Annu 1980; 15:1–22.

20. Breslow A. Prognostic factors in the treatment of cutaneous melanoma. J Cutan Pathol 1979; 6:208–212.

21. Elder DE, Jucovy PM, Tuthill RJ, et al. The classification of malignant melanoma. Am J Dermatopathol 1980; 2:315–320.

22. Gimotty PA, Guerry D, Ming ME, et al. Thin primary cutaneous malignant melanoma: a prognostic tree for 10-year metastasis is more accurate than American Joint Committee on Cancer staging. J Clin Oncol 2004; 22:3668–3676.

23. Kohlmann A, Schoch C, Schnittger S, et al. Molecular characterization of acute leukemias by use of microarray technology. Genes Chromosomes Cancer 2003; 37:396–405.

24. van den Boom J, Wolter M, Kuick R, et al. Characterization of gene expression profiles associated with glioma progression using oligonucleotide-based microarray analysis and real-time reverse transcription–polymerase chain reaction. Am J Pathol 2003; 163:1033–1043.

25. Brafford P, Herlyn M. Gene expression profiling of melanoma cells—searching the haystack. J Transl Med 2005; 3:2.

26. Bagnara JT, Matsumoto J, Ferris W, et al. Common origin of pigment cells. Science 1979; 203:410–415.

27. Nishimura EK, Granter SR, Fisher DE. Mechanisms of hair graying: incomplete melanocyte stem cell maintenance in the niche. Science 2005; 307:720–724.

28. Sieber-Blum M, Grim M, Hu YF, et al. Pluripotent neural crest stem cells in the adult hair follicle. Dev Dyn 2004; 231:258–269.

29. Wellbrock C, Gomez A, Schartl M. Melanoma development and pigment cell transformation in *Xiphophorus*. Microsc Res Tech 2002; 58:456–463.

30. Herlyn M, Berking C, Li G, et al. Lessons from melanocyte development for understanding the biological events in naevus and melanoma formation. Melanoma Res 2000; 10:303–312.

31. Li G, Schaider H, Satyamoorthy K, et al. Downregulation of E-cadherin and desmoglein 1 by autocrine hepatocyte growth factor during melanoma development. Oncogene 2001; 20:8125–8135.

32. Jamal S, Schneider RJ. UV-induction of keratinocyte endothelin-1 downregulates E-cadherin in melanocytes and melanoma cells. J Clin Invest 2002; 110:443–452.

33. Berking C, Takemoto R, Satyamoorthy K, et al. Induction of melanoma phenotypes in human skin by growth factors and ultraviolet B. Cancer Res 2004; 64:807–811.

34. Valyi-Nagy I, Rodeck U, Kath R, et al. The human melanocyte system as a model for studies on tumor progression. Basic Life Sci 1991; 57:315–326; discussion 326–328.

35. Clark WHJ, Herlyn M. Melanocyte differentiation. Lab Invest 1987; 57:600–601.

36. Szabo G. Quantitative histological investigations on the melanocyte system of the human epidermis. In: Gordon M, ed. Pigment Cell Biology. New York: Academic Press, 1959:99–125.

37. Herlyn M, Clark WH, Rodeck U, et al. Biology of tumor progression in human melanocytes. Lab Invest 1987; 56:461–474.

38. Riley PA. Melanogenesis and melanoma. Pigment Cell Res 2003; 16:548–552.

39. Hearing VJ, Jimenez M. Mammalian tyrosinase—the critical regulatory control point in melanocyte pigmentation. Int J Biochem 1987; 19:1141–1147.

40. Elwood JM, Gallagher RP, Hill GB, et al. Pigmentation and skin reaction to sun as risk factors for cutaneous melanoma: western Canada melanoma study. BMJ 1984; 288:99–102.

41. Kollias N, Sayre RM, Zeise L, et al. New trends in photobiology (invited review). J Photochem Photobiol B: Biol 1991; 9:135–160.
42. Hoogduijn MJ, Cemeli E, Ross K, et al. Melanin protects melanocytes and keratinocytes against H_2O_2-induced DNA strand breaks through its ability to bind Ca^{2+}. Exp Cell Res 2004; 294:60–67.
43. De Leeuw SM, Smit NP, Van Veldhoven M, et al. Melanin content of cultured human melanocytes and UV-induced cytotoxicity. J Photochem Photobiol B 2001; 61:106–113.
44. Tsavachidou D, Coleman ML, Athanasiadis G, et al. SPRY2 is an inhibitor of the ras/extracellular signal-regulated kinase pathway in melanocytes and melanoma cells with wild-type BRAF but not with the V599E mutant. Cancer Res 2004; 64:5556–5559.
45. de Gruijl FR, van Kranen HJ, van Schanke A. UV exposure, genetic targets in melanocytic tumors and transgenic mouse models. Photochem Photobiol 2005; 81:52–64.
46. Satyamoorthy K, Li G, Vaidya B, et al. Insulin-like growth factor-1 induces survival and growth of biologically early melanoma cells through both the mitogen-activated protein kinase and beta-catenin pathways. Cancer Res 2001; 61:7318–7324.
47. Satyamoorthy K, Li G, Gerrero MR, et al. Constitutive mitogen-activated protein kinase activation in melanoma is mediated by both BRAF mutations and autocrine growth factor stimulation. Cancer Res 2003; 63:756–759.
48. Goodall J, Wellbrock C, Dexter TJ, et al. The Brn-2 transcription factor links activated BRAF to melanoma proliferation. Mol Cell Biol 2004; 24:2923–2931.
49. Goodall J, Martinozzi S, Dexter TJ, et al. Brn-2 expression controls melanoma proliferation and is directly regulated by beta-catenin. Mol Cell Biol 2004; 24: 2915–2922.
50. Carreira S, Goodall J, Aksan I, et al. Mitf cooperates with Rb1 and activates p21Cip1 expression to regulate cell cycle progression. Nature 2005; 433:764–769.
51. Loercher AE, Tank EM, Delston RB, et al. MITF links differentiation with cell cycle arrest in melanocytes by transcriptional activation of INK4A. J Cell Biol 2005; 168:35–40.
52. Hirobe T. Role of keratinocyte-derived factors involved in regulating the proliferation and differentiation of mammalian epidermal melanocytes. Pigment Cell Res 2005; 18:2–12.
53. Gordon M. The genetics of a viviparous top-minnow *Platypoecilus*; the inheritance of two kinds of melanophores. Genetics 1927; 12:253–283.
54. Kosswig C. Uber bastarde der teleostier *Platypoecilus* und *Xiphophorus*. Zeitschrift fur induktive Abstammungs- und Vererbungslehre 1927; 44:253.
55. Wittbrodt J, Adam D, Malitschek B, et al. Novel putative receptor tyrosine kinase encoded by the melanoma-inducing *Tu* locus in *Xiphophorus*. Nature 1989; 341:415–421.
56. Gomez A, Wellbrock C, Schartl M. Constitutive activation and specific signaling of the Xmrk receptor in Xiphophorus melanoma. Mar Biotechnol 2002; 4:208–217.
57. Gomez A, Volff JN, Hornung U, Schartl M, Wellbrock C. Identification of a second egfr gene in *Xiphophorus* uncovers an expansion of the epidermal growth factor receptor family in fish. Mol Biol Evol 2004 Feb; 21(2):266–275.
58. Wellbrock C, Weisser C, Geissinger E, et al. Activation of p59[Fyn] leads to melanocyte dedifferentiation by influencing MKP-1-regulated mitogen-activated protein kinase signaling. J Biol Chem 2002; 277:6443–6454.

59. Kazianis S, Morizot DC, Coletta LD, et al. Comparative structure and characterization of a *CDKN2* gene in a *Xiphophorus* fish melanoma model. Oncogene 1999; 18:5088–5099.

60. Kazianis S, Khanolkar VA, Nairn RS, et al. Structural organization, mapping, characterization and evolutionary relationships of CDKN2 gene family members in Xiphophorus fishes. Comp Biochem Physiol C Toxicol Pharmacol 2004; 138:291–299.

61. Walter RB, Kazianis S. Xiphophorus interspecies hybrids as genetic models of induced neoplasia. Inst Lab Anim Res 2001; 42:299–321.

62. Kazianis S, Walter RB. Use of platyfishes and swordtails in biological research. Lab Anim 2002; 31:46–52.

63. Patton EE, Widlund HR, Kutok JL, et al. BRAF mutations are sufficient to promote nevi formation and cooperate with p53 in the genesis of melanoma. Curr Biol 2005; 15:249–254.

64. Robinson ES, Hill RH Jr, Kripke ML, et al. The Monodelphis melanoma model: initial report on large ultraviolet A exposures of suckling young. Photochem Photobiol 2000; 71:743–746.

65. Ley RD. Dose response for ultraviolet radiation A-induced focal melanocytic hyperplasia and nonmelanoma skin tumors in Monodelphis domestica. Photochem Photobiol 2001; 73:20–23.

66. Ley RD. Animal models of ultraviolet radiation (UVR)-induced cutaneous melanoma. Front Biosci 7:d1531-4, 2002.

67. Chan J, Robinson ES, Atencio J, et al. Characterization of the CDKN2A and ARF genes in UV-induced melanocytic hyperplasias and melanomas of an opossum (Monodelphis domestica). Mol Carcinog 2001; 31:16–26.

68. Sherburn TE, Gale JM, Ley RD. Cloning and characterization of the *CDKN2A* and *p19ARF* genes from *Monodelphis domestica*. DNA Cell Biol 1998; 17:975–981.

69. Chan J, Robinson ES, Yeh IT, et al. Absence of ras gene mutations in UV-induced malignant melanomas correlates with a dermal origin of melanocytes in Monodelphis domestica. Cancer Lett 2002; 184:73–80.

70. Kusewitt DF, Gale JM, Sherburn TE, et al. H-ras oncogene activation in invasive UVR-induced corneal sarcomas of the opossum Monodelphis domestica. DNA Cell Biol 1997; 16:1217–1222.

71. Samollow PB, Kammerer CM, Mahaney SM, et al. First-generation linkage map of the gray, short-tailed opossum, Monodelphis domestica, reveals genome-wide reduction in female recombination rates. Genetics 2004; 166:307–329.

72. Misfeldt ML, Grimm DR. Sinclair miniature swine: an animal model of human melanoma. Vet Immunol Immunopathol 1994; 43:167–175.

73. Pathak S, Multani AS, McConkey DJ, et al. Spontaneous regression of cutaneous melanoma in sinclair swine is associated with defective telomerase activity and extensive telomere erosion. Int J Oncol 2000; 17:1219–1224.

74. Marshall E. Genome sequencing. Celera assembles mouse genome; public labs plan new strategy. Science 2001; 292:822.

75. Tuveson DA, Jacks T. Technologically advanced cancer modeling in mice. Curr Opin Genet Dev 2002; 12:105–110.

76. Prawitt D, Brixel L, Spangenberg C, et al. RNAi knock-down mice: an emerging technology for post-genomic functional genetics. Cytogenet Genome Res 2004; 105:412–421.

77. Satyamoorthy K, Meier F, Hsu MY, et al. Human xenografts, human skin and skin reconstructs for studies in melanoma development and progression. Cancer Metastasis Rev 1999; 18:401–405.

78. Gruss CJ, Satyamoorthy K, Berking C, et al. Stroma formation and angiogenesis by overexpression of growth factors, cytokines, and proteolytic enzymes in human skin grafted to SCID mice. J Invest Dermatol 2003; 120:683–692.

79. Berking C, Takemoto R, Satyamoorthy K, et al. Basic fibroblast growth factor and ultraviolet B transform melanocytes in human skin. Am J Pathol 2001; 158: 943–953.

80. Gorgoulis VG, Vassiliou LV, Karakaidos P, et al. Activation of the DNA damage checkpoint and genomic instability in human precancerous lesions. Nature 2005; 434:907–913.

81. Bartkova J, Horejsi Z, Koed K, et al. DNA damage response as a candidate anticancer barrier in early human tumorigenesis. Nature 2005; 434:864–870.

82. Stark HJ, Willhauck MJ, Mirancea N, et al. Authentic fibroblast matrix in dermal equivalents normalises epidermal histogenesis and dermoepidermal junction in organotypic co-culture. Eur J Cell Biol 2004; 83:631–645.

83. Valyi-Nagy IT, Murphy GF, Mancianti ML, et al. Phenotypes and interactions of human melanocytes and keratinocytes in an epidermal reconstruction model. Lab Invest 1990; 62:314–324.

84. Meier F, Nesbit M, Hsu MY, et al. Human melanoma progression in skin reconstructs: biological significance of bFGF. Am J Pathol 2000; 156:193–200.

85. Berking C, Herlyn M. Human skin reconstruct models: a new application for studies of melanocyte and melanoma biology. Histol Histopathol 2001; 16:669–674.

86. Whiteman DC, Whiteman CA, Green AC. Childhood sun exposure as a risk factor for melanoma: a systematic review of epidemiologic studies. Cancer Causes Control 2001; 12:69–82.

87. Holman CD, Armstrong BK. Cutaneous malignant melanoma and indicators of total accumulated exposure to the sun: an analysis separating histogenetic types. J Natl Cancer Inst 1984; 73:75–82.

88. Rouzaud F, Kadekaro AL, Abdel-Malek ZA, et al. MC1R and the response of melanocytes to ultraviolet radiation. Mutat Res 2005; 571:133–152.

89. Kanetsky PA, Ge F, Najarian D, et al. Assessment of polymorphic variants in the melanocortin-1 receptor gene with cutaneous pigmentation using an evolutionary approach. Cancer Epidemiol Biomarkers Prev 2004; 13:808–819.

90. Palmer JS, Duffy DL, Box NF, et al. Melanocortin-1 receptor polymorphisms and risk of melanoma: is the association explained solely by pigmentation phenotype? Am J Hum Genet 2000; 66:176–186.

91. Rijken F, Bruijnzeel PL, van Weelden H, et al. Responses of black and white skin to solar-simulating radiation: differences in DNA photodamage, infiltrating neutrophils, proteolytic enzymes induced, keratinocyte activation, and IL-10 expression. J Invest Dermatol 2004; 122:1448–1455.

92. Hu S, Ma F, Collado-Mesa F, et al. UV radiation, latitude, and melanoma in US Hispanics and blacks. Arch Dermatol 2004; 140:819–824.

93. Gandini S, Sera F, Cattaruzza MS, et al. Meta-analysis of risk factors for cutaneous melanoma: II. Sun exposure. Eur J Cancer 2005; 41:45–60.

94. Bulliard JL. Site-specific risk of cutaneous malignant melanoma and pattern of sun exposure in New Zealand. Int J Cancer 2000; 85:627–632.

95. Setlow RB, Grist E, Thompson K, et al. Wavelengths effective in induction of malignant melanoma. Proc Natl Acad Sci USA 1993; 90:6666–6670.
96. Setlow RB, Woodhead AD, Grist E. Animal model for ultraviolet radiation-induced melanoma: platyfish-swordtail hybrid. Proc Natl Acad Sci USA 1989; 86:8922–8926.
97. Setlow RB, Woodhead AD. Temporal changes in the incidence of malignant melanoma: explanation from action spectra. Mutat Res 1994; 307:365–374.
98. Mitchell DL, Meador JA, Byrom M, et al. Resolution of UV-induced DNA damage in Xiphophorus fishes. Marine Biotechnol 2001; 3:S61–S71.
99. Mitchell DL, Scoggins JT, Morizot DC. DNA repair in the variable platyfish (*Xiphophorus variatus*) irradiated in vivo with ultraviolet B light. Photochem Photobiol 1993; 58:455–459.
100. Robinson ES, VandeBerg JL, Hubbard GB, et al. Malignant melanoma in ultraviolet irradiated laboratory opossums: initiation in suckling young, metastasis in adults, and xenograft behavior in nude mice. Cancer Res 1994; 54:5986–5991.
101. Ley RD, Reeve VE, Kusewitt DF. Photobiology of *Monodelphis domestica*. Dev Comp Immunol 2000; 24:503–516.
102. Kannan K, Sharpless NE, Xu J, et al. Components of the Rb pathway are critical targets of UV mutagenesis in a murine melanoma model. Proc Natl Acad Sci USA 2003; 100:1221–1225.
103. Noonan FP, Recio JA, Takayama H, et al. Neonatal sunburn and melanoma in mice. Nature 2001; 413:271–272.
104. Recio JA, Noonan FP, Takayama H, et al. Ink4a/arf deficiency promotes ultraviolet radiation-induced melanomagenesis. Cancer Res 2002; 62:6724–6730.
105. Berking C, Takemoto R, Binder RL, et al. Photocarcinogenesis in human adult skin grafts. Carcinogenesis 2002; 23:181–187.
106. Sayre RM, Dowdy JC, Poh-Fitzpatrick M. Dermatological risk of indoor ultraviolet exposure from contemporary lighting sources. Photochem Photobiol 2004; 80:47–51.
107. De Fabo EC, Noonan FP, Fears T, et al. Ultraviolet B but not ultraviolet A radiation initiates melanoma. Cancer Res 2004; 64:6372–6376.
108. Ikehata H, Nakamura S, Asamura T, et al. Mutation spectrum in sunlight-exposed mouse skin epidermis: small but appreciable contribution of oxidative stress-mediated mutagenesis. Mutat Res 2004; 556:11–24.
109. Sander CS, Chang H, Hamm F, et al. Role of oxidative stress and the antioxidant network in cutaneous carcinogenesis. Int J Dermatol 43:326–335.
110. Ikehata H, Kudo H, Masuda T, et al. UVA induces $C \rightarrow T$ transitions at methyl-CpG-associated dipyrimidine sites in mouse skin epidermis more frequently than UVB. Mutagenesis 2003; 18:511–519.
111. Hussein MR, Haemel AK, Sudilovsky O, et al. Genomic instability in radial growth phase melanoma cell lines after ultraviolet irradiation. J Clin Pathol 2005; 58:389–396.
112. Nghiem DX, Kazimi N, Clydesdale G, et al. Ultraviolet a radiation suppresses an established immune response: implications for sunscreen design. J Invest Dermatol 2001; 117:1193–1199.
113. Kazianis S, Gimenez-Conti IB, Setlow RB, et al. MNU induction of neoplasia in a platyfish model. Lab Invest, 2001. In Press.
114. Kazianis S, Gimenez-Conti I, Trono D, et al. Genetic analysis of neoplasia induced by N-nitroso-N-methylurea in Xiphophorus hybrid fish. Mar Biotechnol (NY) 2001; 3:S37–S43.

115. Takizawa H, Sato S, Kitajima H, et al. Mouse skin melanoma induced in two stage chemical carcinogenesis with 7,12-dimethylbenz[a]anthracene and croton oil. Carcinogenesis 1985; 6:921–923.
116. Arbesman H. UVA, melanoma, and antibacterial soaps. J Am Acad Dermatol 2003; 48:464–465.
117. Arbesman H. Is cutaneous malignant melanoma associated with the use of antibacterial soaps? Med Hypotheses 1999; 53:73–75.
118. http://www.fda.gov/cder/drug/InfoSheets/HCP/ProtopicHCP.htm.
119. Koda T, Umezu T, Kamata R, et al. Uterotrophic effects of benzophenone derivatives and a p-hydroxybenzoate used in ultraviolet screens. Environ Res 2005; 98:40–45.
120. Harvey PW, Darbre P. Endocrine disrupters and human health: could oestrogenic chemicals in body care cosmetics adversely affect breast cancer incidence in women? J Appl Toxicol 2004; 24:167–176.
121. Darbre PD, Byford JR, Shaw LE, et al. Oestrogenic activity of benzylparaben. J Appl Toxicol 2003; 23:43–51.
122. Darbre PD, Aljarrah A, Miller WR, et al. Concentrations of parabens in human breast tumours. J Appl Toxicol 2004; 24:5–13.
123. Davies H, Bignell GR, Cox C, et al. Mutations of the BRAF gene in human cancer. Nature 2002; 417:949–954.
124. Wellbrock C, Ogilvie L, Hedley D, et al. V599EB-RAF is an oncogene in melanocytes. Cancer Res 2004; 64:2338–2342.
125. Casula M, Colombino M, Satta MP, et al. BRAF gene is somatically mutated but does not make a major contribution to malignant melanoma susceptibility: the Italian Melanoma Intergroup Study. J Clin Oncol 2004; 22:286–292.
126. Lang J, Boxer M, MacKie R. Absence of exon 15 BRAF germline mutations in familial melanoma. Hum Mutat 2003; 21:327–330.
127. Laud K, Kannengiesser C, Avril MF, et al. BRAF as a melanoma susceptibility candidate gene? Cancer Res 2003; 63:3061–3065.
128. Meyer P, Klaes R, Schmitt C, et al. Exclusion of BRAFV599E as a melanoma susceptibility mutation. Int J Cancer 2003; 106:78–80.
129. Meyer P, Sergi C, Garbe C. Polymorphisms of the BRAF gene predispose males to malignant melanoma. J Carcinog 2003; 2:7.
130. Pollock PM, Harper UL, Hansen KS, et al. High frequency of BRAF mutations in nevi. Nat Genet 2003; 33:19–20.
131. Uribe P, Wistuba, II, Gonzalez S. BRAF mutation: a frequent event in benign, atypical, and malignant melanocytic lesions of the skin. Am J Dermatopathol 2003; 25:365–370.
132. Yazdi AS, Palmedo G, Flaig MJ, et al. Mutations of the BRAF gene in benign and malignant melanocytic lesions. J Invest Dermatol 2003; 121:1160–1162.
133. Kumar R, Angelini S, Snellman E, et al. BRAF mutations are common somatic events in melanocytic nevi. J Invest Dermatol 2004; 122:342–348.
134. Loewe R, Kittler H, Fischer G, et al. BRAF kinase gene V599E mutation in growing melanocytic lesions. J Invest Dermatol 2004; 123:733–736.
135. Dong J, Phelps RG, Qiao R, et al. BRAF oncogenic mutations correlate with progression rather than initiation of human melanoma. Cancer Res 2003; 63:3883–3885.
136. Shinozaki M, Fujimoto A, Morton DL, et al. Incidence of BRAF oncogene mutation and clinical relevance for primary cutaneous melanomas. Clin Cancer Res 2004; 10:1753–1757.

137. Mihic-Probst D, Perren A, Schmid S, et al. Absence of BRAF gene mutations differentiates spitz nevi from malignant melanoma. Anticancer Res 2004; 24:2415–2418.
138. Turner DJ, Zirvi MA, Barany F, et al. Detection of the BRAF V600E mutation in melanocytic lesions using the ligase detection reaction. J Cutan Pathol 2005; 32:334–339.
139. Miller CJ, Cheung M, Sharma A, et al. Method of mutation analysis may contribute to discrepancies in reports of (V599E)BRAF mutation frequencies in melanocytic neoplasms. J Invest Dermatol 2004; 123:990–992.
140. Saldanha G, Purnell D, Fletcher A, et al. High BRAF mutation frequency does not characterize all melanocytic tumor types. Int J Cancer 2004; 111:705–710.
141. Cruz F 3rd, Rubin BP, Wilson D, et al. Absence of BRAF and NRAS mutations in uveal melanoma. Cancer Res 2003; 63:5761–5766.
142. Omholt K, Platz A, Kanter L, et al. NRAS and BRAF mutations arise early during melanoma pathogenesis and are preserved throughout tumor progression. Clin Cancer Res 2003; 9:6483–6488.
143. Reifenberger J, Knobbe CB, Sterzinger AA, et al. Frequent alterations of Ras signaling pathway genes in sporadic malignant melanomas. Int J Cancer 2004; 109:377–384.
144. Thomas NE, Alexander A, Edmiston SN, et al. Tandem BRAF mutations in primary invasive melanomas. J Invest Dermatol 2004; 122:1245–1250.
145. Kilic E, Bruggenwirth HT, Verbiest MM, et al. The RAS-BRAF kinase pathway is not involved in uveal melanoma. Melanoma Res 2004; 14:203–205.
146. Edmunds SC, Cree IA, Di Nicolantonio F, et al. Absence of BRAF gene mutations in uveal melanomas in contrast to cutaneous melanomas. Br J Cancer 2003; 88:1403–1405.
147. Cohen Y, Goldenberg-Cohen N, Parrella P, et al. Lack of BRAF mutation in primary uveal melanoma. Invest Ophthalmol Vis Sci 2003; 44:2876–2878.
148. Cohen Y, Xing M, Mambo E, et al. BRAF mutation in papillary thyroid carcinoma. J Natl Cancer Inst 2003; 95:625–627.
149. Brose MS, Volpe P, Feldman M, et al. BRAF and RAS mutations in human lung cancer and melanoma. Cancer Res 2002; 62:6997–7000.
150. Schmitz AA, Govek EE, Bottner B, et al. Rho GTPases: signaling, migration, and invasion. Exp Cell Res 2000; 261:1–12.
151. Chin L, Pomerantz J, DePinho RA. The INK4a/ARF tumor suppressor: one gene-two products-two pathways. Trends in Biochemical Sciences 1998, August 23:291–296.
152. Chin L, Merlino G, DePinho RA. Malignant melanoma: modern black plague and genetic black box. Genes Dev 1998; 12:3467–3481.
153. Weber A, Hengge UR, Urbanik D, et al. Absence of mutations of the BRAF gene and constitutive activation of extracellular-regulated kinase in malignant melanomas of the uvea. Lab Invest 2003; 83:1771–1776.
154. Tsao H, Goel V, Wu H, et al. Genetic interaction between NRAS and BRAF mutations and PTEN/MMAC1 inactivation in melanoma. J Invest Dermatol 2004; 122:337–341.
155. Houben R, Becker JC, Kappel A, et al. Constitutive activation of the Ras-Raf signaling pathway in metastatic melanoma is associated with poor prognosis. J Carcinog 2004; 3:6.

156. Eskandarpour M, Hashemi J, Kanter L, et al. Frequency of UV-inducible NRAS mutations in melanomas of patients with germline CDKN2A mutations. J Natl Cancer Inst 2003; 95:790–798.
157. Daniotti M, Oggionni M, Ranzani T, et al. BRAF alterations are associated with complex mutational profiles in malignant melanoma. Oncogene 2004; 23:5968–5977.
158. Sasaki Y, Niu C, Makino R, et al. BRAF point mutations in primary melanoma show different prevalences by subtype. J Invest Dermatol 2004; 123:177–183.
159. Eskandarpour M, Kiaii S, Zhu C, et al. Suppression of oncogenic NRAS by RNA interference induces apoptosis of human melanoma cells. Int J Cancer 2005; 115:65–73.
160. Satyamoorthy K, Herlyn M. p16^{INK4A} and familial melanoma. Methods Mol Biol 2003; 222:185–195.
161. Ruas M, Peters G. The p16INK4a/CDKN2A tumor suppressor and its relatives. Biochim Biophys Acta 1998; 1378:F115–F177.
162. Gruis NA, Sandkujl LA, van der Velden PA, et al. *CDKN2* explains part of the clinical phenotype in Dutch familial atypical multiple-mole melanoma (FAMMM) syndrome families. Melanoma Res 1995; 5:169–177.
163. Rulyak SJ, Brentnall TA, Lynch HT, et al. Characterization of the neoplastic phenotype in the familial atypical multiple-mole melanoma-pancreatic carcinoma syndrome. Cancer 2003; 98:798–804.
164. Barrett JH, Gaut R, Wachsmuth R, et al. Linkage and association analysis of nevus density and the region containing the melanoma gene CDKN2A in UK twins. Br J Cancer 2003; 88:1920–1924.
165. Zhu G, Duffy DL, Eldridge A, et al. A major quantitative-trait locus for mole density is linked to the familial melanoma gene CDKN2A: a maximum-likelihood combined linkage and association analysis in twins and their sibs. Am J Hum Genet 1999; 65:483–492.
166. Pollock PM, Yu F, Qiu L, et al. Evidence for u.v. induction of CDKN2 mutations in melanoma cell lines. Oncogene 1995; 11:663–668.
167. Pollock PM, Pearson JV, Hayward NK. Compilation of somatic mutations of the *CDKN2* gene in human cancers: non-random distribution of base substitutions. Genes Chromosomes Cancer 1996; 15:77–88.
168. Wagner SN, Wagner C, Briedigkeit L, et al. Homozygous deletion of the *p16INK4a* and the *p15INK4b* tumour suppressor genes in a subset of human sporadic cutaneous malignant melanoma. Br J Dermatol 1998; 138:13–21.
169. Funk JO, Schiller PI, Barrett MT, et al. *p16INK4a* expression is frequently decreased and associated with 9p21 loss of heterozygosity in sporadic melanoma (in process citation). J Cutan Pathol 1998; 25:291–296.
170. Fargnoli MC, Chimenti S, Keller G, et al. *CDKN2a/p16INK4a* mutations and lack of *p19ARF* involvement in familial melanoma kindreds. J Invest Dermatol 1998; 111:1202–1206.
171. Hegi ME, zur Hausen A, Ruedi D, et al. Hemizygous or homozygous deletion of the chromosomal region containing the p16INK4a gene is associated with amplification of the EGF receptor gene in glioblastomas. Int J Cancer 1997; 73:57–63.
172. Drexler HG. Review of alterations of the cyclin-dependent kinase inhibitor *INK4* family genes *p15, p16, p18* and *p19* in human leukemia-lymphoma cells. Leukemia 1998; 12:845–859.

173. Gonzalez-Zulueta M, Bender CM, Yang AS, et al. Methylation of the 5′ CpG island of the *p16/CDKN2* tumor suppressor gene in normal and transformed human tissues correlates with gene silencing. Cancer Res 1995; 55:4531–4535.

174. Herman JG, Merlo A, Mao L, et al. Inactivation of the *CDKN2/p16/MTS1* gene is frequently associated with aberrant DNA methylation in all common human cancers. Cancer Res 1995; 55:4525–4530.

175. Pomerantz J, Schreiber A, Liegeois NJ, et al. The *Ink4a* tumor suppressor gene product, p19^Arf, Interacts with MDM2 and Neutralizes MDM2's inhibition of p53. Cell 1998; 92:713–723.

176. Bardeesy N, Bastian BC, Hezel A, et al. Dual inactivation of RB and p53 pathways in RAS-induced melanomas. Mol Cell Biol 2001; 21:2144–2153.

177. Hollstein M, Sidransky D, Vogelstein B, et al. p53 mutations in human cancers. Science 1991; 253:49–53.

178. Weiss J, Schwechheimer K, Cavenee WK, et al. Mutation and expression of the p53 gene in malignant melanoma cell lines. Int J Cancer 1993; 54:693–699.

179. Hartmann A, Blaszyk H, Cunningham JS, et al. Overexpression and mutations of p53 in metastatic malignant melanomas. Int J Cancer 1996; 67:313–317.

180. Satyamoorthy K, Chehab NH, Waterman MJ, et al. Aberrant regulation and function of wild-type p53 in radioresistant melanoma cells. Cell Growth Differ 2000; 11:467–474.

181. Albino AP, Vidal MJ, McNutt NS, et al. Mutation and expression of the p53 gene in human malignant melanoma. Melanoma Res 1994; 4:35–45.

182. Birck A, Ahrenkiel V, Zeuthen J, et al. Mutation and allelic loss of the PTEN/MMAC1 gene in primary and metastatic melanoma biopsies. J Invest Dermatol 2000; 114:277–280.

183. Boni R, Vortmeyer AO, Burg G, et al. The PTEN tumour suppressor gene and malignant melanoma. Melanoma Res 1998; 8:300–302.

184. Tsao H, Zhang X, Benoit E, et al. Identification of PTEN/MMAC1 alterations in uncultured melanomas and melanoma cell lines. Oncogene 1998; 16:3397–3402.

185. Robertson GP, Furnari FB, Miele ME, et al. In vitro loss of heterozygosity targets the PTEN/MMAC1 gene in melanoma. Proc Natl Acad Sci USA 1998; 95:9418–9423.

186. Guldberg P, thor Straten P, Birck A, et al. Disruption of the MMAC1/PTEN gene by deletion or mutation is a frequent event in malignant melanoma. Cancer Res 1997; 57:3660–3663.

187. Stewart AL, Mhashilkar AM, Yang XH, et al. PI3 kinase blockade by Ad-PTEN inhibits invasion and induces apoptosis in RGP and metastatic melanoma cells. Mol Med 2002; 8:451–461.

188. Goding CR. Mitf from neural crest to melanoma: signal transduction and transcription in the melanocyte lineage. Genes Dev 2000; 14:1712–1728.

189. Du J, Miller AJ, Widlund HR, et al. MLANA/MART1 and SILV/PMEL17/GP100 are transcriptionally regulated by MITF in melanocytes and melanoma. Am J Pathol 2003; 163:333–343.

190. Du J, Widlund HR, Horstmann MA, et al. Critical role of CDK2 for melanoma growth linked to its melanocyte-specific transcriptional regulation by MITF. Cancer Cell 2004; 6:565–576.

191. Zhiqi S, Soltani MH, Bhat KM, et al. Human melastatin 1 (TRPM1) is regulated by MITF and produces multiple polypeptide isoforms in melanocytes and melanoma. Melanoma Res 2004; 14:509–516.

192. Miller AJ, Du J, Rowan S, et al. Transcriptional regulation of the melanoma prognostic marker melastatin (TRPM1) by MITF in melanocytes and melanoma. Cancer Res 2004; 64:509–516.
193. Delfgaauw J, Duschl J, Wellbrock C, et al. MITF-M plays an essential role in transcriptional activation and signal transduction in Xiphophorus melanoma. Gene 2003; 320:117–126.
194. McGill GG, Horstmann M, Widlund HR, et al. Bcl2 regulation by the melanocyte master regulator Mitf modulates lineage survival and melanoma cell viability. Cell 2002; 109:707–718.
195. Vachtenheim J, Borovansky J. Microphthalmia transcription factor: a specific marker for malignant melanoma. Prague Med Rep 2004; 105:318–324.
196. Zhu H, Reuhl K, Zhang X, et al. Development of heritable melanoma in transgenic mice. J Invest Dermatol 1998; 110:247–252.
197. Chen S, Zhu H, Wetzel WJ, et al. Spontaneous melanocytosis in transgenic mice. J Invest Dermatol 1996; 106:1145–1151.
198. Cohen-Solal KA, Reuhl KR, Ryan KB, et al. Development of cutaneous amelanotic melanoma in the absence of a functional tyrosinase. Pigment Cell Res 2001; 14:466–474.
199. Marin YE, Chen S. Involvement of metabotropic glutamate receptor 1, a G protein coupled receptor, in melanoma development. J Mol Med 2004; 82:735–749.
200. Flaherty KT. New molecular targets in melanoma. Curr Opin Oncol 2004; 16: 150–154.
201. Danson S, Lorigan P. Improving outcomes in advanced malignant melanoma: update on systemic therapy. Drugs 2005; 65:733–743.
202. Leonard I. Zon, Harvard Medical School, Boston, Massachusetts, U.S.A.
203. Edward S. Robinson, Southwest Foundation for Biomedical Research, San Antonio, Texas, U.S.A.
204. Suzie Chen, Rutgers University, Piscataway, New Jersey, U.S.A.

4

Vitamin D, Moderate Sun Exposure, and Health

Michael F. Holick

Boston University Medical Center, Boston, Massachusetts, U.S.A.

EVOLUTIONARY PERSPECTIVE

When the earth was born and bathed in sunlight, life forms quickly took advantage of the sun's energy by converting it into sugar, which not only sustained life but also helped it to thrive. It is likely that a wide variety of photochemical processes occurred throughout early evolution. One photosynthetic process that has been occurring in phytoplankton for more than 750 million years is the photosynthesis of vitamin D. Although the exact function of vitamin D is unknown in these simple life forms, it has been suggested that the formation of vitamin D in the plasma membrane of these single-celled plants was important for calcium-ion transport into the cell. Also, vitamin D and its photoproducts absorb ultraviolet radiation that is identical to DNA, RNA, and proteins and thus could also have served as a natural sunscreen (1,2).

For whatever reason, vitamin D became critically important for the evolution of vertebrates when they ventured onto land more than 350 million years ago. The oceans contained enough calcium to promote the mineralization of the skeletons of ocean dwelling vertebrates, whereas there was a scarcity of calcium on land. It was locked in the soil and absorbed into plants. In order for land dwelling vertebrates to efficiently absorb calcium from their diet, they were exposed to sunlight and vitamin D was produced, which was essential for the efficient absorption of calcium from their diet (1,2).

HUMAN HISTORICAL PERSPECTIVE

In the mid-1600s, Whistler and Glissen reported that children living in industrialized cities of Great Britain had short stature and had deformities of their skeleton, especially their lower legs. They were the first to recognize this bone deforming disease as a new clinical disease that would plague children for more than 250 years. By the end of the nineteenth century, it was estimated that upwards of 90% of children who lived in the industrialized cities of North America and Europe had skeletal manifestations of rickets (3). These included outward and inward bowing of the legs, hypertrophy of the costalchondral junctions (rachitic rosary), delayed closure of the sutures of the skull bones, and growth retardation (Fig. 1). In addition, the pelvis was not properly formed and was flattened causing high incidence of both maternal and infant morbidity and mortality during birthing. It was for this reason that the cesarean sectioning became popular in the late 1800s.

In 1822, Sniadecki (4) recognized that young patients who lived in Warsaw had a high incidence of rickets, whereas the children in the countryside outside of

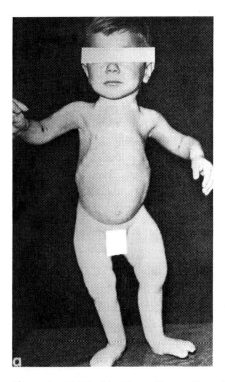

Figure 1   Child with rickets. *Source*: From Ref. 151.

Warsaw had little evidence of this bone deforming disease. He concluded, "strong and obvious is the influence of the sun on the cure of rickets and the frequent occurrence of the disease in densely populated towns where the streets are narrow and poorly lit." It would take 100 years before this insightful observation was fully appreciated. In 1919, Huldschinsky et al. (5) reported that children exposed to a mercury arc lamp twice a week for one hour each time for six weeks had a dramatic cure of rachitic lesions in the hands (Fig. 2). This observation quickly followed by the report of Hess and Unger (6) who took seven children with rickets and exposed them on the roof of a New York City hospital to sunlight. They reported dramatic healing of rachitic lesions and concluded that sun exposure was a reliable treatment for rickets.

The observations that when people (6) and animals (7) were exposed to sunlight and artificial ultraviolet radiation were cured of rickets prompted Hess and Weinstock (8) and Steenbock and Black (9) to irradiate a variety of substances, including grasses, corn, cottonseed oil, and olive oil, and showed that the ultraviolet irradiation of these substances imparted antirachitic activity. It was also known that cod liver oil could often cure rickets, and it was finally demonstrated by Park and coworkers (10) that rats that had rickets had complete healing either by ingesting cod liver oil or by being exposed to ultraviolet radiation. Thus, it was concluded that the antirachitic activity of sunlight was same as the antirachitic activity of the cod liver oil. Originally, it was thought that the vitamin A content in cod liver oil was responsible for promoting bone healing. However, when cod liver oil was exposed to oxygen and heat, which destroyed all vitamin A activity, the antirachitic activity remained active. This led McCollum to announce a new vitamin, which he called vitamin D (11).

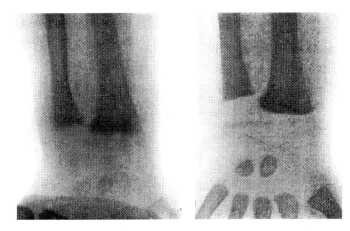

Figure 2   Florid rickets of severe degree. Radiograms taken before (*left*) and after treatment with ultraviolet radiation one hour twice a week for six weeks (*right*). *Source*: From Ref. 152 (now in the public domain).

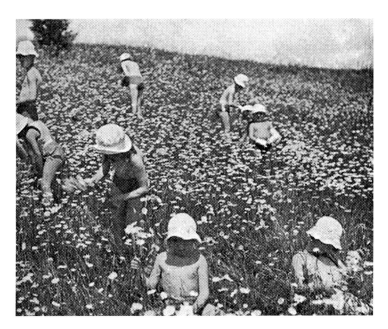

Figure 3   Some of Sir Henry Gauvain's little patients at Alton, Hants (in the public domain). *Source*: From Ref. 152.

It was well documented that cod liver oil was not always a reliable method for treating rickets. As a result, Steenbock (12) introduced the concept of irradiating milk with ultraviolet radiation to promote the production of the antirachitic factor. This simple method was widely adopted, along with the recommendation of guidelines for sensible sun exposure for children (Fig. 3) (13). These two practices quickly eradicated rickets as a worldwide health problem.

In the early 1930s, Windaus et al. (14) structurally identified vitamin D and developed a simple and inexpensive synthesis for it by irradiating the yeast sterol ergosterol. The irradiation of ergosterol was thought to lead to vitamin D. However, it was quickly realized that the resulting product was a mixture of photoproducts. Vitamin D was purified from the mixture and was called vitamin D_2 (Fig. 4).

Originally, it was thought that vitamin D_2 was produced in human skin from sun exposure. However, it was observed that the antirachitic factor in cod liver oil was more effective in preventing rickets in chickens than was vitamin D_2 (15,16). Windaus and Bock (17) finally identified the vitamin D from pig skin labeled as vitamin D_3. The structural differences between vitamin D_2 and vitamin D_3 are that vitamin D_3 has a cholesterol side arm and vitamin D_2 has the cholesterol side arm with the addition of a double bond between carbons 22 and 23 and a methyl group on carbon 24 (Fig. 4).

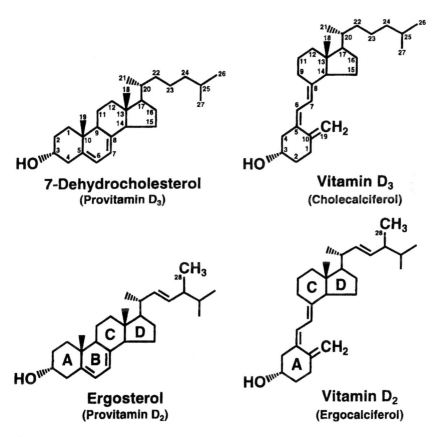

Figure 4 Structure of vitamins D_3 and D_2 and their respective precursors, 7-DHC and ergosterol. The only structural difference between vitamins D_2 and D_3 is their side chains; the side chain for vitamin D_2 contains a double bond among C22, C23, and C24 methyl group. *Source*: From Ref. 153.

PHOTOPRODUCTION OF VITAMIN D_3 IN HUMAN SKIN

When human skin is exposed to sunlight, the solar ultraviolet B (UVB) radiation (290–315 nm) is absorbed by 7-dehydrocholesterol (7-DHC), which is present in the plasma membrane of keratinocytes and fibroblasts (18–20). The absorbed energy causes a rearrangement of the double bonds, leading to a splitting of the B-ring to form previtamin D_3. Previtamin D_3 is unstable to temperature, and its double bonds quickly rearrange to a more stable isomer, that is, vitamin D_3 (Fig. 5) (20,21). During the transformation of previtamin D_3 to vitamin D_3, which occurs within a few hours, the vitamin D_3 is ejected out of the plasma

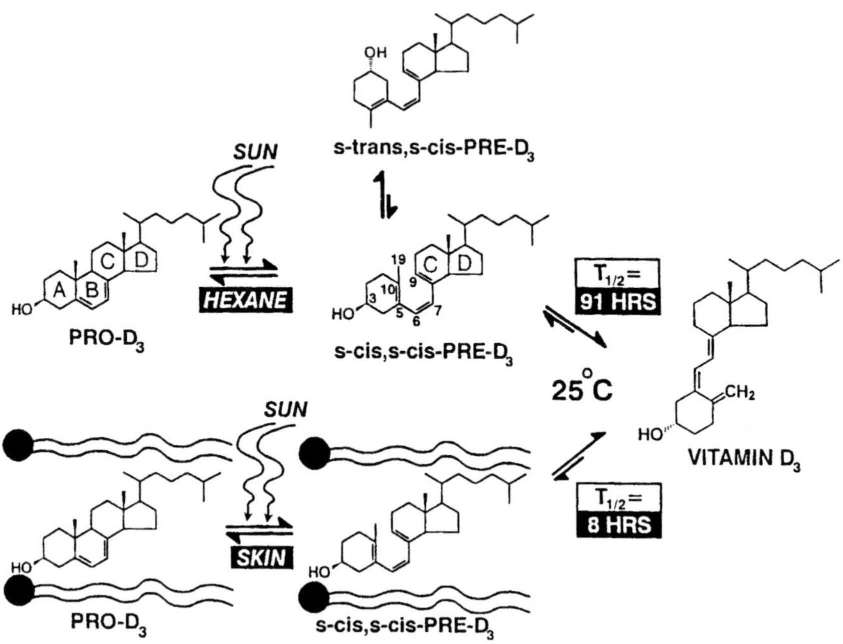

Figure 5 Photolysis of provitamin D_3 (pro-D_3) into previtamin D_3 (pre-D_3) and its thermal isomerization of vitamin D_3 in hexane and in lizard skin. In hexane, pro-D_3 is photolyzed to *s-cis,s-cis*-pre-D_3. Once formed, this energetically unstable conformation undergoes a conformational change to the *s-trans, s-cis*-pre-D_3. Only the *s-cis,s-cis*-pre-D_3 can undergo thermal isomerization to vitamin D_3. The *s-cis,s-cis* conformer of pre-D_3 is stabilized in the phospholipid bilayer by hydrophilic interactions between the 3β-hydroxyl group and the polar head of the lipids, as well as by the van der Waals interactions between the steroid ring and side-chain structure and the hydrophobic tail of the lipids. These interactions significantly decrease the conversion of the *s-cis,s-cis* conformer to the *s-trans,s-cis* conformer, thereby facilitating the thermal isomerization of *s-cis,s-cis*-pre-D_3 to vitamin D_3. *Source*: From Ref. 154.

membrane into the extracellular space. It is drawn into the dermal capillary bed by the vitamin D binding protein (22,23).

FACTORS THAT AFFECT THE CUTANEOUS SYNTHESIS OF VITAMIN D_3

The photosynthesis of previtamin D_3 is dependent on having an adequate source of high-energy UVB photons penetrate into the epidermis. Thus, an increase in skin pigmentation and the topical application of a sunscreen, which absorb solar UVB photons, markedly diminishes the production of previtamin D_3. A sunscreen with a sun protection factor of 8 (SPF8), which reduces the total

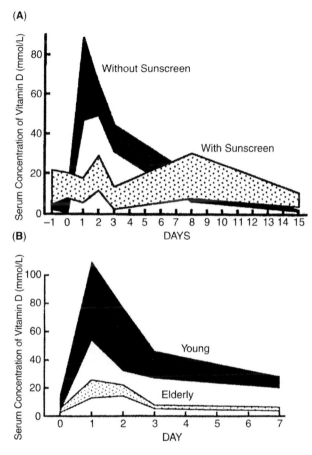

Figure 6 (**A**) Circulating concentrations of vitamin D_3 after a single exposure to 1 MED of simulated sunlight either with a sunscreen, with a SPF-8, or a topical placebo cream. (**B**) Circulating concentrations of vitamin D in response to a whole-body exposure to 1 MED in healthy young and elderly subjects. *Source*: From Ref. 3.

number of UVB photons penetrating into the skin by 95%, also reduces the cutaneous production of vitamin D_3 by the same degree (Fig. 6) (24). People with very dark skin pigmentation (African or Mid-Eastern Asian decent) have skin pigment that is equivalent to at least SPF8 and thus have at least 95% reduction in their capacity to produce vitamin D_3 compared with a light-skinned person exposed to the same amount of sunlight (Fig. 7) (25,26).

The stratospheric ozone layer is extremely efficient in absorbing all of the sun's ultraviolet C radiation and almost all (>99%) of its UVB radiation. Any alteration in the angle at which solar ultraviolet radiation strikes the earth will affect the number of UVB photons that pass through the stratospheric ozone

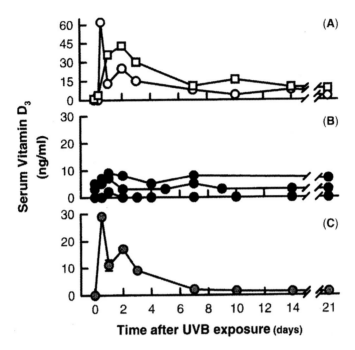

Figure 7 (**A**) Change in serum concentrations of vitamin D in two lightly pigmented white (skin type II) and (**B**) three heavily pigmented black subjects (skin type V) after total-body exposure to 54 mJ/cm² of UVB radiation. (**C**) Serial change in circulating concentrations of vitamin D₃ after re-exposure of one black subject in (**B**) to a 320 mJ/cm² dose of UVB radiation. *Source*: From Ref. 25.

layer. Typically, no more than 1% of the solar UVB photons reach the earth's surface in the summer at the equator. In the winter, the zenith angle is so oblique that essentially all of the UVB photons are absorbed by the stratospheric ozone layer. Thus, people living above a latitude of 37°N, which is around Atlanta, Georgia, and above, have such marked diminishment in UVB photon exposure that they make little, if any, vitamin D_3 from the months of November through February. At higher latitudes, which is typical of Edmonton, Canada, London, Paris, and Bergen, Norway, little vitamin D_3 is produced in the skin from the months of October through April (Fig. 8) (27,28). Similarly, time of day is important, since in the early morning and late afternoon, the sun's angle is oblique and thus little if any vitamin D is produced.

Aging is associated with a decrease in many metabolic functions. Aging also decreases the amount of 7-DHC in the skin (29,30). There is about a four-fold decline in 7-DHC levels in the skin of a 70-year-old and thus vitamin D_3 synthesis in a 70-year old is decreased by approximately 75% compared with a 20-year old (Fig. 6) (31).

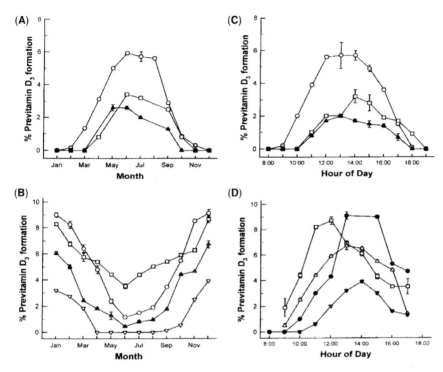

Figure 8 Influence of season, time of day in July, and latitude on the synthesis of previtamin D_3 in northern (**A** and **C**: Boston, -O-; Edmonton, -□-; Bergen, -▲-) and southern hemispheres (**B**: Buenos Aires, -O-; Johannesburg, -□-; Cape Town, -▲-; Ushuala, -▼-; **D**: Buenos Aires, -●-; Johannesburg, -□-; Cape Town, -ρ-; Ushuala, -▼-). The hour indicated in (**C**) and (**D**) is the end of the one-hour exposure time in July. *Source*: From Ref. 155.

MAJOR SOURCES OF VITAMIN D

Cod liver oil, oily fish, irradiated mushrooms, and egg yolks naturally contain vitamin D (D represents either D_2 or D_3). Typically, a serving of salmon and a teaspoon of cod liver oil contain ~400 IU of vitamin D_3 (32). In the United States, Canada, and Sweden, milk is fortified with vitamin D. There is 100 IU of vitamin D in eight ounces. In the United States, orange juice (33), some yogurts, cereals, and breads are fortified with vitamin D. In Europe, very few foods are fortified with vitamin D because of the outbreak of vitamin D intoxication in the 1950s (34). As a result, laws were passed forbidding the fortification of foods, especially dairy products, with vitamin D. In many European countries including France, Germany, England, and Norway, margarine and some cereals are the major fortified food sources.

The major source of vitamin D_3 for children and adults is sensible sun exposure. Both children and adults have seasonal variations in their vitamin D levels (at the highest levels at the end of the summer and at their nadir at the end of the winter) (35–39).

ENDOCRINE, METABOLISM, AND PHYSIOLOGIC FUNCTION OF VITAMIN D ON CALCIUM AND BONE HEALTH

Once vitamin D is ingested or is made in the skin, it enters the circulation and travels to the liver where it is hydroxylated on carbon 25 to 25-hydroxyvitamin D [25(OH)D] (Fig. 9). 25(OH)D is the major circulating form of vitamin D that is used by clinicians to determine a person's vitamin D status. However, 25(OH)D is biologically inert and requires a further hydroxylation on carbon 1 in the kidneys to form 1,25-dihydroxyvitamin D [$1,25(OH)_2D$]. Once it forms, $1,25(OH)_2D$ interacts with its specific nuclear vitamin D receptor (VDR) in the intestine and bone to regulate calcium and bone metabolism (2,28,40–42).

$1,25(OH)_2D$ is solely responsible for regulating the efficiency of intestinal calcium absorption. Increased blood levels of $1,25(OH)_2D$ result in an increase in the efficiency of calcium absorption in the small intestine. The VDR is present in the bone forming cells, osteoblasts. $1,25(OH)_2D$ interacts with its VDR in osteo-blasts to increase the expression of receptor activator of nuclear factor κB ligand (RANKL). This protein, which is expressed on the surface of the plasma mem-brane of osteoblasts, acts as a sentinel for pre-osteoclasts, which has a RANKL receptor known as RANK. When the pre-osteoclast RANK binds the RANKL on the osteoblast, this is the signal for the pre-osteoclast to become a mature osteoclast. Once mature, the osteoclast releases collagenases and hydrochloric acid to dissolve the matrix and mineral to release calcium into the circulation (2,28,43). Thus, the major function of vitamin D_3 is to maintain serum calcium within a very tight physiologic range in order to maintain a multitude of meta-bolic functions and to sustain neuromuscular activity.

CONSEQUENCES OF VITAMIN D DEFICIENCY ON CALCIUM METABOLISM AND BONE HEALTH

Vitamin D deficiency causes a decrease in serum ionized calcium concentrations. The body cannot tolerate this and thus responds by the calcium sensor in the para-thyroid glands recognizing the decrease and signaling the parathyroid glands to express and release parathyroid hormone (PTH). PTH is able to restore the serum calcium to its normal level by stimulating the kidney to produce more $1,25(OH)_2D$ (2,28,40–42). However, in a vitamin D deficient state this cannot occur and thus PTH also enhances tubular re-absorption of calcium in the kidney and therefore decreases the amount of calcium lost in the urine. PTH is also able to stimulate osteoblasts to express RANKL, which is the signal for pre-osteoclasts to become mature, and to mobilize precious calcium stores

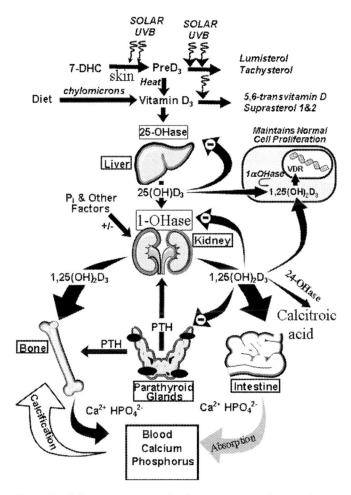

Figure 9 Schematic representation for cutaneous production of vitamin D and its metabolism and regulation for calcium homeostasis and cellular growth. During exposure to sunlight, 7-DHC in the skin absorbs solar ultraviolet (UVB) radiation and is converted to previtamin D_3 (pre-D_3). Once formed, D_3 undergoes thermally induced transformation to vitamin D_3. Further exposure to sunlight converts pre-D_3 and vitamin D_3 to biologically inert photoproducts. Vitamin D coming from the diet or from the skin enters the circulation and is metabolized in the liver by the vitamin D-25-hydroxylase (25-OHase) to 25-hydroxyvitamin D_3 [25(OH)D_3]. 25(OH)D_3 re-enters the circulation and is converted in the kidney by the 25-hydroxyvitamin D_3-1α-hydroxylase (1-OHase) to 1,25-dihydroxyvitamin D_3 [1,25(OH)$_2D_3$]. A variety of factors, including serum phosphorus (P_i) and PTH, regulated the renal production of 1,25(OH)$_2$D. 1,25(OH)$_2$D regulates calcium metabolism through its interaction with its major target tissues, the bone and the intestine. 1,25(OH)$_2D_3$ also induces its own destruction by enhancing the expression of the 25-hydroxyvitamin D-24-hydroxylase (24-OHase). 25(OH)D is metabolized in other tissues for the purpose of regulation of cellular growth. *Source*: From Ref. 2.

from the skeleton. Thus, vitamin D deficiency is initially associated with a normal serum calcium and an increase in PTH levels. However, the skeleton is unable to mineralize the collagen matrix in a vitamin D deficient state because PTH also causes a decrease in renal tubular re-absorption of phosphorus, causing phosphaturia, and a decrease in serum phosphorus levels. Although the serum calcium is normal, the serum phosphorus is low, and there is an inadequate calcium–phosphorus product that is necessary for normal bone mineralization. As a child's skeleton has little calcium, the poor mineralization of the skeleton and the weight of the body with gravity cause the deformation of the lower limbs, resulting in bowed legs or knocked knees (28,44).

Vitamin D deficiency in adults also results in an increase in PTH levels, which increases osteoclastic activity, causing the bones to become more porous, which can lead to osteoporosis (28,44). In addition, the secondary hyperparathyroidism and resultant phosphaturia causes an inadequate calcium–phosphorus product in the circulation, causing a mineralization defect of newly laid down osteoid. Unlike osteoporosis, that is, holes in the bones which do not cause bone pain, osteomalacia causes localized or generalized throbbing, aching bone pain that is often misdiagnosed as fibromyalgia or chronic fatigue syndrome (45–47). It have been estimated that 40% to 60% of patients with fibromyalgic-like symptoms are suffering from vitamin D deficiency (28,48).

Vitamin D deficiency in both children and adults is also associated with muscle weakness (28,49,50). This can be so severe that the disease is misdiagnosed as some type of neurological disorder, such as multiple sclerosis or amyotrophic lateral sclerosis (51).

AUTOCRINE METABOLISM OF VITAMIN D AND ITS PHYSIOLOGIC FUNCTIONS

It is well recognized that essentially every tissue and cell in the body, including the brain, gonads, heart, colon, skin, breast, prostate, activated T and B lymphocytes, and monocytes have a VDR (2,28,40,41,52). Originally, it was thought that circulating levels of $1,25(OH)_2D$ interacted with these receptors to regulate a wide variety of physiologic functions. However, it is now recognized that most of these tissues also express the cytochrome P450 27B (cyp27) enzyme, which is responsible for converting $25(OH)D$ to $1,25(OH)_2D$ in the kidneys. Thus, the colon, breast, skin, lungs, prostate, and monocytes produce $1,25(OH)_2D$ (53–58). Unlike the kidneys, which produce $1,25(OH)_2D$ as an endocrine hormone which leaves the kidney and travels to the intestine and bone to regulate calcium metabolism, the production of $1,25(OH)_2D$ in noncalcemic tissues appears to be important for regulating cellular growth and various cellular activities (2,28,58).

When normal and malignant cells from the colon, breast, prostate, skin, lungs, and melanocytes are incubated with $1,25(OH)_2D_3$, this hormone markedly decreases their proliferative activity and induces them to terminally differentiate

(2,40,41,58–61) $1,25(OH)_2D$ decreases expression of p27 and p21 among other genes that are responsible for the cell cycle. $1,25(OH)_2D$ has also decreased the renal production of renin (62) and increased the β-islet cell production of insulin (63). $1,25(OH)_2D$ also shown marked effects on macrophage activity and regulated both cytokine production and immunoglobulin synthesis in activated T and B lymphocytes (28,41,64).

CONSEQUENCES OF INADEQUATE SUN EXPOSURE AND LIVING AT HIGHER LATITUDES ON HEALTH

In 1941, Apperly (65) reported that if you lived at a higher latitude in the United States such as in Maine, Massachusetts, and Vermont, you had a higher likelihood of dying of cancer than if you lived at lower latitudes in the United States including South Carolina, Georgia, and Texas. He suggested that although living at lower latitudes increases the risk of skin cancer, this disease was much more benign and apparently provided an immunity to the more serious cancers of the solid organs. This insightful observation went unnoticed until the 1980s when Garland et al. (66) reported that there was a higher incidence of colon cancer deaths in both men and women and breast cancer mortality (67) who lived in the northern part of the United States. They suggested that this was likely due to vitamin D deficiency. They speculated that vitamin D deficiency would lead to a decrease in $1,25(OH)_2D$ levels, which was important in preventing cells from becoming malignant. However, it is known that an increase in the production of vitamin D_3 in the skin from sun exposure or increase in the ingestion of vitamin D from the diet would not increase the renal production of $1,25(OH)_2D$ because this calciotropic hormone was extremely potent and therefore its production was tightly regulated (28,41). However, the revelation that many tissues including colon, prostate, breast, and lung could produce $1,25(OH)_2D$ locally, finally, made some sense out of this observation. That is, increased exposure to sunlight increased the blood levels of $25(OH)D$, which bathed all of the cells in the body. These cells could locally produce $1,25(OH)_2D$, which then in turn regulated cellular growth and differentiation decreasing the risk of the cells from becoming malignant (Fig. 10) (2,28).

Over the past two decades, a multitude of reports have linked living at higher latitudes with increased risk of developing and dying of colon, prostate, breast, ovarian, and esophageal cancers among other cancers (66–74). It has also been reported that if a person is diagnosed with lung cancer and has surgery during the summer, they are more likely to survive longer than those with a diagnosis in the winter.

Cancer is not the only chronic disease that has been associated with living at higher latitudes. There is an increased risk of developing autoimmune disorders, including multiple sclerosis, type I diabetes, and Crohn's disease (75–78). In addition, hypertension is more common in people living at higher latitudes (79).

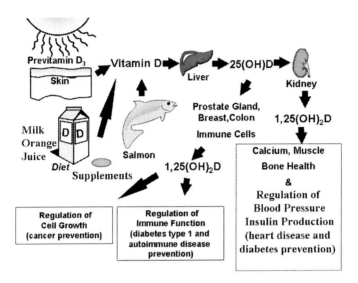

Figure 10 Schematic representation of the multitude of other potential physiologic actions of vitamin D for cardiovascular health, cancer prevention, regulation of immune function, and decreased risk of autoimmune diseases.

When non-obese diabetic mice that typically develop type I diabetes received $1,25(OH)_2D_3$ throughout life, it reduced their risk of developing type I diabetes by 80% (80). Hypponen et al. (81) reported that children who receive 2000 IU of vitamin D at one year of age and followed for the next 25 years had an 80% decrease in risk of developing type I diabetes compared with children who were vitamin D insufficient and did not receive a vitamin D supplement.

There is 100% increase risk of developing multiple sclerosis if you live above $35°$ latitude for the first ten years of your life (77,82,83). $1,25(OH)_2D$ has been shown to prevent development of multiple sclerosis in a mouse model (84). It has also been reported that women who took more than 400 IU of vitamin D, decrease their risk of developing multiple sclerosis by 41% (85). Women who took at least 400 IU of vitamin D daily also had a 42% reduction in risk of developing rheumatoid arthritis (86).

ADEQUATE INTAKE RECOMMENDATIONS FOR VITAMIN D AND WHAT YOU REALLY NEED

The Institute of Medicine in 1997 came out with its new recommendations for vitamin D (87). For all children and adults up to the age of 50, they require 200 IU of vitamin D (1 IU = 25 ng). For adults, 50–70 years and 71+ years, the recommendation was two and three times more or 400 and 600 IU daily, respectively. However, the consensus by most experts is that in order to maintain a healthy level of 25(OH)D of above 30 ng/mL (78 nmol/L) in the absence of adequate sun exposure, 1000 IU of vitamin D_3 a day is required (28,33,88–92).

Originally, it was believed that vitamin D_2 and vitamin D_3 had equal biologic potency in humans. However, it is now recognized that vitamin D_2 is more rapidly metabolized and therefore is only ~30% as effective as vitamin D_3 in maintaining serum 25(OH)D levels (93,94).

PREVENTION AND TREATMENT OF VITAMIN D DEFICIENCY

Sensible sun exposure in the spring, summer, and fall is very effective in not only preventing a deficiency in vitamin D but also helps in maintaining fat stores of vitamin D so that they can be used in the winter when the sun is ineffective in producing vitamin D_3 in the skin. An adult exposed in a bathing suit to simulated sunlight that is equivalent to 1 minimal erythemal dose (MED) raises the blood levels of vitamin D to the same extent as if the person took an oral dose of ~15,000 IU of vitamin D (Fig. 11) (2,28). Thus, the skin has a large capacity to produce vitamin D_3 and a minimum amount of skin surface exposed to a sensible amount of sunlight will satisfy the body's requirement for vitamin D (95). I usually recommend for a Caucasian with skin type II, that is, always burns and sometimes tans, that if they know that their skin will develop a light pinkness

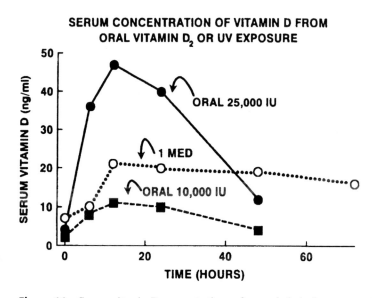

SERUM CONCENTRATION OF VITAMIN D FROM ORAL VITAMIN D_2 OR UV EXPOSURE

Figure 11   Serum vitamin D concentrations after a whole-body exposure to 1 MED (of simulated sunlight in a tanning bed and after a single oral dose of either 10,000 or 25,000 IU vitamin D_2. *Abbreviation*: MED, minimal erythemal dose. *Source*: From Ref. 156.

after being exposed for 30 minutes, exposure to 5 to 10 minutes of arms and legs, or abdomen and back, or arms, hands, and face, two to three times a week, is more than adequate to satisfy the body's requirement.

Lamps that produced UVB radiation were routinely used by both children and adults in the 1930s and 1940s as a guaranteed method to prevent vitamin D deficiency (96). However, with the introduction of vitamin D fortification and concern about skin cancer, these systems lost favor and are no longer available. However, over the past 20 years, there has been an interest by teenagers and adults to enhance their appearance by frequenting tanning salons. Most tanning beds emit UVB radiation. In Europe and the United States, these tanning beds emit between 2% and 5% UVB radiation. As UVB produces vitamin D in the skin, a study was conducted to determine the vitamin D status in healthy, young, non-tanning adults and in healthy adults who frequented a tanning salon at least once a week. Tanners had robust, healthy levels of 25(OH)D in the range of 35–45 ng/mL. The non-tanning adults had 25(OH)D, and were considered on average to be vitamin D deficient with a mean of 17 ± 5 ng/mL (Fig. 12) (97). A bone mineral density study revealed that the tanners had a higher bone density in their total hip compared with the

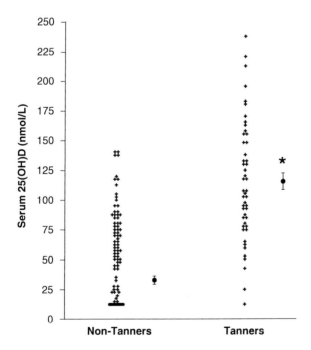

Figure 12   Mean ($\pm$SEM) serum 25-hydroxyvitamin D concentrations in tanners and nontanners. Single points for each category are mean $\pm$ SEM. *Significantly different from nontanners, $P < 0.001$. *Source*: From Ref. 97.

non-tanners. This is consistent with the observation that in both men and women of all ethnicities, bone density was directly related to their serum level of 25(OH)D (98).

Although aging decreases the capacity of the skin to produce vitamin D, elderly still have the ability to make vitamin D in their skin, and when exposed to either sunlight or artificial UVB radiation, they are able to increase their blood levels of 25(OH)D (99,100). Chuck et al. (101) reported that installation of UVB lights in the ceiling of an activity room was the most effective way of maintaining 25(OH)D in nursing home residents. They suggested that installation of UVB lamps in an activity room in a nursing home should be standard of care.

VITAMIN D DEFICIENCY PANDEMIC

It has long been observed that elderly and infirm who are unable to get an adequate amount of sun exposure are at high risk of vitamin D deficiency and fracture (2,28,41,102–105). Upwards of 50% of elders in nursing homes in the United States and Europe have been found to be vitamin D deficient, that is, a 25(OH)D of <20 ng/mL (102–106). More recently, it has been recognized that besides the elderly, children and young and middle-aged adults are also at high risk of vitamin D deficiency (102–132). Tangpricha et al. (35) reported that of the young adults aged 18–20 who often had at least one glass of milk a day and often took a multivitamin containing vitamin D, 32% were vitamin D deficient, that is, a 25(OH)D of <20 ng/mL at the end of the winter. Gordon et al. (107) reported that 52% of adolescent Hispanic and black children in Boston were found to be vitamin D deficient throughout the year. Sullivan et al. reported that of the young white girls aged 9–11 who lived in Maine, 48% were vitamin D deficient at the end of the winter. Many of these young girls went to summer camp, but always wore sun protection. An analysis of their 25(OH)D at the end of the summer revealed that 17% had blood levels of 25(OH)D of <20 ng/mL (36). Vitamin D deficiency is equally common even in sunny areas of the world. In Saudi Arabia, where often both children and women avoid all direct sun exposure, both rickets and osteomalacia and vitamin D deficiency are common (133,134). In Lebanon, Fuleihan et al. (37) reported that 32% of children were vitamin D deficient. Even in India, 25% of children living in New Delhi were found to be vitamin D deficient (135).

CONCLUSION

We need to appreciate that humans have depended on sun exposure for their vitamin D requirement throughout evolution. The industrialization of northern Europe and the northeastern United States markedly diminished exposure to solar UVB radiation, leading to vitamin D deficiency and an epidemic of rickets and osteomalacia.

Sensible sun exposure is the best method of guaranteeing adequate vitamin D. People with increased skin pigmentation need to be aware that they need longer exposures compared with Caucasians to produce the same amount of vitamin D_3. It is almost impossible to obtain the recommended 1000 IU of vitamin D_3 a day from dietary sources. It would require that a person eat oily fish at least five times a week, drink at least four glasses of vitamin D fortified beverages such as milk and orange juice in the United States, and take a multi-vitamin that contains 400 IU of vitamin D. Vitamin D as a single supplement is often hard to find in the United States, although is more commonly found in Canada and in Europe. However, 1000 IU of vitamin D_3 is needed every day. It is often difficult for both children and older adults to remember to take an additional pill once a day. This is why the recommendation that you can get all of your vitamin D from dietary sources and do not need to be exposed to sunlight (136) is not only naive but also puts people's lives at risk for metabolic bone disease and other more serious and chronic illnesses, including common cancers, autoimmune diseases and cardiovascular heart disease, osteoporotic fractures, and periodontal disease (137–144).

To put this into perspective, there is no question that excessive exposure to sunlight increases risk of nonmelanoma, squamous, and basal cell cancers (145). However, melanoma, the most deadly form of skin cancer, often occurs on the least sun-exposed areas, and evidence suggests that casual and occupational sun exposure decreases risk of developing malignant melanoma (145,146). It was reported that people who develop melanoma are more likely to survive if they had good sun exposure as children and young adults (147). There is also evidence that more sun exposure during childhood and adolescence decreases risk of developing non-Hodgkin's lymphoma by as much as 40% (148).

It is a mistake to recommend abstinence from all direct sun exposure. Even in Australia, vitamin D deficiency is becoming a problem because of the campaign to encourage wearing sun protection at all times (149). This may be especially true for children. There is concern that vitamin D deficiency during childhood could imprint on them for the rest of their lives and increase risk of developing deadly cancers, autoimmune diseases, and cardiovascular heart disease (28,150). The recommendation by the New Zealand Bone and Mineral Society in conjunction with the Australian College of Dermatologists and the Cancer Council of Australia is more reasonable and realistic, that is, that caution is needed to prevent too much sun exposure and increased risk of skin cancer, but that there needs to be sensible recommendation for limited sun exposure to promote vitamin D synthesis, and satisfy the body's vitamin D requirement. This recommendation is not only sensible but also highly desirable and should be adopted worldwide.

ACKNOWLEDGMENTS

This work was supported in part by NIH grants MOIRR00533 and AR36963 and the UV Foundation.

REFERENCES

1. Holick MF. Phylogenetic and evolutionary aspects of vitamin D from phytoplankton to humans. In: Pang PKT, Schreibman MP, eds. Vertebrate Endocrinology: Fundamentals and Biomedical Implications. Vol. 3. Orlando, FL: Academic Press, 1989:7–43.
2. Holick MF. Vitamin D: a millennium perspective. J Cell Biochem 2003; 88:296–307.
3. Holick MF. Vitamin D: new horizons for the 21st century. Am J Clin Nutr 1994; 60:619–630.
4. Sniadecki J. Jerdrzej Sniadecki (1768–1838) on the cure of rickets (1840). Cited by W. Mozolowski. Nature 1939; 143:121–124.
5. Huldschinsky K. Heilung von Rachitis durch Kunstliche Hohensonne. Deutsche Med Wochenschr 1919; 45:712–713.
6. Hess AF, Unger LJ. The cure of infantile rickets by sunlight. JAMA 1921; 77:39–41.
7. Mellanby T. The part played by an "accessory factor" in the production of experimental rickets. J Physiol 1918; 52:11–14.
8. Hess AF, Weinstock M. Antirachitic properties imparted to inert fluids and to green vegetables by ultraviolet irradiation. J Biol Chem 1924; 62:301–313.
9. Steenbock H, Black A. The reduction of growth promoting and calcifying properties in a ration by exposure to ultraviolet light. J Biol Chem 1924; 61:408–422.
10. Powers GF, Park EA, Shipley PG, et al. The prevention of rickets in the rat by means of radiation with the mercury vapor quartz lamp. Proc Soc Exp Biol Med 1921; 19:120–121.
11. McCollum EF, Simmonds N, Becker JE, et al. Studies on experimental rickets; and experimental demonstration of the existence of a vitamin which promotes calcium deposition. J Biol Chem 1922; 53:293–312.
12. Steenbock H. The induction of growth-prompting and calcifying properties in a ration exposed to light. Science 1924; 60:224–225.
13. Eliot MM. The control of rickets: preliminary discussion of the demonstration in new haven. JAMA 1925; 85(9):656–663.
14. Windaus A, Luttringhaus A, Deppe M. Uber das krystallisierte vitamin D. Justus Liebig's Ann Chem 1931; 489:252–269.
15. Steenbock H, Kletzien SWF. The reaction of chicken to irradiated ergosterol and irradiated yeast as contrasted with the natural vitamin D in fish liver oil. J Biol Chem 1932; 97:249–264.
16. Massengale ON, Nussmeier M. The action of activated ergosterol in the chicken. J Biol Chem 1930; 87:423–425.
17. Windaus A, Bock F. Uber das provitamin aus dem sterin der schweineschwarte. Hoppe-Seyler's Z Physiol Chem 1937; 245:168.
18. Holick MF, MacLaughlin JA, Clark MB, et al. Photosynthesis of previtamin D_3 in human skin and the physiologic consequences. Science 1980; 210:203–205.
19. MacLaughlin JA, Anderson RR, Holick MF. Spectral character of sunlight modulates photosynthesis of previtamin D_3 and its photoisomers in human skin. Science 1982; 216:1001–1003.
20. Holick MF, Tian XQ, Allen M. Evolutionary importance for the membrane enhancement of the production of vitamin D_3 in the skin of poikilothermic animals. Proc Natl Acad Sci USA 1995; 92:3124–3126.
21. Tian XQ, Holick MF. A liposomal model that mimics the cutaneous production of vitamin D3. J Biol Chem 1999; 274(7):4174–4179.

22. Tian XQ, Chen TC, Lu Z, et al. Characterization of the translocation process of vitamin D_3 from the skin into the circulation. Endocrinology 1994; 135:655–661.

23. Haddad JG, Matsuoka LY, Hollis BW, et al. Human plasma transport of vitamin D after its endogenous synthesis. J Clin Invest 1993; 91:2552–2555.

24. Matsuoka LY, Ide L, Wortsman J, et al. Sunscreens suppress cutaneous vitamin D_3 synthesis. J Clin Endocrinol Metab 1987; 64:1165–1168.

25. Clemens TL, Henderson SL, Adams JS, et al. Increased skin pigment reduces the capacity of skin to synthesize vitamin D_3. Lancet 1982; 6:74–76.

26. Lo CW, Paris PW, Holick MF. Serum vitamin D in response to ultraviolet irradiation in Asians. In: Norman AW, ed. Proceedings of Sixth Workshop on Vitamin D, Merano, Italy. Walter de Gruyter, Berlin, 1985:709–710.

27. Webb AR, Kline L, Holick MF. Influence of season and latitude on the cutaneous synthesis of vitamin D_3: exposure to winter sunlight in Boston and Edmonton will not promote vitamin D_3 synthesis in human skin. J Clin Endocrinol Metab 1988; 67:373–378.

28. Holick MF. Sunlight and vitamin D for bone health and prevention of auto-immune diseases, cancers, and cardiovascular disease. Am J Clin Nutr 2004; 80:1678S–1688S.

29. MacLaughlin J, Holick MF. Aging decreases the capacity of human skin to produce vitamin D_3. J Clin Invest 1985; 76:1536–1538.

30. Need AG, Morris HA, Horowitz M, et al. Effects of skin thickness, age, body fat, and sunlight on serum 25-hydroxyvitamin D. Am J Clin Nutr 1993; 58:882–885.

31. Holick MF, Matsuoka LY, Wortsman J. Age, vitamin D, and solar ultraviolet. Lancet 1989; 2(8671):1104–1105.

32. United States Food and Drug Administration Web site. Reference daily intakes, recommended dietary allowances. Available at: http://www.fda.gov/fdac/special/foodlabel/rditabl.html. Accessed July 27, 2004.

33. Tangpricha V, Koutkia P, Rieke SM, et al. Fortification of orange juice with vitamin D: a novel approach to enhance vitamin D nutritional health. Am J Clin Nutr 2003; 77:1478–1483.

34. British Pediatric Association. Hypercalcemia in infants and vitamin D. Brit Med J 1956; 2:149–151.

35. Tangpricha V, Pearce EN, Chen TC, et al. Vitamin D insufficiency among free-living healthy young adults. Am J Med 2002; 112:659–662.

36. Sullivan SS, Rosen CJ, Halteman WA, et al. Adolescent girls in Maine at risk for vitamin D insufficiency. J Am Diet Assoc 2005; 105:971–974.

37. Fuleihan GEH, Nabulsi M, Choucair M, et al. Hypovitaminosis D in healthy school-children. Pediatrics 2001; 107:53–59.

38. Outila TA, Karkkainen MU, Lamberg-Allardt CJ. Vitamin D status affects serum parathyroid hormone concentrations during winter in female adolescents: associations with forearm bone mineral density. Am J Clin Nutr 2001; 74:206–210.

39. Krall EA, Sahyoun N, Tannenbaum S, et al. Effect of vitamin D intake on seasonal variations in parathyroid hormone secretion in postmenopausal women. N Engl J Med 1989; 321:1777–1783.

40. DeLuca H. Overview of general physiologic features and functions of vitamin D. Am J Clin Nutr 2004; 80(suppl):1689S–1696S.

41. Bouillon, R. Vitamin D: from photosynthesis, metabolism, and action to clinical applications. In: DeGroot LJ, Jameson JL, eds. Endocrinology. Philadelphia: WB Saunders, 2001:1009–1028.

42. Christakos S, Dhawan P, Liu Y, et al. New insights into the mechanisms of vitamin D action. J Cell Biochem 2003; 88:695–705.

43. Khosla S. The OPG/RANKL/RANK system. Endocrinology 2001; 142(12): 5050–5055.

44. Holick MF. Vitamin D. The underappreciated D-lightful hormone that is important for skeletal and cellular health. Curr Opin Endocrinol Diabetes 2002; 9:87–98.

45. Plotnikoff GA, Quigley JM. Prevalence of severe hypovitaminosis D in patients with persistent, nonspecific musculoskeletal pain. Mayo Clin Proc 2003; 78: 1463–1470.

46. Holick MF. Vitamin D deficiency: what a pain it is. Mayo Clin Proc 2003; 78: 1457–1459.

47. Glerup H, Mikkelsen K, Poulsen L, et al. Commonly recommended daily intake of vitamin D is not sufficient if sunlight exposure is limited. J Intern Med 2000; 247:260–268.

48. Malabanan AO, Turner AK, Holick MF. Severe generalized bone pain and osteoporosis in a premenopausal black female: effect of vitamin D replacement. J Clin Densitometer 1983; 1:201–204.

49. Bischoff-Ferrari HA, Dietrich T, Orav EJ, et al. Higher 25-hydroxyvitamin D concentrations are associated with better lower-extremity function in both active and inactive persons aged ≥60 y. Am J Clin Nutr 2004; 80:752–758.

50. Visser M, Deeg DJ, Lips P. Low vitamin D and high parathyroid hormone levels as determinants of loss of muscle strength and muscle mass (sarcopenia): Longitudinal Aging Study Amsterdam. J Clin Endocrinol Metab 2003; 88:5766–5772.

51. Whitaker CH, Malchoff CD, Felice KJ. Treatable lower motor neuron disease due to vitamin D deficiency and secondary hyperparathyroidism. Amyotroph Lateral Scler Other Motor Neuron Disord 2005; 1:283–286.

52. Stumpf WE, Sar M, Reid FA, et al. Target cells for 1,25-dihydroxyvitamin D3 in intestinal tract, stomach, kidney, skin, pituitary, and parathyroid. Science 1979; 206:1188–1190.

53. Bikle DD. Vitamin D: role in skin and hair. In: Feldman et al., eds. Vitamin D. New Jersey: Elsevier Academic Press, 2005:609–630.

54. Tangpricha V, Flanagan JN, Whitlatch LW, et al. 25-Hydroxyvitamin D-1α-hydroxylase in normal and malignant colon tissue. Lancet 2001; 357:1673–1674.

55. Cross HS, Bareis P, Hofer H, et al. 25-Hydroxyvitamin D_3-1-α-hydroxlyase and vitamin D receptor gene expression in human colonic mucosa is elevated during early carcinogenesis. Steroids 2001; 66:287–292.

56. Schwartz GG, Whitlatch LW, Chen TC, et al. Human prostate cells synthesize 1,25-dihydroxyvitamin D_3 from 25-hydroxyvitamin D_3. Cancer Epidemiol Biomarkers Prev 1998; 7:391–395.

57. Mawer EB, Hayes ME, Heys SE, et al. Constitutive synthesis of 1,25-dihydroxyvitamin D3 by a human small cell lung cell line. J Clin Endocrinol Metab 1994; 79:554–560.

58. Zhao XY, Feldman D. The role of vitamin D in prostate cancer. Steroids 2001; 66:293–300.

59. Spina C, Tangpricha V, Yao M, et al. Colon cancer and solar ultraviolet B radiation and prevention and treatment of colon cancer in mice with vitamin D and its Gemini analogs. J Steroid Biochem Mol Biol 2005; 97:111–120.
60. Chen TC, Holick MF. Vitamin D and prostate cancer prevention and treatment. Trends Endocrinol Metab 2003; 14:423–430.
61. Nagpal S, Na S, Rathnachalam R. Noncalcemic actions of vitamin D receptor ligands. Endocrine Rev 2005; 26:662–687.
62. Li YC. Vitamin D regulation of the renin–angiotensin system. J Cell Biochem 2003; 88:327–331.
63. Chiu KC, Chu A, Go V, et al. Hypovitaminosis D is associated with insulin resistance and β cell dysfunction 44. Am J Clin Nutr 2004; 79:820–825.
64. Mathieu C, Adorini L. The coming of age of 1,25-dihydroxyvitamin D3 analogs as immunomodulatory agents. Trends Mol Med 2002; 8(4):174–179.
65. Apperly FL. The relation of solar radiation to cancer mortality in North America. Cancer Res 1941; 1:191–195.
66. Garland CF, Comstock GW, Garland FC, et al. Serum 25-hydroxyvitamin D and colon cancer: eight-year prospective study. Lancet 1989; 2:1176–1178.
67. Garland FC, Garland CF, Gorham ED, et al. Geographic variation in breast cancer mortality in the United States: a hypothesis involving exposure to solar radiation. Prev Med 1990; 19:614–622.
68. Grant WB. An estimate of premature cancer mortality in the U.S. due to inadequate doses of solar ultraviolet-B radiation. Cancer 2002; 94:1867–1875.
69. Freedman DM, Dosemeci M, McGlynn K. Sunlight and mortality from breast, ovarian, colon, prostate, and non-melanoma skin cancer: a composite death certificate based case–control study. Occup Environ Med 2002; 59:257–262.
70. Gorham ED, Carland CF, Garland FC, et al. Vitamin D and prevention of colorectal cancer. J Steroid Biochem Mol Biol 2005; 97:179–194.
71. Grant WB, Holick MF. Benefits and requirements of vitamin D for optimal health: a review. Altern Med Rev 2005; 10:94–111.
72. Moan J, Porojnicu AC, Robsahm TE, et al. Solar radiation, Vitamin D and survival rate of colon cancer in Norway. J Photochem Photobiolol B 2005; 78:189–193.
73. Luscombe CJ, Fryer AA, French ME, et al. Exposure to ultraviolet radiation: association with susceptibility and age at presentation with prostate cancer. Lancet 2001; 358(9282):641–642.
74. Ahonen MH, Tenkanen L, Teppo L, Hakama, et al. Prostate cancer risk and prediagnostic serum 25-hydroxyvitamin D levels (Finland). Cancer Causes Control 2000; 11:847–852.
75. Zella JB, DeLuca HF. Vitamin D and autoimmune diabetes. J Cell Biochem 2003; 88:216–222.
76. Cantorna MT, Munsick C, Bemiss C, et al. 1,25-Dihydroxycholecalciferol prevents and ameliorates symptoms of experimental murine inflammatory bowel disease. J Nutr 2000; 130:2648–2652.
77. Hernán MA, Olek MJ, Ascherio A. Geographic variation of MS incidence in two prospective studies of US women. Neurology 1999; 51:1711–1718.
78. Ponsonby AL, McMichael A, van der Mei I. Ultraviolet radiation and autoimmune disease: insights from epidemiological research. Toxicology 2002; 181: 71–78.

79. Rostand SG. Ultraviolet light may contribute to geographic and racial blood pressure differences. Hypertension 1997; 30:150–156.

80. Mathieu C, Badenhoop K. Vitamin D and type 1 diabetes mellitus: state of the art. Trends Endocrinol Metab 2005; 16:261–266.

81. Hypponen E, Laara E, Reunanen A, et al. Intake of vitamin D and risk of type 1 diabetes: a birth-cohort study. Lancet 2001; 358:1500–1503.

82. van der Mei I, Ponsonby AL, Dwyer T, et al. Past exposure to sun, skin phenotype, and risk of multiple sclerosis: case–control study. Br Med J 2003; 327: 316–317.

83. Embry AF, Snowdon LR, Vieth R. Vitamin D and seasonal fluctuations of gadolinium-enhancing magnetic resonance imaging lesions in multiple sclerosis. Ann Neurol 2000; 48:271–272.

84. Cantorna MT, Humpal-Winter J, DeLuca HF. *In vivo* upregulation of interleukin-4 is one mechanism underlying the immunoregulatory effects of 1,25-dihydroxyvitamin D_3. Arch Biochem Biophys 2000; 377:135–138.

85. Munger KL, Zhang SM, O'Reilly E, et al. Vitamin D intake and incidence of multiple sclerosis. Neurology 2004; 62:60–65.

86. Merlino LA, Curtis J, Mikuls TR, et al. Vitamin D intake is inversely associated with rheumatoid arthritis: results from the Iowa Women's Health Study. Arthritis Rheum 2004; 50:72–77.

87. Standing Committee on the Scientific Evaluation of Dietary Reference Intakes Food and Nutrition Board Institute of Medicine 1997 Vitamin D. Dietary Reference Intakes for Calcium, Phosphorus, Magnesium, Vitamin D, and Fluoride. Washington, DC, National Academy Press, 1997:250–287.

88. Heaney RP, Davies KM, Chen TC, et al. Human serum 25-hydroxycholecalciferol response to extended oral dosing with cholecalciferol. Am J Clin Nutr 2003; 77:204–210.

89. Heaney RP, Dowell MS, Hale CA, et al. Calcium absorption varies within the reference range for serum 25-hydroxyvitamin D. J Am Coll Nutr 2003; 22:142–146.

90. Dawson-Hughes B, Heaney RP, Holick MF, et al. Estimates of optimal vitamin D status. Osteoporos Int (Editorial) 2005; 16:713–716.

91. Hollis BW. Circulating 25-hydroxyvitamin D levels indicative of vitamin D sufficiency: implications for establishing a new effective dietary intake recommendation for vitamin D. J Nutr 2005; 135:317–322.

92. Vieth R. The pharmacology of vitamin D, including fortification strategies. In: Feldman D, Pike JW, Glorieux FH, eds. Vitamin D. 2nd ed. Elsevier Academic Press, 2005.

93. Tang HM, Cole DEC, Rubin LA, et al. Evidence that vitamin D_3 increases serum 25-hydroxyvitamin D more efficiently than does vitamin D_2. Am J Clin Nutr 1998; 68:854–858.

94. Armas LAG, Hollis B, Heaney RP. Vitamin D2 is much less effective than vitamin D3 in humans. J Clin Endocrinol Metab 2004; 89:5387–5391.

95. Holick MF, Jenkins M. The UV Advantage. New York, NY: iBooks, 2003.

96. Holick MF. Vitamin D: importance for bone health, cellular health and cancer prevention. In: Holick MF, ed. Biologic Effects of Light 2001 (Proceedings of a Symposium, Boston, MA). Kluwer Academic Publishing: Boston, 2002:155–173.

97. Tangpricha V, Turner A, Spina C, et al. Tanning is associated with optimal vitamin D status (serum 25-hydroxyvitamin D concentration) and higher bone mineral density. Am J Clin Nutr 2004; 80:1645–1649.

98. Bischoff-Ferrari HA, Dietrich T, Orav J, et al. Positive association between 25-hydroxyvitamin D levels and bone mineral density: a population-based study of younger and older adults. JAMA 2004; 116:634–639.

99. Chel VGM, Ooms ME, Popp-Snijders C, et al. Ultraviolet irradiation corrects vitamin D deficiency and suppresses secondary hyperparathyroidism in the elderly. J Bone Miner Res 1998; 13:1238–1242.

100. Chen TC, Perez A, Lu Z, et al. Effect of sunscreen use and clothing on the circulating concentrations of vitamin D_3. In: Holick MF, Jung EG, eds. Proceedings, Symposium on the Biological Effects of Light, Berlin, Walter De Gruyter & Co., 1996:83–86.

101. Chuck A, Todd J, Diffey B. Subliminal ultraviolet-B irradiation for the prevention of vitamin D deficiency in the elderly: a feasibility study. Photochem Photoimmun Photomed 2001; 17(4):168–171.

102. Kauppinen-Mäkelin R, Tähtelä R, Löyttyniemi E, et al. High prevalence of hypovitaminosis D in Finnish medical in- and outpatients. J Intern Med 2001; 249: 559–563.

103. Chapuy MC, Preziosi P, Maamer M, et al. Prevalence of vitamin D insufficiency in an adult normal population. Osteoporos Int 1997; 7:439–443.

104. Webb AR, Pilbeam C, Hanafin N, et al. A one-year study to evaluate the roles of exposure to sunlight and diet on the circulating concentrations of 25-OH-D in an elderly population in Boston. Am J Clin Nutr 1990; 51(6):1075–1081.

105. Gloth FM III, Gundberg CM, Hollis BW, et al. Vitamin D deficiency in homebound elderly persons. JAMA 1995; 274:1683–1686.

106. Isaia G, Giorgino R, Rini GB, et al. Prevalence of hypovitaminosis D in elderly women in Italy: clinical consequences and risk factors. Osteoporos Int 2003; 14:577–582.

107. Gordon CM, DePeter KC, Feldman HA, et al. Prevalence of vitamin D deficiency among healthy adolescents. Arch Pediatr Adolesc Med 2004; 158:531–537.

108. Lips P, Duong T, Oleksik A, et al. A global study of vitamin D status and parathyroid function in postmenopausal women with osteoporosis: baseline data from the multiple outcomes of raloxifene evaluation clinical trial. J Clin Endocrinol Metab 2001; 86:1212–1221.

109. Looker AC, Dawson-Hughes B, Calvo MS, et al. Serum 25-hydroxyvitamin D status of adolescents and adults in two seasonal subpopulations from NHANES III. Bone 2002; 30:771–777.

110. Malabanan A, Veronikis IE, Holick MF. Redefining vitamin D insufficiency. Lancet 1998; 351:805–806.

111. Kinyamu HK, Gallagher JC, Rafferty KA, et al. Dietary calcium and vitamin D intake in elderly women: effect on serum parathyroid hormone and vitamin D metabolites. Am J Clin Nutr 1998; 67:342–348.

112. Lips P. Vitamin D deficiency and secondary hyperparathyroidism in the elderly: consequences for bone loss and fractures and therapeutic implications. Endocr Rev 2001; 22:477–501.

113. Heaney RP. Functional indices of vitamin D status and ramifications of vitamin D deficiency. Am J Clin Nutr 2004; 80(suppl):1706S–1709S.

114. McKenna MJ, Freany R. Secondary hyperparathyroidism in the elderly: means to defining hypovitaminosis D. Osteoporos Int 1998; 8(suppl):S3–S6.
115. Kinyamu HK, Gallagher JC, Balhorn KE, et al. Serum vitamin D metabolites and calcium absorption in normal young and elderly free-living women and in women living in nursing homes. Am J Clin Nutr 1997; 65:790–797.
116. Gaugris S, Heaney RP, Boonen S, et al. Vitamin D inadequacy among post-menopausal women: a systematic review. Q J Med 2005; 98:667–676.
117. Harwood RH, Sahota O, Gaynor K, et al. The Nottingham Neck of Femur (NONOF) Study: a randomized, controlled comparison of different calcium and vitamin D supplementation regimens in elderly women after hip fracture. Age Ageing 2004; 33:45–51.
118. Glowacki J, Hurwitz S, Thornhill TS, et al. Osteoporosis and vitamin D deficiency among postmenopausal women with osteoarthritis undergoing total hip arthroplasty. J Bone Joint Surg Am 2003; 85A:2371–2377.
119. Blau EM, Brenneman SK, Bruning AL, et al. Prevalence of vitamin D insufficiency in an osteoporosis population in Southern California. J Bone Miner Res 2004; 19(suppl 1):S342.
120. Simonelli C, Weiss TW, Morancey J, et al. Prevalence of vitamin D inadequacy in a minimal trauma fracture population. Curr Med Res Opin 2005; 21:1069–1074.
121. Nesby-O'Dell S, Scanlon KS, Cogswell ME, et al. Hypovitaminosis D prevalence and determinants among African American and white women of reproductive age: third National Health and Nutrition Examination Survey, 1988–1994. Am J Clin Nutr 2002; 76:187–192.
122. Hanley DA, Davison KS. Vitamin D insufficiency in North America. J Nutr 2005; 135:332–337.
123. Romagnoli E, Caravella P, Scarnecchia L, et al. Hypovitaminosis D in an Italian population of healthy subjects and hospitalized patients. Br J Nutr 1999; 81: 133–137.
124. van der Wielen RPJ, de Groot LCPG, van Staveren WA, et al. Serum vitamin D concentrations among elderly people in Europe. Lancet 1995; 346:207–210.
125. Passeri G, Pini G, Troiano L, et al. Low vitamin D status, high bone turnover, and bone fractures in centenarians. J Clin Endocrinol Metab 2003; 88:5109–5115.
126. Harris SS, Soteriades E, Coolidge JA, et al. Vitamin D insufficiency and hyper-parathyroidism in a low income, multiracial, elderly population. J Clin Endocrinol Metab 2000; 85:4125–4130.
127. Thomas MK, Lloyd-Jones DM, Thadhani RI, et al. Hypovitaminosis D in medical inpatients. N Engl J Med 1998; 338:777–783.
128. McKenna MJ. Differences in vitamin D status between countries in young adults and the elderly. Am J Med 1992; 93:69–77.
129. Simonelli C, Morancey JA, Swanson L, et al. A high prevalence of vitamin D insufficiency/deficiency in a minimal trauma fracture population. J Bone Miner Res 2004; 19(suppl1):S433.
130. LeBoff MS, Kohlmeier L, Hurwitz S, et al. Occult vitamin D deficiency in post-menopausal US women with acute hip fracture. JAMA 1999; 281:1505–1511.
131. Aaron JE, Gallagher JC, Anderson J, et al. Frequency of osteomalacia and osteo-porosis in fractures of the proximal femur. Lancet 1974; 1:229–233.
132. Hordon LD, Peacock M. Osteomalacia and osteoporosis in femoral neck fracture. Bone Miner 1990; 11:247–259.

133. Taha SA, Dost SM, Sedrani SH. 25-Hydroxyvitamin D and total calcium: extraordinarily low plasma concentrations in Saudi mothers and their neonates. Pediatr Res 1984; 18:739–741.

134. Sedrani SH. Low 25-hydroxyvitamin D and normal serum calcium concentrations in Saudi Arabia: Riyadh region. Ann Nutr Metab 1984; 28:181–185.

135. Marwaha RK, Tandon N, Reddy D, et al. Vitamin D and bone mineral density status of healthy schoolchildren in northern India. Am J Clin Nutr 2005; 82:477–482.

136. Wolpowitz D, Gilchrest BA. The vitamin D questions: how much do you need and how should you get it? J Am Acad Dermatol 2005; 11:1057.

137. Chapuy MC, Arlot ME, Duboeuf F, et al. Vitamin D_3 and calcium to prevent hip fractures in elderly women. N Engl J Med 1992; 327:1637–1642.

138. Trivedi DP, Doll R, Khaw KT. Effect of four monthly oral vitamin D_3 (cholecalciferol) supplementation on fractures and mortality in men and women living in the community: randomized double blind controlled trial. BMJ 2003; 326:469–475.

139. Bischoff-Ferrari HA, Willet WC, Wong JB, et al. Fracture prevention with vitamin D supplementation: a meta-analysis of randomized controlled trials. JAMA 2005; 293:2257–2264.

140. Dawson-Hughes B, Dallal GE, Krall EZ, et al. Effect of vitamin D supplementation on wintertime and overall bone loss in healthy postmenopausal women. Ann Intern Med 1991; 115:505–512.

141. Krause R, Buhring M, Hopfenmuller W, et al. Ultraviolet B and blood pressure. Lancet 1998; 352:709–710.

142. Dietrich T, Joshipura KJ, Dawson-Hughes B, et al. Association between serum concentrations of 25-hydroxyvitamin D_3 and periodontal disease in the US population. Am J Clin Nutr 2004; 80:108–113.

143. Zittermann A, Schleithoff SS, Tenderich G, et al. Low vitamin D status: a contributing factor in the pathogenesis of congestive heart failure? J Am Coll Cardiol 2003; 41:105–112.

144. Holick M. The vitamin D epidemic and its health consequences. J Nutr 2005; 135:2739S–2748S.

145. Kennedy C, Bajdik CD, Willemze R, et al. The influence of painful sunburns and lifetime of sun exposure on the risk of actinic keratoses, seborrheic warts, melanocytic nevi, atypical nevi and skin cancer. J Invest Dermatol 2003; 120(6): 1087–1093.

146. Garland FC, Garland CF. Occupational sunlight exposure and melanoma in the U.S. Navy. Arch Environ Health 1990; 45:261–267.

147. Berwick M, Armstrong BK, Ben-Porat L, et al. Sun exposure and mortality from melanoma. J Natl Cancer Inst 2005; 97:195–199.

148. Chang ET, Smedby KE, Hjalgrim H, et al. Family history of hematopoietic malignancy and risk of lymphoma. J Natl Cancer Inst 2005; 97:1466–1474.

149. McGrath JJ, Kimlin MG, Saha S, et al. Vitamin D insufficiency in south-east Queensland. Med J Aust 2001; 174:150–151.

150. McGrath J. Does "imprinting" with low prenatal vitamin D contribute to the risk of various adult disorders? Med Hypotheses 2001; 56(3):367–371.

151. Fraser D and Scriver CR. Disorders associated with hereditary or acquired abnormalities of vitamin D function: hereditary disorders associated with vitamin D

resistance or defective phosphate metabolism. In: De Groot LJ et al., eds. Endocrinology. New York: Grune and Stratton, 797–808.
152. Gamgee KML. The Artificial Light Treatment of Children. New York: Paul B. Hoeber, 1927.
153. MacLaughlin JA, Holick MF. Mediation of cutaneous vitamin D_3 synthesis by UV radiation. In: Goldsmith LA, ed. Biochemistry and Physiology of the Skin. New York: Oxford University Press, 1983.
154. Holick MF. Evolution, biologic functions, and recommended dietary allowances for vitamin D. In: Holick MF, ed. Vitamin D: Physiology, Molecular Biology and Clinical Applications. NJ: Humana Press, 1998:1–16.
155. Lu Z, Chen T, Kline L, et al. Photosynthesis of previtamin D3 in cities around the world. In Holick M, Kligman A, eds. Biologic Effects of Light. Proceedings. Berlin: Walter De Gruyter, 1992:48–51.
156. Darwish H, DeLuca HF. Vitamin D regulated gene expression. Crit Rev Eukaryot Gene Expr 1993; 3:89–116.

5

Ultraviolet Radiation Risks to the Eye

David H. Sliney

*U.S. Army Center for Health Promotion and Preventive Medicine,
Aberdeen Proving Ground, Maryland, U.S.A.*

INTRODUCTION

The human eye is exquisitely sensitive to light (i.e., visible radiant energy), and when dark-adapted, the retina can detect a few photons of blue-green light (1). It is therefore not at all surprising that ocular tissues are also more vulnerable to ultraviolet radiation (UVR) damage than the skin. For this reason, we have evolved with certain anatomical, physiological, and behavioral traits that protect this critical organ from UV damage that would otherwise be certain from the intense bath of overhead solar UVR when we are outdoors during daylight. For example, the UV exposure threshold dose for photokeratitis (also known as "snow blindness" or "welder's flash")—if measured by an outdoor, global UVR meter designed to respond as the action spectrum for photokeratitis—would be reached in <10 minutes around midday in the summer sun. There are three critical ocular structures that could be affected by UV exposure: the cornea, the lens, and the retina. Figure 1 shows a simple diagram of the human eye and points to these three critical and complex ocular tissues. The eye is ~25 mm in diameter and has an effective focal length in air of ~17 mm. Very little UV reaches the retina. The cornea transmits radiant energy only at 295 nm and above. The crystalline lens absorbs almost all incident energy to wavelengths of ~400 nm. In youth, a very small amount of UVA reaches the retina, but the lens becomes more absorbing with age. Thus, there are intraocular filters that effectively filter different parts of the UV spectrum and allow only of the order of 1% or less to actually reach the retina (1).

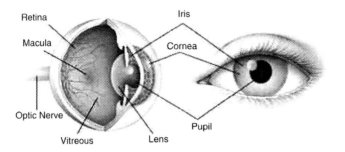

Figure 1 The human eye.

The acute phototoxic effect of UVR on the eye, photokeratitis, has long been recognized. Less obvious are potential hazards to the eye from chronic exposure. Certain age-related changes to the cornea, conjunctiva, and lens have also been thought to be related to chronic exposure to solar UVR in certain climates. Determining environmental ocular exposure can be quite difficult, and this exposure to sunlight has been misjudged in many epidemiological studies. There are many occasions where one views bright light sources such as the sun, arc lamps, and welding arcs. But such viewing is normally only momentary, as the aversion response to bright light and discomfort glare limits exposure to a fraction of a second. Delayed effects are almost exclusively considered to result from environmental UVR exposure. Hence, the increased terrestrial UVR related to ozone depletion has been one cause for health concern.

EFFECTS FROM ENVIRONMENTAL EXPOSURE

Human exposure to sunlight, particularly the UVB component, is believed to be associated with a variety of eye disorders, including damage to the cornea, lens, and retina (2). Photokeratitis (snow blindness) is clearly related to UVR exposure, whereas, cataracts (opacities of the lens) are the most frequently cited delayed consequence. Certain keratopathies (corneal degenerations) and pterygium (a fleshy growth on the conjunctiva) also are believed to result from excessive UVB exposures. Cataracts are a major cause of blindness in both developed and developing countries. However, the relative importance of different wavelengths in cataractogenesis, as well as the dose–response curve, remains uncertain.

The geographical variation in the incidence of age-related ocular changes such as presbyopia and cataracts, and diseases such as pterygium and droplet keratopathies, have led to theories pointing to sunlight, UVR exposure, and ambient temperature as potential etiological factors (3–5). Some epidemiological evidence also point to an association of age-related macular degeneration (AMD) to sunlight (particularly blue light) exposure (6). The actual distribution of sunlight exposure of different tissues within the anterior segment of the eye is more difficult to assess than one would expect. Of greatest importance are the geometrical factors that influence the selective UVR exposure to different segments of the lens, cornea, and retina. Studies show that sunlight exposure to local areas of the cornea, lens, and retina varies greatly in different environments. Perhaps for this reason, the epidemiological studies of the potential role of environmental UVR in the development of ocular diseases such as cataract, pterygium, droplet keratopathies, and AMD have produced surprisingly inconsistent findings (3,7–9). All of these ocular diseases vary geographically; however, the lack of consistent epidemiological results is almost certainly the result of either incomplete or erroneous estimates of outdoor UVR exposure dose (5,10–14). Geometrical factors dominate the determination of UVR exposure of the eye. The degree of lid opening limits ocular exposure to rays entering at angles near the horizon. Clouds redistribute overhead UVR to the horizon sky. Mountains, trees, and buildings shield the eye from direct sky exposure. Most ground surfaces reflect only a small fraction of incident UVR. The result is that the highest UVR exposure appears to occur during light overcast where the horizon is visible and ground surface reflection is high. By contrast, exposure in a high mountain valley (lower ambient temperature) with green foliage results in a much lower ocular dose. Other findings of these studies show that retinal exposure to light and UVR in daylight occurs largely in the superior retina (15).

Epidemiological Evidence

So why is it important to study the spectral and geometrical exposures of the human eye from solar UVR? It has long been suggested that the great latitudinal variation of "the world's most blinding disease," cataract (3), is strongly suggestive (as in the case of skin cancers) to result from UVR. World Health Organization (WHO) estimates that the worldwide prevalence of cataract exceeds 50 million (3). Indeed, if this dependence is examined along with a wide variety of laboratory studies, it suggests that environmental factors surely plays a major role in the time of onset of lenticular opacities. However, most epidemiological evidence point to UVR in sunlight as a significant risk factor only in one type of cataract, i.e., cortical cataract (16). The evidence for UVR as an etiological factor in at least two adverse changes in the cornea, that is, droplet keratopathies and pterygium, is much stronger (3,17). Furthermore, the environmental studies of Sasaki (4) have provided very important insights into the geographical variations in the incidence of cataract by examining the different types of cataract characteristic of different latitudes (4). Nuclear cataract was shown to be more common in the tropics; cortical cataract, more common in mid-latitudes, and posterior sub-capsular cataract was not so clearly related to latitude. Despite this latitudinal variation, some other published epidemiological studies do not appear to show a relation between UVR and cataract. Nevertheless, a wide variety of scientific evidence, from laboratory studies of the UV photochemistry of lens proteins to a number of different animal exposure studies, all provide support for the hypothesis that UVR should play a far greater role in cataracto-genesis. Most age-related changes in the skin (from accelerated aging to skin cancer) have been conclusively shown to result from excessive exposure to solar UVR (or "sunlight exposure"). Although no one questions that UVR exposure produces the acute effects of "sunburn" (erythema) and snow blindness (photokeratitis), some have questioned whether pterygium and droplet keratopa-thies are clearly related to UVR exposure (3,7). Even more under debate are the-ories that suggest that UVR and light may affect retinal diseases such as AMD (3). A better resolution of these questions requires far better ocular dosimetry.

With the strong geographical variations in the incidence of nuclear catar-act (4), it is surprising that most epidemiological studies show only weak or no apparent relation between UV or sunlight exposure and the incidence of nuclear cataract (9). Perhaps, it is necessary to consider the other important environmental parameter—environmental temperature. Both sunlight and ambient temperature have been cited as potential etiological factors in several age-related ocular dis-eases (5). However, the combined role of these physical factors and their possible synergisms generally has not been carefully examined. These environmental co-factors, together with geometrical factors, have recently been examined to give some suggestions about the etiology of these ocular diseases (14).

Animal Studies

Injury thresholds for acute UVR injury to the cornea, conjunctiva, lens, and retina in experimental animals have been corroborated for the human eye from labora-tory and accidental injury data. Guidelines for human health and safety limits for exposure to UVR are based upon this knowledge (18–20).

There are several types of hazards to the eye from intense UVR exposure, and the dosimetric concepts applicable to the anterior segment differ from quan-tities applicable to retinal exposure. The following effects are considered in current safety standards, which depend upon the spectrum of the UVR exposure and the temporal and geometrical characteristics of the exposure (1,11,18–23).

Photokeratoconjunctivitis

UV photokeratoconjunctivitis (more simply, "photokeratitis," also known as "welder's flash" or "snow blindness"—180 to 400 nm) is a temporary photoche-mical injury of the cornea (photokeratitis) and conjunctiva (photoconjunctivitis) that appears several hours after the acute exposure; symptoms generally last for only 24 to 48 hours (24–27). Due to the very superficial nature of the corneal injury and the rapid turnover of surface epithelial cells of the cornea (~48-hour cycle), the effect is transient.

The symptoms of photokeratitis are severe pain and, in some cases, blepharospasm (uncontrolled blinking). The onset of symptoms, like erythema, is delayed for several hours after the UVR exposure. The signs and symptoms last for a day or two, and the haze appears in the region of the cornea (the superficial surface layer of the eye) within the palpebral fissure (i.e., within the lid opening). The condition is almost always reversible and it has generally been accepted that the condition is without sequelae. However, the laboratory studies of Ringvold (26) show damage of both keratinocytes and endothelial cells of the cornea, and it could be speculated that repeated, severe episodes of snow blindness may well increase the risk of delayed corneal pathologies such as pterygium and droplet keratopathies.

Lenticular Opacities

As noted earlier, the epidemiological evidence for the role of ambient UVR report varying results. Some research studies related to UVR and cataract are of interest, as exposures of all other anterior structures would also be revealed in such research, and all animal studies showed that the cornea was injured at lower exposures than the lens. UV cataract can be produced in animals from acute exposures to UVR of wavelengths between 295 and 325 nm (and perhaps to 400 nm). Action spectra can only be obtained from animal studies, and the cataract is generally anterior sub-capsular, produced by intense exposures delivered over a period of days (25,28,29). Human cortical cataract has been linked to chronic, life-long UVA radiation exposure (2,3,5,16). These suggest that it is primarily UVB radiation in sunlight, and not UVB, that is most injurious to the lens. Biochemical studies suggest that UVA radiation may also contribute to accelerated ageing of the lens (3).

One area of UV cataract research is of note when considering lens exposure geometry of the crystalline lens. As the only direct pathway of UVR to the inferior germinative area of the lens is from the extreme temporal direction, it has been speculated that side exposure is particularly hazardous (30,31).

Ophthalmoheliosis—The Coroneo Effect

For any greatly delayed health effect, such as pterygium, droplet keratopathies, cataract, or retinal degeneration, it is critical to determine the actual dose distribution at critical locations. A factor of great practical importance is the actual UVR that reaches the germinative layers of any tissue structure. In the case of the lens, the germinative layer where lens fiber cell nuclei are located is of great importance. The DNA in these cells is normally well shielded by the parasol effect of the irises. However, Coroneo (30) has suggested that focusing of peripheral rays by the temporal edge of the cornea—those which do not even reach the retina—can enter the pupil and reach the equatorial region, as shown in Figure 2. He terms this effect, which can also produce a concentration of UVR at the nasal side of the limbus and lens, "ophthalmoheliosis." He notes the more frequent onset of cataract in the nasal quadrant of the lens and the

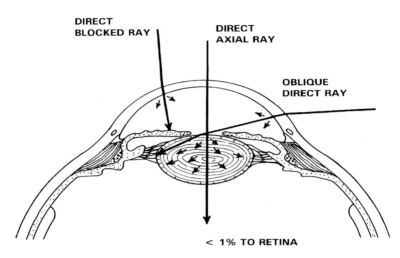

Figure 2 Coroneo effect. Oblique rays striking the peripheral cornea can be refracted into the pupil and irradiate the sensitive germinative equatorial region of the human lens. It is this region where cell nuclei with DNA reside.

formation of pterygium (described subsequently) in the nasal region of the cornea (31).

Pterygium and Droplet Keratopathies

The possible role of UVR in the etiology of a number of age-related ocular diseases has been the subject of many medical and scientific papers. However, there is still a debate as to validity of these arguments. Although photokeratitis is unquestionably caused by UVR reflection from the snow (5,32,33), pterygium and droplet keratopathies are less clearly related to UVR exposure (3). Pterygium, a fatty growth originating in the conjunctiva that produces visual loss as it progresses over the cornea, is most common in ocean island residents (where both UVR and wind exposure is prevalent). UVR is a likely etiologic factor (2,3,31,34), and the Coroneo effect may also play a role (31).

Erythema

UV erythema ("sunburn" or reddening of the skin—200 to 400 nm) applies to the lids of the eye. This effect appears several hours after an acute exposure and generally lasts eight to 72 hours depending upon degree of exposure and spectral region. Thresholds are higher than those for producing photokeratoconjunctivitis (1,2,35). The American Conference of Governmental Industrial Hygienists (ACGIH) and International Commission for Non-Ionizing Radiation Protection (ICNIRP) occupational exposure limits for UVR also protect against erythema with an added safety factor for all skin types.

Ocular Cancers

Cancers arising from chronic exposure to UVR, particularly from UVB (280–315 nm), have been demonstrated for the skin (2,36–39); however, little is known about the potential contribution of UVR to ocular cancers and ocular melanoma. It is interesting to note that while corneal cancers do occur in cattle, they are almost unknown in humans (40). Current theory holds that uveal melanomas are not related to UVR exposure. In any case, there is no evidence suggesting that single, acute exposures can produce skin or ocular tumors; chronic, repeated exposures are always required.

Retinal Effects

Theories which suggest that UVR (and even light) may contribute to some age-related retinal diseases are very much in debate (1–3,31,34). Acute exposure to light can produce a photochemical injury to the retina. This effect is principally from visible 400 to 550 nm blue light, with generally only a small UV contribution in the phakic eye. This often is referred to as "blue light" photoretinitis, for example, solar retinitis that may lead to a permanent scotoma (41–44). Prior to conclusive animal experiments two decades ago, solar retinitis was thought to be a thermal injury mechanism (1). Unlike thermal retinal injury, there is no image-size dependence. The ICNIRP/ACGIH $B(\lambda)$ weighted integrated radiance limit L_B is 20 J/cm^2 sr, averaged over a right circular cone of 0.011 radian for durations up to 10^4 seconds (2.8 hours), although a larger averaging angle is generally used for durations of the order of 1000 seconds or greater where a non-fixation visual task is involved. Normally, the cornea, aqueous, and crystalline lens absorb 99% or more of the UVR that could enter the eye (as shown in Fig. 3), although it may be higher in youth. The $B(\lambda)$ function has a value of 0.01 from 310 to 380 nm (44); hence, the hazardous integrated radiance

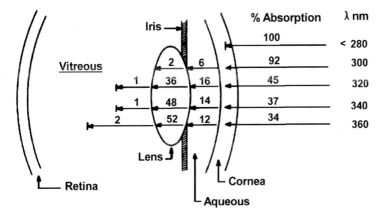

Figure 3 Spectral absorption of UV radiant energy within ocular structures.

for a pure UVB source is $\sim 2\ \mathrm{kJ/cm^2}$ sr for the phakic eye. However, in infancy or during cataract surgery after the cataractous lens has been removed (aphakia) and before a UV absorbing intra-ocular lens implant has been placed in the eye (pseudophakia), the retina can receive considerable UV exposure. The aphakic hazard spectrum $A(\lambda)$ can be applied for a hazard analysis.

GUIDELINES FOR HUMAN EXPOSURE

Based upon the extensive research carried out during the last few decades on both acute and delayed effects resulting from UV exposure of the eye, safety guidelines for limiting UVR exposure to protect the eye have been developed. The guidelines were fostered to a large extent by the growing use of lasers and the quickly recognized hazard posed by viewing laser sources. To assess potential hazards, one must not only consider the optical and radiometric parameters of the optical source in question, but also the geometrical exposure factors. This knowledge is required to accurately determine the irradiances (dose rates) to exposed tissues. Thermal injury is rare unless the UV source is pulsed or nearly in contact with the tissue. Generally, photochemical interaction mechanisms dominate in the UV spectrum where photon energies are sufficient to alter key biological molecules. A characteristic of photochemically initiated biological damage is the reciprocity of exposure dose rate and duration of exposure (the Bunsen–Roscoe Law), and acute UV effects are therefore most readily observed for lengthy exposure durations of many minutes or hours. The current guidance for UV exposure at wavelengths >315 nm (UVB) is 1 J/ $\mathrm{cm^2}$, and this was based upon conservative assumptions designed to protect the intact crystalline lens from both thermal and photochemical stress.

As with any photochemical injury mechanism, one must consider the action spectrum, which describes the relative effectiveness of different wavelengths in causing a photobiological effect (1,2,45–48). The relative action spectra for both the UV hazards to the eye, acute cataract and photokeratitis, are shown in Figure 4 (24–27,49). The UV safety function $S_{UV}(\lambda)$ is also an action spectrum, which is an envelope curve for protection of both eye and skin (Fig. 4).

The $S_{UV}(\lambda)$ curve of Figure 4 is an action spectrum, which is used to spectrally weigh the incident UVR to determine an effective irradiance for comparison with the threshold value or exposure limit (18). With modern computer spreadsheet programs, one can readily develop a method for spectrally weighing a lamp's spectrum by a variety of photochemical action spectra.

$$E_{\mathrm{eff}} = \sum E_\lambda \cdot S_{UV}(\lambda) \cdot \Delta\lambda \qquad (1)$$

The exposure limit is then expressed as a permissible effective irradiance E_{eff} or an effective radiant exposure. One then can compare different sources to determine relative effectiveness of the same irradiance from several lamps for a given action spectrum.

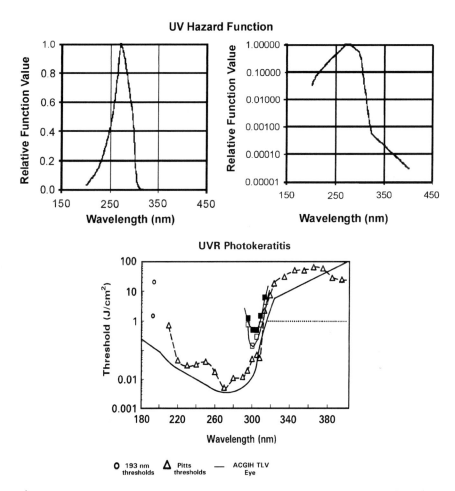

Figure 4 Action spectra. Top is the UV hazard action spectrum $S(\lambda)$ used for safety assessments of both eye and skin hazards. The action spectrum expressed as an absolute threshold is shown in the lower panel, with threshold data of Pitts (Δ) and Sliney et al. (o).

A number of national and international groups have recommended virtually the same occupational or public exposure limits for UVR. The guidelines of the ICNIRP (18,44,50) and the ACGIH (19) are by far the widest known. Both groups have recommended essentially the same limit based in large part on ocular injury data from animal studies and human accidental injury studies. The guideline to protect the skin, lens, and cornea is an $S_{UV}(\lambda)$-weighted daily (8 hours) exposure H_{eff} of 3 mJ/cm^2 or 30 J/m^2 normalized at 270 nm. This corresponds to a limit of 27 J/cm at 365 nm. This limit is just below the level that produces a barely detectable increase in corneal light scatter and substantially below levels that produce clinically significant photokeratitis at 270 nm.

The daily exposure limit is also about one-third to one-fourth of a minimal erythemal dose and less than half the exposure necessary for clinically reported keratitis. Annex 1 provides the ACGIH/ICNIRP human exposure limits based upon $S_{UV}(\lambda)$.

A number of field survey measuring instruments have been developed, which employ detectors matching the $S_{UV}(\lambda)$ action spectrum shown in Figure 4 (see Table 1 in Annex for listed values). However, the geometry of the measurement is also of enormous importance when assessing risk of UV exposure to the eye. Outdoor safety assessments and epidemiologic studies can arrive at erroneous conclusions if measurements ignore geometrical factors and epidemiological assignments of exposure are seriously in error. A number of "reasonable" assumptions previously made by some epidemiologists regarding relative exposures have been shown to be false (10,15).

Challenge of Measuring Actinic UVR in Sunlight

Both the quantity (irradiance) and quality (spectrum) of terrestrial UVR varies with the solar zenith angle (Z), that is, the angular position of the sun below the zenith, where $Z = 90°$ is $0°$ elevation angle above the horizon. The sun's position varies with time-of-day, the day of the year, and latitude. This variation is particularly striking in the UVB spectral region (280–315 nm) because of the greater atmospheric attenuation along the direct atmospheric path. Stratospheric ozone absorption and molecular (Rayleigh) scattering by atmospheric N_2 and O_2 combine to attenuate the global UVR in this spectral region. However, in the troposphere, further absorption by air pollutants such as the oxides of nitrogen, sulfur dioxide, and ozone, and Mie scattering by water vapor in clouds and particulates can significantly add to the attenuation. Clouds and haze reduce the global UV (ground, horizontal) irradiance. However, haze and clouds redistribute the UVR, so that the UVR (i.e., the sky "brightness," or more correctly, radiance) of the horizon-sky can actually increase in comparison to a clear, blue-sky day. As water vapor in clouds greatly attenuates infrared radiation, but does not significantly attenuate ground-level UVR, the warning sensation of heat to reduce the risk of sunburn can be absent on an overcast day. A light overcast, or light clouds scattered over a blue sky, do little to attenuate the UV global irradiance (unless a dense cloud lies directly over the sun), and severe sunburns occur at the beach under such conditions. A light cloud cover may reduce the terrestrial global UVR (measured on a horizontal surface) to about half of that from a clear sky, although the horizon-sky UVR radiance does not decrease—and can even increase. Even under a heavy cloud-cover, the scattered UV component of sunlight (termed the diffuse component, or "skylight") is seldom <10% of that under a clear sky (51). Only very heavy storm clouds can virtually eliminate terrestrial UV during summertime conditions. Although a higher global erythemal effective irradiance is measured at high altitude (52), the atmospheric scatter (diffuse component) is less, and the horizon-sky UVR does not increase by climbing mountains (5). All of these observations point to the complex geometrical factors that challenge any outdoor UVR measurements.

As the eye receives most of its outdoor UVR exposure from ground reflectance, the proper measurement of reflected sunlight adds a further challenge. The ground reflection of solar UVB radiation varies >100-fold. Green grass reflects <1% and most artificial surfaces and rock normally reflect <10%. Two exceptions are ocean surf and white, gypsum sand, which reflect ~20% to 25%. Fresh snow reflects ~85%, thus producing "snow blindness." Open water reflects the entire sky (diffuse plus direct component) and can be of the order of 20%, although the direct, specular reflection from the sun's image is only ~2% to 3% of the incident, direct UV radiation when the sun is high in the sky. Table 1 provides more detailed values for ground reflectance.

Ocular exposure is far more affected than skin exposure by these geometrical factors. For an industrial UV source such as a welding arc, the cornea is shown to be more sensitive to UVR injury than the skin, but photokeratitis seldom accompanies summer sunburn of the skin. This seeming paradox is explained by the fact that people do not look directly overhead when the sun is very hazardous to view, while most people may stare at the sun when it is comfortable to observe near the horizon. Fortunately, at sunset, the filtering of UVR and blue light by the atmosphere allows us to directly view the sun. When the solar elevation angle exceeds 10° above the horizon, strong squinting is observed, which effectively shields the cornea and retina from most direct exposure. These factors reduce the exposure of the cornea to a maximum 5% of that falling on the exposed top of the head. However, if the ground reflectance exceeds 15%, photokeratitis may be produced after a few hours of exposure. If one were to ignore the squinting factor and proper instrument field-of-view, the photokeratitis threshold would be achieved in <15 minutes for midday summer sunlight.

When wearing sunglasses, the pupil dilates proportionally to the darkness of the sunglasses (53). Coroneo et al. (31,54) have shown that very oblique temporal rays can be refracted into the critical nasal equatorial region of the lens, and this could explain the increased incidence of opacification originating in the nasal sector of the lens in cortical cataract. The protective value of upper and lower lids, when they close down during squinting, determines the ocular UVR exposure dose in different environments. A brimmed hat or other headwear—associated with or without dark sunglasses—will modify greatly the UVR exposure dose. The geometrical factors that should be modeled by a radiometer now begin to appear as almost insurmountable. What can be done? Even geometrical positioning of the body greatly affects the solar exposure of human skin.

Biologically Relevant Measurements

With ocular UVR exposure so dependent upon geometry, the measurement challenge is not only to employ detectors with a spectral response that matches the action spectrum for the biological effect, but also provide a match of the geometry. Several types of badges that measure total effective irradiance on the badge surface have been developed and can match the geometry of the skin, but not the eye.

Polysulfone Film-Badge Dosimeters

To date, the most widely used UV film-badge dosimeter has been the thermoplastic film, polysulfone. When polysulfone is exposed to UVR (particularly UVB), its UV absorption (generally calibrated at 330 nm) increases. This increase in absorbance has a useful linear-response range. Most typically, a 40-μm thick piece of polysulfone film is mounted in a cardboard or plastic mount, and these are worn by the experimental subjects on anatomic sites of interest. Sydenham constructed contact lenses of polysulfone and was able to corroborate the low UV exposure compared with that of the skin (55).

Direct Clinical Measurement of UVR Exposure

The action spectrum and threshold for photokeratitis (snow blindness) has been carefully studied, and was the basis of the action spectrum, $S_{UV}(\lambda)$, hence, where individuals develop a threshold, just-detectable photokeratitis, the cornea itself is acting as a dosimeter. Sliney used this approach to estimate UV exposure to the crystalline lens or intra-ocular lens implant, and showed it to be an extremely small dose compared with that of the skin (56). Erythema has long been used as a measure of individual, acute exposure of the skin to UVR (57), and dermatologists routinely examine benign markers of sun damage of skin on the face and on the back of the hands to judge the accelerated aging of the skin, and thereby estimate the risk for nonmelanoma skin cancer. However, previous attempts to correlate the incidence of cataract with the skin-exposure estimates have been unsuccessful, presumably because of the lack of any direct relation between skin exposure and direct ocular exposure with the lids open. Another factor of interest is the impact of hats. Hats (particularly with wide brims) and other headwear greatly affect exposure to the face; however, hats which shade the eyes may actually lead to greater lid opening, rendering the eye more vulnerable to ground reflections (58–59).

Ocular Exposure Dosimetry

Very pertinent data could be given by UV-sensitive contact lens dosimeters (55), but most of the pertinent data will come from studies of lid-opening conditions combined with directional field measurements and different environmental conditions. Also, the ground reflection will enter in these evaluations. Tables 1 and 2 from Sliney (5) provide information on the reflectance of ACGIH/ICNIRP-weighted solar UVB and the measured ACGIH/ICNIRP-effective UVR (60–64) from the sky with a 40° cone field-of-view. He effectively measured the UV radiance over a 40° averaging (acceptance) angle. This was later used to calculate ocular dose. Note that the relative effective UV irradiance

Table 1 Reflectance of ACGIH/ICNIRP-Effective Solar UV-B from Terrain Surfaces

Terrain surfaces	Diffuse reflectance effective solar UV-B (ACGIH/ICNIRP spectral weighting) (%)
Green mountain grassland	0.8–1.6
Dry grassland	2.0–3.7
Wooden boat dock	6.4
Black asphalt	5–9
Concrete pavement	8–12
Atlantic beach sand (dry)	15–18
Atlantic beach sand (wet)	7
Sea foam (surf)	25–30
Dirty snow	59
Fresh snow	88

Abbreviations: ACGIH, American Conference of Governmental Industrial Hygienists; ICNIRP, International Commission for Non-Ionizing Radiation Protection. *Source*: Adapted from Ref. 5.

near the horizon (i.e., within the eye's field-of-view) did not show big variations if the sky was visible and could increase with haze. Indeed, on an overcast day with the eyelids more open, the actual UVB dose rate to the eye from the sky scatter can increase.

Table 2 Measured ACGIH Effective UV-B from the Sky with a 40° Cone Field of View

Sky conditions location, elevation	Zenith reading (μW cm^{-2} sr^{-1})	Direct sun (μWcm^{-2} sr^{-1})	Opposite to sun (μWcm^{-2}sr^{-1})	Horizon sky (μWcm^{-2} sr^{-1})
Clear sky, dry, sea level	0.1	1.4, Z = 70°	0.22	0.27
Clear sky, humid, sea level	0.27	4.1, Z = 50°	0.27	0.24
Ground fog, sea level	0.04	0.19, Z = 75°	0.04	0.03
Hazy humid, sea level	0.014	1.4, Z = 70°	0.22	0.54
Cloudy bright, 700 m	0.54	0.44, Z = 45°	0.27	0.05 (tree-line)
Hazy beach	0.54	0.60, Z = 75°	0.54	0.60
Hazy beach	0.38	3.5, Z = 40°	0.54	0.44
Clear mountain top 2750 m	0.54	1.6, Z = 25°	0.82	0.08

Source: Adapted from Ref. 5.

The natural protection against overhead UVR afforded to the eye by the upper lid and brow ridge may be of little value for exposure to open-arc sources in the work place, because the source may frequently be within the normal horizontal line-of-sight. Hence, greater eye protection is routinely required in industrial applications. Goggles and face shields are required when working around electric arc welding, which produces high levels of all UVR wavelengths. Close-fitting facemasks with low transmittance to UV, visible, and infrared radiations are used for protection (1,33).

CONCLUSIONS

A considerable range of studies have examined the potential risk factors associated with age-related diseases of the eye—including uvcal melanoma and corneal neoplasias (59–158). However, the interpretation of the varying findings of these studies are not always consistent. Better ocular UV dosimetry is needed.

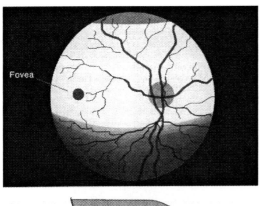

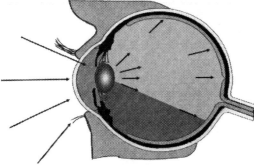

Figure 5 Retinal illumination pattern. During most outdoor conditions, much of the inferior retina is shaded, and only under conditions of bright sand or snow do both lids close to allow only the illumination of the macula and a horizontal band on either side.

The design of instrumentation intended to measure the photobiological dose to ocular tissues must take into account a number of geometrical shading factors, such as the eyelids and brow ridge, as well as behavioral aspects of vision. These geometrical and imaging factors challenge the task of attempting to accurately measure the photobiologically significant exposure of the cornea, lens, and retina to UV, visible, and infrared (IR) radiations. The human eye is actually exposed to a very small fraction of the global UV irradiance (diffuse plus direct radiation incident upon a horizontal surface). Therefore, the acceptance angle (field-of-view) should mimic that of the human eye. However, this acceptance angle varies with sky brightness. Thus, the instrument field-of-view must be adjustable in an instrument designed to really measure the UVR exposure dose to the cornea and lens. The UV exposure to the anterior segment of the eye can be measured in a mannequin fitted with UV detectors at the ocular positions, and measurements can be made with and without UV-absorbing spectacles, or as would occur when a person wears different types of sunglasses. The exposure is greatly affected by the type of sunglass frame and partially by the UV transmittance of the sunglass lenses. In some instances, UV exposures of some specific ocular tissues can actually equal or exceed those when not wearing sunglasses.

The retina is exposed to visible light and some IR-A radiant energy within an imaged scene. Although the lid opening varies with ambient scene luminance (brightness), it is possible to mathematically predict the opening of the lids and the angular field-of-view from studies of lid opening. The light exposure to the retina is not at all uniform in outdoor daylight conditions. The central and superior regions of the retina receive much more light than the inferior retina (Fig. 5). Thus, instrumentation should simulate these geometrical factors.

REFERENCES

1. Sliney DH, Wolbarsht ML. Safety with Lasers and Other Optical Sources. New York: Plenum Publishing Corp, 1980.
2. World Health Organization (WHO). Environmental Health Criteria No. 160, Ultraviolet Radiation. Joint publication of the United Nations Environmental Program, the International Radiation Protection Association and the World Health Organization. Geneva: WHO, 1994.
3. World Health Organization. The Effects of Solar UV Radiation on the Eye, Report of an Informal Consultation, Geneva 30 August–September 1993. Publication WHO/PBL/EHG/94.1. Geneva: Program for the Prevention of Blindness Program, World Health Organization, 1995.
4. Sasaki K, Sasaki H, Kojima M, et al. Epidemiological studies on UV-related cataract in climatically different countries. J Epidemiol (Japan) 1999; 9:S33–S38.
5. Sliney DH. Physical factors in cataractogenesis: ambient ultraviolet radiation and temperature. Invest Ophthalmol Vis Sci 1986; 27(5):781–790.
6. West SK, Rosenthal FS, Bressler NM, et al. Exposure to sunlight and other risk factors for age-related macular degeneration. Arch Ophthalmol 1989; 107:875–879.

7. Dolin PJ. Ultraviolet radiation and cataract: A review of the epidemiological evidence. Br J Ophthalmol 1994; 78(6):478–482.

8. Klein BEK, Klein R, Linton KLP. Prevalence of age-related lens opacities in a population, the Beaver Dam eye study. Ophthalmology 1992; 44(4):546–552.

9. Taylor HR. Ultraviolet light exposure and risk of posterior subcapsular cataracts. Arch Ophthalmol 1989; 107:369–372.

10. Sliney DH. Photoprotection of the eye—UV radiation and sunglasses. J Photochem Photobiol B: Biol 2001; 64:166–175.

11. Sliney DH. UV radiation ocular exposure dosimetry. J Photochem Photobiol B: Biol 1995; 31:69–77.

12. Sliney DH. Epidemiological studies of sunlight and cataract: the critical factor of ultraviolet exposure geometry. Ophthalmic Epidemiol 1994; 1(2):107–119.

13. Sliney DH. Ultraviolet radiation exposure criteria. Radiation Protection Dosimetry 2000; 91(1–3):213–222.

14. Sliney DH. Geometrical gradients in the distribution of temperature and absorbed ultraviolet radiation in ocular tissues. Dev Ophthalmol 2002; 35:40–59.

15. Sliney DH. Ocular exposure to environmental light and ultraviolet—the impact of lid opening and sky condition. In: Sasaki K, Hockwin O, eds. Cataract Epidemiology. Basel, Switzerland: Karger, 2000.

16. Taylor HR, West SK, Rosenthal FS, et al. Effect of ultraviolet radiation on cataract formation New Engl J Med 1988; 319:1429–1433.

17. Taylor HR (ed.) Pteryguim. The Netherlands: Kugler Publications, 2000.

18. International Commission on Non-Ionizing Radiation Protection (ICNIRP). Guidelines on limits of exposure to ultraviolet radiation of wavelengths between 180 nm and 400 nm (Incoherent Optical Radiation). Health Phys 2004; 87(2):171–186.

19. American Conference of Governmental Industrial Hygienists (ACGIH). TLV's, Threshold Limit Values and Biological Exposure Indices for 2001. Cincinnati: ACGIH, 2001.

20. ACGIH. Documentation for the Threshold Limit Values. 4th ed. Cincinnati: American Conference of Governmental Industrial Hygienists, 1992.

21. Sliney DH. Measurement of light and the geometry of exposure of the human eye. In: Marshall J, ed. The Susceptible Visual Apparatus. Vol. 16. in series on Visual and Visual Dysfunction. New York: McMillan Press, 1991:23–39.

22. Sliney DH, Armstrong BC. Radiometric evaluation of surgical microscope lights for hazards analyses. Applied Opt 1986; 25(12):1882–1889.

23. Sliney DH, Campbell CE. Ophthalmic instrument safety standards. Laser Light Ophthalmol 1994; 6(4):207–215.

24. Pitts DG. The human ultraviolet action spectrum Am J Optom Physiol Optics 1974; 51(12):946–960.

25. Pitts DG, Cullen AP, Hacker PD. Ocular effects of ultraviolet radiation from 295 to 365 nm. Invest Ophthalmol Vis Sci 1977; 16(10):932–939.

26. Ringvold A. Damage of the cornea epithelium caused by ultraviolet radiation. Acta Ophthalmologica 1983; 61:898–907.

27. Sliney DH, Krueger RR, Trokel SL, Rappaport KD. Photokeratitis from 193-nm argon–fluoride laser radiation. Photochem Photobiol 1991; 53(6):739–744.

28. Bachem A. Ophthalmic ultraviolet action spectra. Am J Ophthalmol 1956; 41: 969–975.

29. Jose JG, Pitts DG. Wavelength dependency of cataracts in albino mice following chronic exposure. Exp Eye Res 1985; 41:545–563.
30. Coroneo MT, Müller-Stolzenburg NW, Ho A. Peripheral light focussing by the anterior eye and the ophthalmohelioses. Ophthalmic Surg 1991; 22:705–711.
31. Coroneo MT. Pterygium as an early indicator of ultraviolet insolation: an hypothesis. Brit J Ophthalmol 1993; 77:734–739.
32. Hedblom EE. Snowscape eye protection. Arch Environ Health 1961; 2:685–704.
33. Sliney DH. Eye protective techniques for bright light. Ophthalmology 1983; 90(8):937–944.
34. Sliney DH. Epidemiological studies of sunlight and cataract: the critical factor of ultraviolet exposure geometry. Ophthalmic Epidemiol 1994; 1(2):107–119.
35. Parrish JA, Jaenicke KF, Anderson R. Erythema and melanogenesis action spectra of normal human skin. Photochem Photobiol 1982; 36(2):187–191.
36. Urbach F, Gange RW, eds. The Biological Effects of UVA Radiation. Westport: Praeger Publishers, 1986.
37. Passchier WF, Bosnjakovic BFM, eds. Human Exposure to Ultraviolet Radiation: Risks and Regulations. New York: Excerpta Medica Division, Elsevier Science Publishers, 1987.
38. Cole CA, Forbes DF, Davies PD. An action spectrum for UV photocarcinogenesis. Photochem Photobiol 1986; 43(3):275–284.
39. DeGruijl FR, van der Leun JC. Estimate of the wavelength dependency of ultraviolet carcinogenesis in humans and its relevance to the risk assessment of stratospheric ozone depletion. Health Phys 1994; 67:317–323.
40. Taylor HR. Pterygium. Amsterdam: Kugler, 2000.
41. Ham WT Jr. The photopathology and nature of the blue-light and near-UV retinal lesion produced by lasers and other optical sources. In: Wolbarsht ML, ed. Laser Applications in Medicine and Biology. New York: Plenum Publishing Corp, 1983.
42. Ham WT, Mueller HA, Ruffolo J, Guerry D III, Guerry RK. Action spectrum for retinal injury from near ultraviolet radiation in the aphakic monkey. Am J Ophthalmol 1982; 93(3):299–306.
43. Mainster MA. Spectral transmission of intraocular lenses and retinal damage from intense light sources. Am J Ophthalmol 1978; 85:167–170.
44. International Commission on Non-Ionizing Radiation Protection (ICNIRP). Guidelines on limits of exposure to optical radiation from 0.38 to 3.0 µm. Health Phys 1997; 73(3):539–554.
45. Grossweiner LI. Photochemistry of proteins: a review. Curr Eye Res 1984; 3(1):137–144.
46. Smith KC. The Science of Photobiology. New York: Plenum Press, 1988.
47. Diffey BL. Ultraviolet Radiation in Medicine. Bristol: Adam Hilger, 1982.
48. Forbes PD, Davies PD. Factors that influence photocarcinogenesis. Chapter 7. In: Parrish JA, Kripke ML, Morison WL, eds. Photoimmunology. New York: Plenum Publishing Corp, 1982.
49. Zuclich JA. Ultraviolet-induced photochemical damage in ocular tissues. Health Phys 1989; 56(5):671–682.
50. Rosenthal FS, Bakalian AE, Taylor HR. The effect of prescription eyewear on ocular exposure to ultraviolet radiation. Amer J Publ Health 1988; 78:72–74.

51. Sliney DH, Wood RL, Moscato PM, Marshall WJ, Eriksen P. Ultraviolet exposure in the outdoor environment. In: Grandolfo, Rindi, Sliney, eds. Light, Lasers, and Synchrotron Radiation—A Health Risk Assessment. New York: Plenum Press, 1991:169–180.

52. Blumthaler M, Ambach W. Solar UVB-albedo of various surfaces. Photochem Photobiol 1988; 48(1):85–88.

53. Deaver DM, Davis J, Sliney DH. Vertical visual fields-of-view in outdoor daylight. Lasers Light Ophthalmol 1996; 7(2/3):121–125.

54. Coroneo MT. Peripheral light focusing by the anterior eye and the ophthalmohelioses. Opthalmic Surg 1991; 22(12):705–711.

55. Sydenham MM, Collins MJ, Hirst LW. Measurement of ultraviolet radiation at the surface of the eye. Invest Ophthalmol Vis Sci 1997; 38(8):1485–1492.

56. Sliney DH. Estimating the solar ultraviolet radiation exposure to an intraocular lens implant. J Cataract Refract Surg 1987; 13:296–301.

57. CIE. Erythemal reference action spectrum and standard erythemal dose, CIE Standard S007-1998. Vienna: CIE, 1998 (also available as ISO 17166:1999).

58. Sliney DH. The focusing of ultraviolet radiation in the eye and ocular exposure. In: Taylor HR, ed. Pterguim. The Netherlands: Kugler Publications, 2000, Chapter 3.

59. Sliney DH. Eye protective techniques for bright light. Ophthalmology 1983; 90(8):937–944.

60. CIE. Standardization of the terms UVA1, UVA2 and UVB, Report CIE-134/1. Vienna: CIE, 1999.

61. Cogan DG, Kinsey VE. Action spectrum of keratitis produced by ultraviolet radiation. Arch Ophthalmol 1946; 35:617–670.

62. International Commission on Non-Ionizing Radiation Protection (ICNIRP). Guidelines on UV Radiation Exposure Limits. Health Phys 1996; 71(6):978.

63. Sliney DH. The merits of an envelope action spectrum for ultraviolet radiation exposure criteria. Amer Industr Hyg Assn J 1972; 33(10):646–653.

64. Sliney DH, Matthes R, eds. The Measurement of Optical Radiation Hazards. ICNIRP Publication 6/98; CIE Publication CIE-x016-1998. Munich: ICNIRP and Vienna: CIE, 1999.

65. Wulf HC. Effects of ultraviolet radiation from the sun on the Inuit population. In: Petursdottir G, Sigurdsson SB, Karlsson MM, Axelsson J, eds. Circumpolar Health '93 Arctic Medical Research 1994; 53:416–422.

66. Commission International de l'Eclairage (International Commission on Illumination). International Lighting Vocabulary. 4th ed. Pub. CIE No. 17 (E–1.1). Vienna: CIE, 1987.

67. Parrish JA, Anderson RR, Urbach F, Pitts D. UVA, Biological Effects of Ultraviolet Radiation with Emphasis on Human Responses to Longwave Radiation. New York: Plenum Press, 1978.

68. Taylor HR, ed. Pterygium. The Hague: Kugler Publications, 2000.

69. Anderson JR. A pterygium map. Acta Ophthalmol 1954; 3:1631–1642.

70. Baasanhu J, Johnson GJ, Burendei G, Minassian DC. Prevalence and Causes of Blindness and Visual Impairment in Mongolia. Bull WHO 1994; 72(5):771–776.

71. Bergmanson JP, Pitts DG, Chu LW. Protection from harmful UV radiation by contact lens. J Am Optom Assoc 1988; 59:178–182.

72. Bhatnagar R, West KP, Vitale S, Sommer A, Joshi S, Venkataswamy G. Risk of cataract and history of severe diarrheal disease in Southern India. Arch Ophthalmol 1991; 109:696–699.

73. Blumthaler M, Ambach W, Daxecker F. On the threshold radiant exposure for keratitis solaris. Invest Ophthalmol Vis Sci 1987; 28:1713–1716.
74. Bochow TW, West SK, Azar A, Munoz B, Sommer A, Taylor HR. Ultraviolet light exposure and risk of posterior subcapsular cataracts. Arch Ophthalmol 1989; 107:369–372.
75. Boettner EA, Wolter JR. Transmission of the ocular media. Invest Ophthalmol Vis Sci 1962; 1:776–783.
76. Booth F. Heredity in one hundred patients admitted for excision of pterygia. Aust NZ J Ophthalmol 1985; 13:59–61.
77. Brilliant LB, Grasset NC, Pokhrel RP, et al. Associations among cataract prevalence, sunlight hours, and altitude in the Himalayas. Am J Epidemiol 1983; 118:250–264.
78. Cameron ME. Pterygium throughout the World. Springfield, IL: Charles Thomas, 1965.
79. Chatterjee A, Milton RC, Thyle S. Prevalence and aetiology of cataract in Punjab. Br J Ophthalmol 1982; 66:35–42.
80. Colin J, Bonissent JF, Resnikoff S. Epidemiology of the exfoliation syndrome. Proc 17th Congr European Soc Ophthalmol Helsinki 1985; 230–231.
81. Collman GW, Shore DL, Shy CM, Checkoway H, Luria AS. Sunlight and other risk factors for cataract: an epidemiological study. Am J Public Health 1988; 78:1459–1462.
82. Cruickshanks KJ, Klein R, Klein BE. Sunlight and age-related macular degeneration: the Beaver Dam Eye Study. Arch Ophthalmol 1993; 111:514–518.
83. Darrell RW, Bachrach CA. Pterygium among veterans. Arch Ophthalmol 1963; 70:158–169.
84. Detels R, Dhir SP. Pterygium: a geographical study. Arch Ophthalmol 1967; 78:485–491.
85. Dhir SP, Detels R, Alexander ER. The role of environmental factors in cataract, pterygium and trachoma. Am J Ophthalmol 1967; 64:128–135.
86. Dolezal JM, Perkins ES, Wallace RB. Sunlight, skin sensitivity, and senile cataract. Am J Epidemiol 1989; 129:559–568.
87. Doll R. Urban and rural factors in the aetiology of cancer. Int J Cancer 1991; 47:803–810.
88. Elliott R. The aetiology of pterygium. Trans Ophthalmol Soc NZ 1961; 13: 22–41.
89. Eye Disease Case-Control Study Group. Risk factors for neovascular age-related macular degeneration. Arch Ophthalmol 1992; 110:1701–1708.
90. Fitzpatrick TB, Pathak MA, Harber LC, Seiji M, Kukita A. Sunlight and Man. Tokyo: University of Tokyo Press, 1974.
91. Forsius H. Exfoliation syndrome in various ethnic populations. Acta Ophthalmol 1988; 68(suppl 184):71–85.
92. Gallagher RP, Elwood JM, Rootman J, et al. Risk factors for ocular melanoma: western Canada melanoma study. J Natl Cancer Inst 1985; 74:775–778.
93. Garner A. The pathology of tumours at the limbus. Eye 1989; 3:210–217.
94. Gray RH, Johnson GJ, Freedman A. Climatic droplet keratopathy. Surv Ophthalmol 1992; 36:241–253.
95. Guex-Crosier Y, Herbort CP. Presumed corneal intraepithelial neoplasia associated with contact lens wear and intense ultraviolet light exposure. Br J Ophthalmol 1993; 77:191–192.

96. Ham WT Jr, Ruffolo JJ Jr, Mueller HA, et al. Histologic analysis of photochemical lesions produced in rhesus retina by short wavelength light. Invest Ophthalmol 1978; 17:1029–1035.

97. Hiller R, Giacometti L, Yuen K. Sunlight and cataract: an epidemiologic investigation. Am J Epidemiol 1977; 105:450–459.

98. Hiller R, Sperduto RD, Ederer F. Epidemiologic associations with cataract in the 1971–1972 national health and nutrition examination survey. Am J Epidemiol 1983; 118:239–249.

99. Hiller R, Sperduto RD, Ederer F. Epidemiologic associations with nuclear, cortical, and posterior subcapsular cataracts. Am J Epidemiol 1986; 124:916–925.

100. Hollows F, Moran D. Cataract—the ultraviolet risk factor. Lancet 1981; 2:1249–1250.

101. Holly EA, Aston DA, Char DH, Kristiansen JJ, Ahn DK. Uveal melanoma in relation to ultraviolet light exposure and host factors. Cancer Res 1990; 50:5773–5777.

102. Hyman LG, Lilienfeld AM, Ferris FL, Fine SL. Senile macular degeneration: a case-control study. Am J Epidemiol 1983; 118:213–227.

103. International Agency for Research on Cancer. IARC monographs on the evaluation of carcinogenic risk to humans. Vol. 55. Solar and Ultraviolet Radiation. Lyon: IARC, 1992.

104. Italian–American Cataract Study Group. Risk factors for age-related cortical, nuclear, and posterior subcapsular cataracts. Am J Epidemiol 1991; 133:541–553.

105. Johnson GJ. Aetiology of spheroidal degeneration of the cornea in Labrador. Br J Ophthalmol 1981; 65:270–283.

106. Johnson GJ, Overall M. Histology of spheroidal degeneration of the cornea in Labrador. Br J Ophthalmol 1978; 62:53–61.

107. Johnson GJ, Paterson GD, Green JS, Perkins ES. Ocular conditions in a Labrador community. In: Harvald B, Hansen JP, eds. Circumpolar Health 81. Copenhagen: Nordic Council for Arctic Medical Research, 1981.

108. Johnson GJ, Minassian DC, Franken S. Alterations of the anterior lens capsule associated with climatic keratopathy. Br J Ophthalmol 1989; 73:229–234.

109. Jose JG. Posterior cataract induction by UVB radiation in albino mice. Exp Eye Res 1986; 42:11–20.

110. Karai I, Horiguchi S. Pterygium in welders. Br J Ophthalmol 1984; 68:347–349.

111. Kinsey VE. Spectral transmission of the eye to ultraviolet radiation. Arch Ophthalmol 1948; 39:505–513.

112. Lee GA, Hirst LW. Incidence of ocular surface epithelial dysplasia in metropolitan Brisbane: a 10-year survey. Arch Ophthalmol 1992; 110:525–527.

113. Lerman S. Human ultraviolet radiation cataracts. Ophthalmic Res 1980; 12: 303–314.

114. Leske MC, Chylack LT, Wu S, The Lens Opacities Case-Control Study Group. The lens opacities case-control study: risk factors for cataract. Arch Ophthalmol 1991; 109:244–251.

115. Lindberg JG. Kliniska undersökningar över depigmenteringen av pupillarranden och genomlysbarheten av iris vid fall av åldstarr samt i normala ögon hos gamla personer. Dissertation, Helsingfors, Finland, 1917.

116. Lischko AM, Seddon JM, Gragoudas ES, Egan KM, Glynn RJ. Evaluation of prior primary malignancy as a determinant of uveal melanoma. A case-control study. Ophtalmology 1989; 96:1716–1721.

117. Mack TM, Floderus B. Malignant melanoma risk by nativity, place of residence at diagnosis, and age at migration. Cancer Causes Control 1991; 2:401–411.
118. Mackenzie FD, Hirst LW, Battistutta D, Green A. Risk analysis in the development of pterygia. Ophthalmol 1992; 99:1056–1061.
119. Mainster MA, Ham WT, Delori FC. Potential retinal hazards, instrument and environmental light sources. Ophthalmology 1983; 90:927–931.
120. Mao W, Hu T. An epidemiologic survey of senile cataract in China. Chinese Med J 1982; 95:813–818.
121. Milham S Jr. Occupational Mortality in Washington State 1950–1979. DHSS (NIOSH) Publ. No. 83-116. Cincinnati, OH: National Institute for Occupational Safety and Health, 1983.
122. Minassian DC, Mehra V, Johnson GJ. Mortality and cataract: findings from a population-based longitudinal study. Bull WHO 1992; 70:219–223.
123. Mohan M, Sperduto RD, Angra SK, et al. India–US case-control study of age-related cataracts. Arch Ophthalmol 1989; 107:670–676.
124. Moran DJ, Hollows FC. Pterygium and ultraviolet radiation: a positive correlation. Br J Ophthalmol 1984; 68:343–346.
125. Nachtwey DB, Rundel RD. A photobiological evaluation of tanning booths. Science 1981; 211:405–407.
126. Naumann GOH, Apple D. Pathology of the Eye. New York: Springer-Verlag, 1986.
127. Noell WK, Walker VS, Kang BS. Retinal damage by light in rats. Invest Ophthalmol Vis Sci 1966; 5:450–473.
128. Norn MS. Spheroid degeneration, pinguecula, and pterygium among Arabs in the Red Sea Territory, Jordan. ACTA Ophthalmol 1982; 60:949–954.
129. Office of Population Censuses and Surveys. Occupational Mortality: the Registrar General's Decennia Supplement for Great Britain 1979–80, 1982–83 (Series DS No. 6). London: Her Majesty's Stationary Office, 1986.
130. Oldenburg JB, Gritz DC, McDonnell PJ. Topical ultraviolet light-absorbing chromophore protects against experimental photokeratitis. Arch Ophthalmol 1990; 108:1142–1144.
131. Ostendfeld-Åkerblom A. Pseudoexfoliation in Eskimos (Inuit) in Greenland. Acta Ophthalmol 1988; 66:467–468.
132. Østerlind A. Trends in incidence of ocular malignant melanoma in Denmark 1943–1982. Int J Cancer 1987; 40:161–164.
133. Østerlind A, Olsen JH, Lynge E, Ewertz M. Second cancer following cutaneous melanoma and cancers of the brain, thyroid, connective tissue, bone, and eye in Denmark, 1943–80. Natl Cancer Inst Monogr 1985; 68:361–388.
134. Parkin DM, Muir CS, Whelan SL, Gao Y-T, Ferlay J, Powell J, eds. Cancer Incidence in Five Continents. Vol. 6. IARC Scientific Publications No. 120. Lyon: International Agency for Research on Cancer, 1992.
135. Pitts DG. The ocular effects of ultraviolet radiation. Am J Optom Phys Optics 1978; 55:19–35.
136. Ringvold A, Davangar M. Changes in the rabbit corneal stroma caused by UV irradiation. Acta Ophthalmol 1985; 63:601–606.
137. Rosen ES. Filtration of non-ionizing radiation by the ocular media. In: Cronley-Dillon J, Rosen ES, Marshall J, eds. Hazards of Light: Myths and Realities of Eye and Skin. Oxford: Pergamon Press, 1986:145–152.
138. Saftlas AF, Blair A, Cantor KP, Hanrahan L, Anderson HA. Cancer and other causes of death among Wisconsin farmers. Am J Ind Med 1987; 11:119–129.

139. Schwartz SM, Weiss NS. Place of birth and incidence of ocular melanoma in the United States. Int J Cancer 1988; 41:174–177.
140. Seddon JM, Gragoudas ES, Glynn RJ, Egan KM, Albert DM, Blitzer PH. Host factors, UV radiation, and risk of uveal melanoma: a case-control study. Arch Ophthalmol 1990; 108:1274–1280.
141. Shibata T, Katoh N, Hatano T, Sasaki K. Population based case-control study of cortical cataract in the Noto area, Japan. Dev Ophthalmol 1994; 26:25–33.
142. Siemiatycki J. Risk Factors for Cancer in Workplace. Boca Raton, Florida: CRC Press, 1991.
143. Taylor HR. Pseudoexfoliation, an environmental disease? Trans Ophthalmol Soc UK 1979; 99:302–307.
144. Taylor HR. Aetiology of climatic droplet keratopathy and pterygium. Br J Ophthalmol 1980; 64:154–163.
145. Taylor HR The environment and the lens. Br J Ophthalmol 1980; 64:303–310.
146. Taylor HR, West SK, Rosenthal FS, Munoz B, Newland HS, Emmett EA. Corneal changes associated with chronic UV irradiation. Arch Ophthalmol 1989; 107:1481–1484.
147. Taylor HR, West S, Munoz B, Rosenthal FS, Bressler SB, Bressler NM. The long-term effects of visible light on the eye. Arch Ophthalmol 1992; 110:99–104.
148. Tucker MA, Shields JA, Hartge P, Augsburger J, Hoover RN, Fraumeni J. Sunlight exposure as risk factor for intraocular malignant melanoma. New Engl J Med 1985; 313:789–792.
149. Turner BJ, Siatkowski RM, Augsburger JJ, Shields JA, Lustbader E, Mastrangelo MJ. Other cancers in uveal melanoma patients and their families. Am J Ophtalmol 1989; 107:601–608.
150. Vitale S, West S, Munoz B, et al. Watermen Study II: mortality and baseline prevalence of nuclear opacity. Invest Ophthalmol Vi Sci 1992; 33:1097.
151. Waring GO, Roth AM, Ekins MB. Clinical and pathological description of 17 cases of corneal intraepithelial neoplasia. Am J Ophthalmol 1984; 97:547–559.
152. Wittenberg S. Solar radiation and the eye: a review of knowledge relevant to eye care. Am J Optom Physiol Optics 1986; 63:676–689.
153. Wong L, Ho SC, Coggon D, et al. Sunlight exposure, antioxidant status, and cataract in Hong Kong fishermen. J Epidemiol Comm Health 1993; 47:46–49.
154. Yannuzzi L, Fisher Y, Slakter J, Krueger A. Solar retinipathy. A photobiologic and geophysical analysis. Retina 1989; 9:28–43.
155. Young RW. Age-related Cataract. New York: Oxford University Press, 1991.
156. Zaunuddin D, Sasaki K. Risk factor analysis in a cataract epidemiology survey in West Sumatra, Indonesia. Dev Ophthalmol 1991; 21:78–86.
157. Zigman S, Yulo T, Schultz J. Cataract induction in mice exposed to near UV light. Ophthalmol Res 1974; 6:259–270.
158. Zigman S, Graff J, Yulo T, Vaughen T. The response of mouse ocular tissue to continuous near-UV light exposure. Invest Ophthalmol 1975; 14:710–713.

APPENDIX: APPLYING THE UVR EXPOSURE LIMITS

The ACGIH/ICNIRP Exposure Limit for exposure to the eye and skin to UVR is 3 mJ/cm^2 effective, when the spectral irradiance E_8 at the eye or skin surface is mathematically weighted against the hazard sensitivity spectrum $S(\lambda)$ from 180 to 400 nm as follows:

$$E_{\text{eff}} = \sum E_\lambda \cdot S(\lambda) \cdot \Delta\lambda \tag{1}$$

The permissible exposure duration, t_{max}, in seconds, to the spectrally weighted UVR is calculated by

$$t_{\text{max}} = \frac{3 \text{ mJ/cm}^2}{E_{\text{eff}} \text{W/cm}^2} \tag{2}$$

In addition to the above requirement, the ocular exposure is also limited to 1 J/cm^2 for periods up to 1000 seconds (16.7 min) by ACGIH and to 30,000 seconds by ICNIRP. ACGIH limits the total irradiance to 1 mW/cm^2 for periods greater than 1000 seconds. For this requirement, the total irradiance, E_{UVA}, in the UVA spectral region is summed from 315 to 400 nm (Table A1)

$$E_{\text{UVA}} = \Sigma E_\lambda \cdot \Delta\lambda \tag{3}$$

where E_λ is the spectral irradiance in $\text{W/(cm}^2 \text{ nm)}$.

One way to express the ACGIH limit for the UVA is: If the total irradiance exceeds the 8-hour criterion of 1 mW/cm^2, the maximum exposure must also be less than

$$t_{\text{max}} = \frac{1 \text{ J/cm}^2}{E_{\text{UVA}}(\text{W/cm}^2)} \tag{4}$$

Equation (4) applies to all periods up to 8 hours for the ICNIRP guidelines.

Table A1 UVR Hazard Spectral Weighting Function

Wavelength (nm)	UVR hazard function ($S_{UV}(\lambda)$)	Wavelength (nm)	UVR hazard function ($S_{UV}(\lambda)$)
180	0.012	295	0.540
190	0.019	300	0.300
200	0.030	305	0.060
205	0.051	310	0.014
210	0.075	315	0.003
215	0.095	320	0.001
220	0.012	325	0.0005
225	0.015	330	0.00041
230	0.019	335	0.00034
235	0.240	340	0.00028
240	0.300	345	0.00024
245	0.360	350	0.00020
250	0.430	355	0.00016
254[a]	0.500	360	0.00013
255	0.520	365	0.00011
260	0.650	370	0.000093
265	0.810	375	0.000077
270	1.000	380	0.000064
275	0.960	385	0.000053
280	0.880	390	0.000044
285	0.770	395	0.000036
290	0.640	400	0.000030

[a]Low-pressure mercury germicidal lamp emission.

6

Histopathology Standards: Nonmelanoma Skin Cancer

Nigel Kirkham

Department of Cellular Pathology, Royal Victoria Infirmary
Newcastle upon Tyne, U.K.

INTRODUCTION

In this chapter, the two main types of nonmelanoma skin cancer, squamous cell carcinoma and basal cell carcinoma, will be described and the histopathological features of the tumors, which are of clinical relevance, will be enumerated. These tumors are mainly associated with adverse effects of sun exposure.

The histopathology of nonmelanoma skin cancer is related to the accurate recognition and classification of these tumors and their differentiation from benign lesions such as viral warts and from a range of adnexal skin tumors. The main aim of the histopathology biopsy report is the clear communication of this diagnostic and prognostic information to the clinicians who are directly involved in managing the patient.

The classification of these tumors has recently been formulated in a new edition of the World Health Organization Blue Book on Skin Cancer (1). In an attempt to establish some standards for reporting of skin cancers, the Royal College of Pathologists has produced a minimum data set document that aims to provide an evidence-based foundation for histopathological reporting (2). Clinical guidelines on recommended care have also been published (3,4).

SQUAMOUS CELL CARCINOMA

Squamous cell carcinoma is an archetypical tumor characterized as it is by evidence of squamous differentiation with tumor cells which resemble the normal epithelial cells of the prickle cell layer of the epidermis and by keratinization of the tumor cells, which typically results in the development of keratin pearls (Fig. 1) (5).

The aim of treatment is usually to eradicate the tumor, typically by excision. Complete primary excision of a squamous cell carcinoma is a desirable aim, because the majority of cutaneous squamous cell carcinomas are cured this way, with a subsequent metastasis, an unusual event except in special circumstances. Local recurrence of tumor is one such circumstance that can be associated with a less-favorable prognosis. Both Mohs' micrographic surgery and better training of surgeons have been advocated as a way of ensuring completeness of excision with a subsequent reduction in local tumor recurrences (6,7).

Differential Diagnosis

In most cases, the diagnosis of squamous cell carcinoma does not present any great difficulty to the pathologist. When the diagnosis is uncertain, the epithelial nature of the tumor can be established using immunohistochemical markers for cytokeratin. The distinction between some examples of squamous cell carcinoma from basal cell carcinoma may be a problem. The use of the Ber EP4, together with epithelial membrane antigen (EMA), has been advocated in this situation: basal cell carcinomas show much greater immunoreactivity for Ber EP4 than most squamous cell carcinomas whereas the reverse is true for EMA (8).

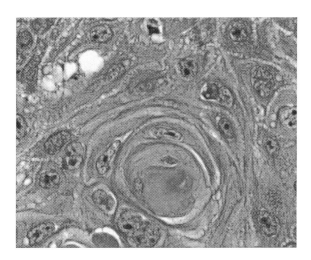

Figure 1   Squamous cell carcinoma, Grade 1 well differentiated, showing keratinization and intercellular prickles.

The distinction between squamous cell carcinoma and keratoacanthoma is sometimes problematic. In diagnosing keratoacanthoma, it is important to have full clinical details and to know if the lesion has only been present for a relatively short time and has grown rapidly. This usual history of rapid proliferation, taken together with typical architectural and cytological features should enable a diagnosis to be made, but there is a clear overlap in histopathological features with well-differentiated squamous cell carcinoma. Immunohistochemical staining with markers such as p16 has not provided any further assistance in making this differential diagnosis (9).

Tumor Site

Tumor site also plays a part in determining prognosis. While the majority of squamous cell carcinomas arising in sun-exposed sites are cured by complete primary excision, tumors arising on the lips and ears are associated with more recurrent disease and metastasis to regional lymph nodes and distant sites (6,10).

Anogenital tumors are more likely to be associated with infection with human papilloma virus, rather than sun exposure, and have the potential to behave more aggressively with the potential for a poor prognosis (11).

Tumor Size and Thickness

Tumor size is a another factor in prognosis. Primary tumors <2 cm in diameter are less likely to recur or to metastasize. Tumor thickness also appears to give an indication of likely behavior. Tumors with a thickness of <2 cm diameter are rarely associated with metastasis, tumors between 2 and 6 cm in diameter are rarely associated with metastasis, and tumors >6 cm in diameter carry a high risk of metastasis (8).

Tumor Type

Of the major subtypes of squamous cell carcinoma, spindle cell and pseudoangiomatous tumors are of high histopathological grade and are associated with higher rate of metastasis and death from disease (12,13).

Verrucous carcinomas have a higher rate of local recurrence but metastasis is rare. The diagnosis of verrucous carcinoma is fraught with difficulty. These tumors lack the cytological atypia that is so useful in facilitating the diagnosis of squamous cell carcinoma of the usual type. Initial biopsies will often show benign viral warts, with the eventual diagnosis of verrucous carcinoma only established being repeated recurrence, repeated biopsy, and repeated clinico-pathological debate.

Tumor Grade

Tumor grade was first propounded by Broders, who showed that grade was related to prognosis, with high-grade tumors having a worse prognosis (14).

This grading system was described 85 years ago and has had little substantial scrutiny since that time. It is a grading system based on degrees of differentiation within the tumor but with differentiation being poorly defined. In current practice, differentiation is taken to be the degree of keratinization. Thus, a Grade 1 tumor is well differentiated, showing >75% keratinization (Fig. 1). Grade 2 is moderately differentiated, showing between 25% and 75% keratinization (Figs. 2 and 3). Grade 3 is poorly differentiated, showing <25% keratinization. Grade 4 is undifferentiated, showing no keratinization (Fig. 4).

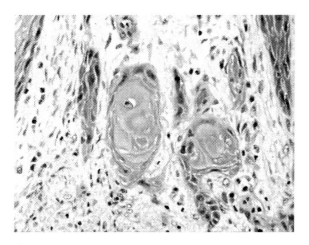

Figure 2 Squamous cell carcinoma, Grade 1 well differentiated, showing keratinization and an invasive growth pattern with occasional eosinophils in the surrounding stroma.

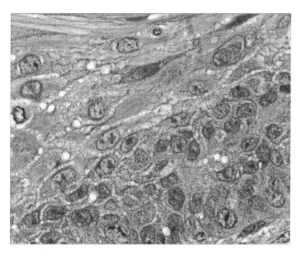

Figure 3 Squamous cell carcinoma, Grade 2 moderately differentiated showing more cellular pleomorphism and less keratinization than a Grade 1 tumor.

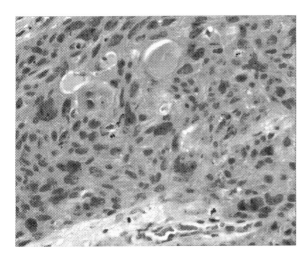

Figure 4 Squamous cell carcinoma, Grade 3 poorly differentiated showing little keratinization and marked cellular and nuclear pleomorphism.

Excision Margins

There has not been the same debate about excision margins for squamous cell carcinoma as has been experienced with melanoma. The distance between the edge of the tumor and the deep and lateral excision margins, expressed in millimeters, will normally form part of the histopathology report and minimum data set.

Perineural invasion is uncommon in squamous cell carcinoma but may be associated with an increased rate of local recurrence and metastasis (15). There does not appear to be any good evidence that vascular invasion is associated with increased local recurrence or metastasis and does not appear to be an independent prognostic variable.

Recommended Standards

On the basis of this evidence it is recommended that histopathology reports should include information about the following features:

1. tumor site,
2. tumor diameter, probably measured macroscopically and tumor thickness, measured microscopically,
3. tumor type,
4. tumor grade,
5. the presence or absence of vascular or perineural invasion, and
6. tumor excision margins measured laterally and at the base of the tumor.

BASAL CELL CARCINOMA

Basal cell carcinomas form a group of related subtypes that have in common the cytological appearance of basaloid cells (Fig. 5). Like squamous cell carcinomas, they mainly develop in sun-damaged skin. The basal cell nevus syndrome is a rare autosomal dominant condition in which patients have multiple basal cell carcinomas, which may start to appear in childhood. The syndrome is associated with abnormalities of the hedgehog signalling pathway. Sporadic basal cell carcinomas also appear to show related abnormalities (16).

Tumor Site

The importance of tumor site in basal cell carcinoma is mainly related to problems and difficulties in treating the tumors. Thus sites such as the nose, nasolabial fold, eyes, inner canthus, lip, and ear, are more difficult to treat than areas such as the back because of the need to optimize the cosmetic result and to avoid damage to adjacent normal structures. Tumors at these sites are, therefore, associated with a higher local recurrence rate.

Tumor Size

With increasing tumor size, there is a tendency for tumors more likely to recur, especially if the primary tumor is >2 cm in diameter (17). Metastasis is an exceedingly rare event with basal cell carcinoma, but metastasis may be associated with larger primary tumors. Most metastases are said to arise from primary tumors >3 cm in diameter, where a metastatic rate of 1.9% has been reported. For morpheaform tumors, an overall metastatic rate of 1% has been claimed

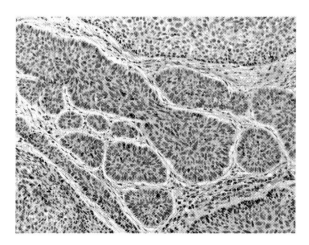

Figure 5 Basal cell carcinoma of archetypical type showing islands of basaloid cells with peripheral palisading.

(18–20). The rare giant cell variant of basal cell carcinoma is an example of a tumor which may become aggressive and metastatic when the primary tumor is >3 cm in diameter (21).

Tumor Type

The subtypes of basal carcinoma are particularly important to recognize and to classify accurately. The subtypes can be divided into those that are associated with a low risk of recurrence and those with a high risk.

Low-risk histological types include the nodular (Figs. 6 and 7) and fibroepithelial (fibroepithelioma of Pinkus) types (Fig. 8). These tumors are well circumscribed and easily seen clinically. They do not have a tendency for an invasive or infiltrative growth pattern or perineural invasion. As a consequence, they are usually excised completely on the first occasion.

High-risk histological types include the superficial subtype, which is characterized by lobules of tumor lying at the base of the epidermis and usually limited to the papillary dermis (Figs. 9 and 10). The reason for the high risk of recurrence is that they are typically multifocal and are more difficult to see clinically than a nodular basal cell carcinoma. Excision is therefore more likely to be incomplete, with residual disease leading to local recurrence.

Other high-risk subtypes owe their notoriety to their growth pattern. The infiltrating subtype produces tumors that typically form a plaque with ill-defined edges (Figs. 11, 12, and 13). The tumors mainly occur on the face and upper trunk. When perineural invasion is present, this may cause paraesthesia. Because of the infiltrative growth pattern, the size of the tumor may be underestimated resulting in involvement of the excision margins by tumor. Histologically, the tumors show infiltration of the dermis by cords and strands of tumor cells, with little in the way

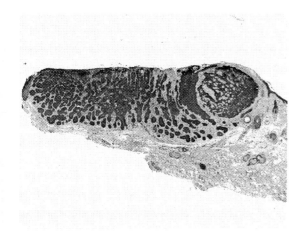

Figure 6 Nodular basal cell carcinoma of low-risk type, with a well-circumscribed tumor and no infiltrative growth pattern.

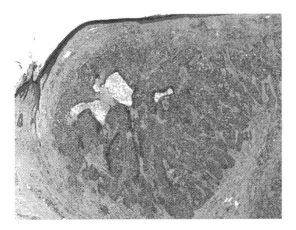

Figure 7 Nodular basal cell carcinoma of low-risk type, with a well-circumscribed tumor, central cystic change, and no infiltrative growth pattern.

of reactive dermal fibrosis or sclerosis. Staining of sections for low-molecular weight cytokeratin may serve to emphasize the smaller groups of cells at the periphery of the tumor and aid in assessing completeness of excision.

The related morphoeic subtype shares an infiltrative growth pattern, but with the addition of a densely collagenized tumor-associated stroma.

Less well recognized, but more important in the group of high-risk basal cell carcinomas, is the micronodular subtype (Figs. 14 and 15). In contrast to infiltrative and morphoeic tumors, where the importance of dermal infiltration by slender cords and columns of cells is well known to pathologists, the

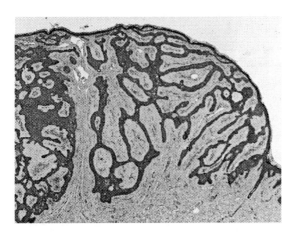

Figure 8 Fibroepitheioma of Pinkus: a well-circumscribed low-risk tumor with characteristic architecture and no infiltrative growth pattern.

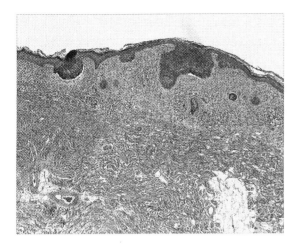

Figure 9 Superficial multicentric basal cell carcinoma, a tumor of high-risk type because of its multicentricity.

micronodular basal cell carcinoma has a much more innocent appearance. Small nodules of basal cells lie in the reticular dermis, often without any obvious stromal reaction or fibrosis. These micronodules have a fairly innocent appearance, but often may extend deeply into the dermis, even into the subcutis and often invade around and into nerves.

In practice, many basal cell carcinomas show a mixed growth pattern. This is especially true with micronodular differentiation, where the micronodular

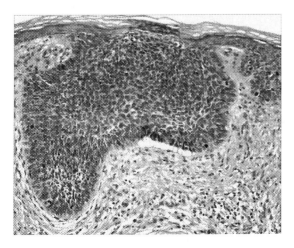

Figure 10 Superficial multicentric basal cell carcinoma, with nests of tumor cells attached to the base of the epidermis.

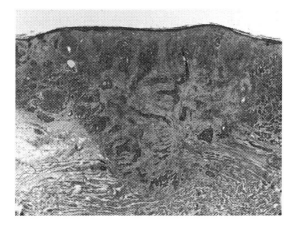

Figure 11 Basal cell carcinoma with a prominent infiltrative growth pattern and extension deep into the dermis.

element often lies at the base of an otherwise unremarkable nodular basal cell carcinoma.

The relative proportions of the subtypes and the frequency of mixed subtypes were emphasized in a study by Saxton et al., who found that in a series of 1039 consecutive cases of basal cell carcinoma, five major patterns of differentiation were identified: 21% nodular, 17% superficial, 15% micronodular, 7% infiltrative, and 1% morphoeic. Importantly, they found that 38.5% of tumors showed a mixed growth pattern (22).

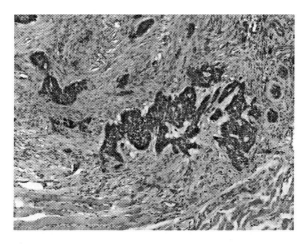

Figure 12 High-power view of the tumor seen in Figure 11, with infiltrating tumor deep in the dermis.

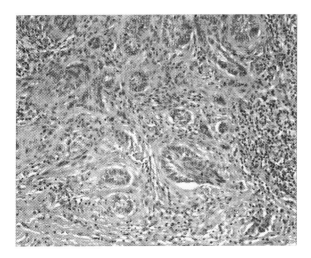

Figure 13 Basal cell carcinoma with infiltrating growth pattern. Cords and strands of tumor infiltrate the dermis.

Tumor Margins

The successful excision of a basal cell carcinoma is mainly dependent on the site and the presence or absence of anatomical difficulties and on the tumor type, with positive margins being more likely in high-risk subtypes. Mohs' micrographic surgery has been developed as a way of ensuring that excision margins are free of tumor (23).

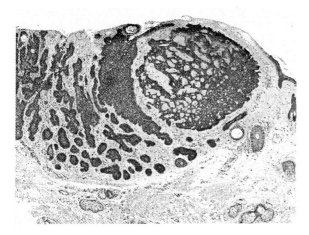

Figure 14 Micronodular basal cell carcinoma with micronodules of tumor cells, particularly prominent toward the base of the tumor.

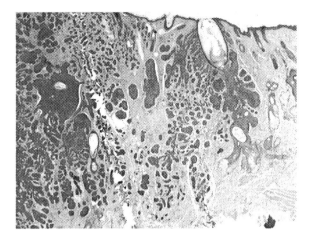

Figure 15   Micronodular basal cell carcinoma with micronodules of tumor cells infiltrating deeply into the dermis.

Recommended Standards

On the basis of this evidence, it is recommended that histopathology reports on excision specimens of basal cell carcinoma should include information about the following features:

1. tumor site,
2. tumor type, especially to distinguish high-risk from low-risk tumor types,
3. the presence or absence of perineural invasion, and
4. tumor excision margins measured laterally and at the base of the tumor.

CONCLUSION

Squamous cell carcinoma and basal cell carcinoma are malignant tumors that arise from the malignant proliferation of epidermal cells. In the past, this malignancy was more apparent. Tumors that were not treated early could progress to widespread local tissue destruction or to distant metastasis. With current trends toward earlier treatment, this aspect of the natural history of these tumors is seen less often (24).

The pathologist is an important member of the multidisciplinary team involved in the treatment of patients with skin cancer. For both squamous and basal cell carcinomas, there are important elements of prognostic information that must be included in the histopathology report on biopsy and excision specimens so as to identify high-risk tumors and to advise upon the completeness of tumor removal (25,26).

The histopathological diagnosis and differential diagnosis of these tumors still relies to a large extent upon the use of hematoxylin and eosin-stained tissue sections. Immunohistochemical markers have some value in differential diagnosis, but these adjuncts still have their limitations (6,27).

The application of minimum data sets in the histopathological reporting of biopsy specimens provides robust standards that allow for greater uniformity of practice both nationally and internationally (2). These pathology standards form an integral part of multidisciplinary standards of practice such as those published in the United Kingdom by the National Institute for Health and Clinical Excellence (28).

REFERENCES

1. LeBoit PE, Burg G, Weedon D, Sarasin A, eds. Pathology and Genetics of Skin Tumours. Lyon: IARC Press, 2006.
2. Royal College of Pathologists. Standards and minimum datasets for reporting cancers. Minimum dataset for histopathological reporting of common skin cancers. 2002. www.rcpath.org.
3. Guidelines of care for cutaneous squamous cell carcinoma. Committee on Guidelines of Care. Task force on cutaneous squamous cell carcinoma. J Am Acad Dermatol 1993; 28:628–631.
4. Motley R, Kersey P, Lawrence C. Multiprofessional guidelines for the management of the patient with primary cutaneous squamous cell carcinoma. Br J Dermatol 2002; 146:18–25.
5. Alam M, Ratner D. Cutaneous squamous-cell carcinoma. N Engl J Med 2001; 344:975–983.
6. Rowe DE, Carroll RJ, Day CL Jr. Prognostic factors for local recurrence, metastasis, and survival rates in squamous cell carcinoma of the skin, ear, and lip. Implications for treatment modality selection. J Am Acad Dermatol 1992; 26:976–990.
7. Talbot S, Hitchcock B. Incomplete primary excision of cutaneous basal and squamous cell carcinomas in the Bay of Plenty. N Z Med J 2004; 117:U848.
8. Beer TW, Shepherd P, Theaker JM. Ber EP4 and epithelial membrane antigen aid distinction of basal cell, squamous cell and basosquamous carcinomas of the skin. Histopathology 2000; 37:218–223.
9. Kaabipour E, Haupt HM, Stern JB, Kanetsky PA, Podolski VF, Martin AM. p16 expression in keratoacanthomas and squamous cell carcinomas of the skin: an immunohistochemical study. Arch Pathol Lab Med 2006; 130:69–73.
10. Holmkvist KA, Roenigk RK. Squamous cell carcinoma of the lip treated with Mohs micrographic surgery: outcome at 5 years. J Am Acad Dermatol 1998; 38:960–966.
11. Johnson TM, Rowe DE, Nelson BR, Swanson NA. Squamous cell carcinoma of the skin (excluding lip and oral mucosa). J Am Acad Dermatol 1992; 26:467–484.
12. Petter G, Haustein UF. Rare and newly described histological variants of cutaneous squamous epithelial carcinoma. Classification by histopathology, cytomorphology and malignant potential. Hautarzt 2001; 52:288–297.
13. Schmults CD. High-risk cutaneous squamous cell carcinoma: identification and management. Adv Dermatol 2005; 21:133–152.

14. Broders AC. Squamous-cell epithelioma of the skin. Ann Surg 1921; 63:141–160.
15. Lawrence N, Cottel WI. Squamous cell carcinoma of skin with perineural invasion. J Am Acad Dermatol 1994; 31:30–33.
16. Rubin AI, Chen EH, Ratner D. Basal-cell carcinoma. N Engl J Med 2005; 353: 2262–2269.
17. Walling HW, Fosko SW, Geraminejad PA, Whitaker DC, Arpey CJ. Aggressive basal cell carcinoma: presentation, pathogenesis, and management. Cancer Metastasis Rev 2004; 23:389–402.
18. Snow SN, Sahl W, Lo JS, Mohs FE, Warner T, Dekkinga JA, Feyzi J. Metastatic basal cell carcinoma. Report of five cases. Cancer 1994; 73:328–335.
19. Ting PT, Kasper R, Arlette JP. Metastatic basal cell carcinoma: report of two cases and literature review. J Cutan Med Surg 2005; 9:10–15.
20. Ionescu DN, Arida M, Jukic DM. Metastatic basal cell carcinoma: four case reports, review of literature, and immunohistochemical evaluation. Arch Pathol Lab Med 2006; 130:45–51.
21. Sahl WJ Jr, Snow SN, Levine NS. Giant basal cell carcinoma. Report of two cases and review of the literature. J Am Acad Dermatol 1994; 30:856–859.
22. Sexton M, Jones DB, Maloney ME. Histologic pattern analysis of basal cell carcinoma. Study of a series of 1039 consecutive neoplasms. J Am Acad Dermatol 1990; 23:1118–1126.
23. Batra RS, Kelley LC. Predictors of extensive subclinical spread in nonmelanoma skin cancer treated with Mohs micrographic surgery. Arch Dermatol 2002; 138: 1043–1051.
24. Perez GL, Randle HW. Natural history of squamous cell carcinoma of the skin: case report. Cutis 1995; 55:34–36.
25. Barksdale SK, O'Connor N, Barnhill R. Prognostic factors for cutaneous squamous cell and basal cell carcinoma. Determinants of risk of recurrence, metastasis, and development of subsequent skin cancers. Surg Oncol Clin N Am 1997; 6:625–638.
26. Friedman NR. Prognostic factors for local recurrence, metastases, and survival rates in squamous cell carcinoma of the skin, ear, and lip. J Am Acad Dermatol 1993; 28:281–282.
27. Swanson PE, Fitzpatrick MM, Ritter JH, Glusac EJ, Wick MR. Immunohistologic differential diagnosis of basal cell carcinoma, squamous cell carcinoma, and trichoepithelioma in small cutaneous biopsy specimens. J Cutan Pathol 1998; 25:153–159.
28. National Institute for Health and Clinical Excellence. Improving outcomes for people with skin tumours including melanoma. 2006. www.nice.org.uk/csgstim.

7

Pathology of Skin Cancer with Particular Reference to Melanoma

David E. Elder

Department of Pathology and Laboratory Medicine, Hospital of the University of Pennsylvania, Philadelphia, Pennsylvania, U.S.A.

INTRODUCTION

Despite recent efforts at high throughput molecular characterization of tumors, histopathology remains the gold standard for diagnosis of cancer in general, and of cancer in the skin in particular. Skin cancers, like other cancers, are classified largely on the basis of their cell or tissue of origin (1). Cancers of the skin can arise from any of the many cell types that are present within skin, and are thus very diverse. The most important skin cancer, in terms of mortality, is melanoma. However, squamous cell and basal cell carcinomas (often lumped together as "nonmelanoma skin cancer") are much more common than melanomas in Caucasian populations. Squamous cell carcinoma, which may arise from surface epidermis, usually with an associated precursor lesion called an actinic keratosis, is perhaps the prototypic skin cancer (2). Actinic keratoses are potential precursors of squamous cell carcinoma and are also markers of individuals at increased risk of skin cancer (including melanoma) (3). Basal cell carcinoma, more common than squamous cell carcinoma, usually does not arise in association with an evident precursor. These lesions can be divided into subtypes that correlate with risk of local recurrence and, rarely, metastasis (4). Basal cell and squamous cell carcinoma are exceedingly common in populations with susceptible fair skin who live in sunny climates or work or vacation in the sun. These nonmelanoma skin cancers are often not collected by tumor registries, and are often treated locally, yet because of their large numbers, they contribute substantially to morbidity and also to mortality from skin cancer.

Other types of carcinomas, much less common, can arise from skin appendages, presenting with varying degrees of glandular and squamoid differentiation. These are rare, and their biologic behavior is difficult to predict, but tend to be correlated with histopathologic grade and, of course, with stage at diagnosis (5). Basal cell and squamous cell carcinomas, like most melanomas, are caused by sun exposure. Human papilloma virus is the cause of carcinomas in genital sites, including vulvar skin, but it is not a common cause of cancer in non-genital skin (3,6). The etiology of most sweat gland carcinomas is unknown. Of the epithelial cancers, the two that are most likely to be lethal are malignant melanoma, which will be discussed extensively in this chapter, and Merkel cell tumor (7). The latter arises from neuroendocrine cells in the skin and has a relatively high mortality with a propensity to spread to regional lymph nodes and to distant metastasis. In addition to the epithelial tumors, sarcomas can occur in the skin, of which the most common potentially lethal example is angiosarcoma (8). Kaposi's sarcoma, once a rare locally endemic disease in elderly patients, has increased in incidence as a part of the AIDS epidemic, and has recently been related to a viral etiology (HHV8) (9). This chapter will concentrate on the pathology of malignant melanoma, because of its higher mortality rate than that of the other common skin cancers.

MALIGNANT MELANOMA

Malignant melanoma is a malignant neoplasm of melanocytes. This simple definition conceals numerous ambiguities and uncertainties. The term "malignancy" is primarily a clinical concept, yet the "gold standard" for diagnosis of melanoma, like most malignancies, is histopathology. The term "malignancy" implies a neoplasm that has the capacity to cause death of a patient. This capacity may be inherent in the neoplasm at the time of diagnosis ("neoplasms with competence for metastasis"), or it may be merely a potential outcome in the future evolution of a neoplasm ("neoplasms without competence for metastasis") (10–12). Even in the case of neoplasms with competence for metastasis, metastasis and death of patients are not usually inevitable outcomes, at least when one is dealing with a localized primary "malignant" neoplasm that has been completely resected. As Leslie Foulds observed many years ago (13), the histopathologic diagnosis of cancer or "malignancy" is inferential, and at best imperfectly predictive. Today, with modern high throughput molecular techniques, efforts are being undertaken to improve the predictive capacity of diagnostic tests, in order to better classify the tumors and identify those patients prospectively who are fated to either live, or to die from their neoplasm (14). At the present time, these efforts are in their infancy, and traditional histopathologic diagnosis remains the gold standard.

Clinical and Gross Morphology

The clinical morphology of malignant melanoma corresponds to the gross pathology. Malignant melanoma, like other cancers, evolves through stages of neoplasia without and with competence for metastasis, and these stages are evident both clinically and histologically. In the early stages of this evolution, a melanoma presents as a patch in the skin, which is usually hyperpigmented and, with time, becomes progressively more variegated in color and more irregular in outline. These properties have been summarized as the "A, B, C, D" rule for clinical diagnosis of melanoma (15). "A" stands for "asymmetry," where one half of the lesion is different from the other half in terms of color, outline, or texture and so on. "B" stands for "border irregularity," like the indented coastline of a small island. "C" stands for "color variegation," with shades of tan, brown, gray, blue-black, black, and red (the "red, white, and blue" lesion). "D" stands, in the original description, for "diameter" >6 mm; however, today, convincing melanomas are being recognized when they are considerably less than this size. To these criteria, change in size and in elevation may be added, and, and in more advanced lesions, ulceration and bleeding (16). If "E" for "enlargement" is added to the "ABCDE" criteria, the sensitivity and specificity of diagnosis of melanoma are 65.5% and 81%, respectively, if three of the five criteria are present (17). In addition, it has been demonstrated that experienced clinicians look for a lesion that is "out of step" with other lesions in the same patient—the "ugly duckling sign" (18). An important indicator of a potential melanoma is a history of change or growth, compared with benign nevi, which are typically stable. Any lesion giving rise to such a history that cannot be confidently assigned to a benign category should be excised for histological examination.

During the period of growth of a melanoma as an enlarging variegated pigmented patch in the skin, the lesion enlarges as it were among the radii of an imperfect circle, and for this reason the term "radial growth phase (RGP)" has been applied to this phase of progression (10). During this period, the prognosis for cure is very good if the lesion is excised before progression occurs to the next phase, the "vertical growth phase (VGP)," where an expansile mass is formed which tends to elevate the lesion perpendicular to the skin surface, and to infiltrate the underlying dermis "vertically." Compared with the RGP, the VGP is often quite symmetrical, may be uniformly pigmented, and may be a relatively small lesion, of the order of a few millimeters in diameter and depth, yet can have significant potential for metastasis and causing the death of the patient. In some melanomas, called "nodular melanomas," a nodule of tumorigenic VGP is present without an adjacent RGP. Thus, these lesions lack the diagnostically helpful ABCDE criteria of the RGP. Diagnosis may therefore be delayed until advanced symptoms, such as ulceration, bleeding, oozing, or even the development of satellite metastases occur (19).

Microscopic Morphology

The microscopic morphology of malignant melanoma parallels the clinical morphology. Thus, two components of melanomas can be recognized, paralleling RGPs and VGPs (20). In RGP melanoma, the lesion is "nontumorigenic" because the lesional cells lack the capacity for proliferation to form a mass in the dermis, and this fact can be recognized histologically (10,12). VGP melanomas, on the other hand, have capacity for proliferation in the dermis and are usually "tumorigenic" (10,12).

Nontumorigenic Melanoma (Radial Growth Phase)

In the nontumorigenic melanomas, there is evidence that proliferation occurs in the epidermis, where lesional cells remained confined at least for a time as "in situ" melanoma (MIS) (21). After a variable period of confinement to the epidermis, lesional cells may migrate from the epidermis into the dermis, a process often termed "invasion." This process, however, may be considered to parallel the process of migration of benign nevus cells from a junctional nevus into the dermis to form a "compound nevus" (22). Thus, the property of migration from the epidermis into the dermis is apparently inherent in neoplastic melanocytes, whether they are benign or malignant. Neoplastic melanocytes in the epidermis tend to form nests, either in a nevus or in a melanoma, and as these cells descend into the dermis they appear to do so in the form of nests that had originally been formed in the epidermis. If these melanocytes lack the capacity for proliferation in the dermis, there will be no mitotic activity in the dermis, and the nests of cells in the dermis, having been formed in the epidermis, will not be larger than those that remained in the overlying or adjacent epidermis. Thus, the presence of a tumorigenic VGP in a thin melanoma is recognized by the presence of nests in the dermis that are larger than the largest intraepidermal nest, while a mitogenic VGP is recognized by the presence of even a single mitosis in the dermis (Fig. 1). Metastasis is very rare in melanomas that lack either tumorigenic or mitogenic VGP (12,23,24).

Most of the best-known diagnostic attributes of melanomas are properties of the RGP or nontumorigenic compartment. These properties can be divided into architectural and cytologic properties (25). The most important architectural property is the presence of increased cellularity of neoplastic melanocytes, which may be arranged in one of the two major patterns, with considerable overlap. In the "lentiginous" pattern, lesional cells are arranged mainly as single cells, mainly near the dermal–epidermal junction, in contiguity with one another, and in a "continuous" pattern between rete ridges and along the junction. The term "lentiginous" apparently derives from the clinical morphology of the lentigo simplex, a small, lentil seed-like lesion, in which single cells are present around the tips and sides of elongated rete ridges, but not in a continuous pattern between the rete. In the other major pattern, there is "pagetoid"

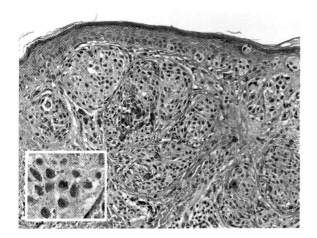

Figure 1   Early tumorigenic and mitogenic vertical growth phase in a thin melanoma. There are several clusters of neoplastic melanocytes in the papillary dermis that are larger than the largest intraepidermal clusters. One of these clusters, from the top left of the image, contains a lesional cell mitosis (enlarged in the inset).

proliferation (26), usually of large epithelioid cells, within the epidermis in a pattern that has been graphically described as "buckshot scatter" (27).

These abnormalities of growth control are of primary importance in the diagnosis of a nontumorigenic melanoma. In addition, there are cytologic features and there are stromal responses. Cytologically, the lesional cells exhibit varying degrees of atypia in the form of nuclear enlargement, irregularity, hyperchromatism, nucleolation, and/or mitotic activity. Importantly, in our view, this atypia is "uniform" involving a majority of the lesional cells in contrast to the "random" atypia that may be seen in dysplastic nevi, which are the major simulants of nontumorigenic melanomas (25,28). Paracrine responses that may be seen in nontumorigenic melanomas include a pattern of irregular epidermal thickening and thinning, the presence of diffuse fibroplasia and a band-like lymphocytic infiltrate, and of increased vessels in the papillary dermis (25).

Clinicopathologic subtypes of melanoma: There are variations among the nontumorigenic melanomas, based on histopathology and also on clinicopathologic characteristics. The molecular underpinning of some of these differences is now beginning to be understood, and has etiologic significance (29). Melanomas can be characterized according to the presence or absence of a nontumorigenic compartment. Tumorigenic melanomas that lack an adjacent nontumorigenic compartment are termed "nodular melanomas" (10). Their biological behavior may be the same once other prognostic factors are controlled, but the diagnosis may be made more difficult by the absence of the adjacent component (19). Melanomas that contain a nontumorigenic compartment can be classified on the basis of its morphology.

The most common melanomas, termed superficial spreading or "pagetoid" melanomas, occur on intermittently sun-exposed skin in relatively young people, who have relatively little evidence of sun damage. This form of melanoma is most likely to be associated with a nevus and with a family history (30). Melanomas with a predominantly lentiginous component, termed "lentigo maligna melanoma," occur in chronically exposed skin, in more elderly subjects who often have a lifetime history of outdoor work, and are less likely to be associated with nevi (31). Melanomas of acral skin also tend to have a lentiginous pattern of the nontumorigenic compartment. Recent studies by comparative genomic hybridization (CGH) have demonstrated that melanomas of acral sites tend to have non-random amplification of chromosome 11q at the locus of cyclin D1 (32,33). Molecular differences between lentigo maligna and superficial spreading melanomas are also becoming apparent; no doubt these genetic variants are associated with different etiologic agents and/or patterns of exposure (29).

Simulants of nontumorigenic melanomas: The most common clinically important simulants of melanomas are nevi, and the most important simulants of nontumorigenic melanomas are dysplastic nevi (34–36). Dysplastic nevi are distinguished from the in-situ component of melanomas by the lack of continuous basal or extensive pagetoid proliferation of melanocytes, the lack of uniform cytologic atypia, and by the lack of mitotic activity. In contrast, in a dysplastic nevus, the lesional cells are distributed, with nests predominating, predominantly near the dermo–epidermal junction, mainly around the tips and sides of elongated rete ridges, with some nests that bridge between adjacent rete. In the dermis, there is concentric fibroplasia and a patchy lymphocytic infiltrate rather than the diffuse fibroplasia with a band-like lymphocytic infiltrate that characterizes many melanomas.

Dysplastic nevi have primary significance as markers of individuals at increased risk for melanoma (37–46). The risk for an individual with one dysplastic nevus is elevated about two-fold, and when ten or more dysplastic nevi are present there is a twelve-fold elevated risk (47). These risk elevations are even greater when there is a personal or family history of melanoma (48,49). In addition, the degree of atypia in a dysplastic nevus has been correlated with melanoma risk (42,50). If a histologic diagnosis of a dysplastic nevus or of a "nevus with dysplastic features" is made, the clinician, in our opinion, should evaluate the patient's other risk factors and if the patient has other clinically dysplastic nevi, especially if there is a family or personal history of melanoma, periodic surveillance may be indicated. Even in the absence of these factors, a patient with a severely dysplastic nevus should likely be offered follow-up.

Junctional and "pagetoid" Spitz nevi (51) and the pigmented spindle cell nevus of Reed (52–54) are additional benign lesions that may simulate a nontumorigenic melanoma. These lesions have no significance as risk markers.

Tumorigenic and/or Mitogenic Melanomas
(Vertical Growth Phase)

The key attribute of VGP melanoma cells compared with those of the RGP is the ability to not only survive but also to proliferate in the dermis. In melanomas thicker than about 1 mm, the presence of a tumorigenic component is patently obvious. In thinner melanomas, the presence of a dermal nest larger than the largest intraepidermal nest defines an early tumorigenic VGP (55,56). A few melanomas lack a tumorigenic component as just defined, yet are distinguished by the presence of mitotic activity in the dermis. The presence of a dermal mitosis clearly indicates that the lesion has capacity for proliferation in the dermis. Therefore, the presence of VGP is recognized by either the property of "tumorigenicity" (clusters or nests of tumor cells in the dermis larger than the largest intraepidermal nests) or by the property of "mitogenicity" (the presence of any dermal mitoses) (55,56). Melanomas that are tumorigenic and/or mitogenic may have competence for metastasis, the likelihood of which depends on a number of different "prognostic attributes."

Most tumorigenic melanomas have an adjacent nontumorigenic compartment, and the diagnostic attributes of the nontumorigenic compartment are helpful in diagnosis of the melanoma. In nodular melanomas, there is no nontumorigenic compartment and diagnosis is more difficult (19). In the tumorigenic compartment of a melanoma, whether it is of the nodular type or of another subtype, there is contiguous sheet-like proliferation of uniformly atypical melanocytes, usually with mitotic activity. Cytologic atypia, in comparison with the nontumorigenic melanomas, is typically more severe and is uniform. In advanced melanoma, there may be ulceration and satellites may be present (56).

Simulants of tumorigenic melanomas: The tumorigenic compartment of melanomas needs to be distinguished from benign nevi, and from other tumors that may simulate melanomas, such as histiocytomas, sarcomas, and carcinomas. Immunohistochemistry may be very helpful for making the latter distinctions. However, the distinction between a benign nevus and a melanoma may be very difficult. Spitz nevi are lesions that are particularly difficult to distinguish from melanomas, because they are comprised of large, spindle, and/or epithelioid melanocytes, which may have large nuclei with prominent nucleoli (29,57–61). Nevoid melanomas, although fortunately rare, also present difficulties because they simulate a benign nevus at least at scanning magnification (62–65). The key distinguishing features are the greater cellularity of nevoid melanomas compared with benign nevi and the presence of dermal mitoses. Ki-67 staining may also be helpful. In addition to these lesions, other "tumorigenic," but benign or low malignant potential, lesions need to be distinguished from melanomas. These include cellular blue nevi (66,67), deep penetrating nevi (68–70), and pigmented epithelioid melanocytomas (71). In some lesions, a diagnostic distinction is difficult or impossible to make. In these circumstances, we use a descriptive term, "melanocytic tumor of uncertain potential (MELTUMP)" (72,73).

Metastatic Melanoma

Although metastasis of a melanocytic lesion might be thought to be a defining characteristic of malignant melanoma, there are some "benign" lesions that have been found to be associated with lymph node metastases, followed by prolonged survivals. This phenomenon has been described in association with cellular blue nevi and with Spitz nevi. In some of these cases, we have made a diagnosis of "metastatic melanocytic tumors of uncertain potential." Management of these lesions, like those of primary melanocytic tumors of uncertain malignant potential, should take into account the "worst-case scenario," namely the differential diagnosis of malignant melanoma.

PROGNOSTIC ATTRIBUTES FOR MELANOMA

In addition to making an accurate histologic diagnosis, an important role of pathology is in the prediction of outcome by characterizing these prognostic attributes for individual cases.

Clark's Levels

In 1967, Wallace Clark described "Clark's levels" of invasion, which became the first widely used prognosticating or "microstaging" attribute for melanoma (10). The Clark's levels also have descriptive value (20,74,75). In Clark level 1, the melanoma cells are confined to the epidermis, above the basement membrane, and there is theoretically no competence for metastasis whatsoever. In Clark level 2, their lesional cells are present in the papillary dermis, which may be expanded but is not filled by a dermal tumor. In Clark level 3, the papillary dermis is both filled and expanded by the tumor. A few Clark level 2 tumors may meet the definition of "tumorigenic" provided; however, most Clark level 2 melanomas are nontumorigenic. In contrast, most Clark level 3 melanomas are tumorigenic. In Clark level 4, the lesional cells invade beyond the papillary dermis, which is a loose and vascular structure specialized to support epithelium, and infiltrate the less-hospitable environment of the reticular dermis. In Clark level 5, there is infiltration of the subcutaneous fat. The progression through the levels, perhaps with the exception of the last, likely represents the acquisition of new properties of the lesional cells, which correlate with increasing competence for metastasis.

Breslow's Thickness

In 1970, Alexander Breslow described a system for prognostication of melanoma based on the thickness of the melanoma from the top of the granular layer to the deepest invasive tumor cell (76). Although this exact measurement technique is somewhat counterintuitive (because in a thin melanoma a hyperplastic epidermis may contribute disproportionately to the apparent thickness), Breslow's thickness is highly predictive of the likelihood of metastasis. In his original papers, Breslow identified a subset of cases thinner than 0.76 mm, in which the probability of metastasis was close to zero (76–78). Today, in the 2002 American Joint Committee on Cancer (AJCC) classification, a cutpoint of 1.0 mm is used. Using this cutpoint, the probability of metastasis for "thin" melanomas is ~12% at 10 years (79).

Mitotic Rate

Mitotic rate was first used for prediction of survival by Alistair Cochran in 1969 (79). Schmoeckel, in 1978, described a "mitotic index" representing the product of mitotic rate and Breslow thickness (80). In the 1989 Clark model, mitotic rate was the single strongest predictor of survival in VGP melanomas (81). More recent studies have confirmed the importance of mitotic rate as a predictor of disease-free survival and of regional lymph node metastasis (23,82–85). In addition, as already discussed, the property of "mitogenicity" defines VGP in a thin melanoma even in the absence of tumorigenicity.

Tumor-Infiltrating Lymphocytes

First described in the 1989 Clark model, tumor-infiltrating lymphocytes (TIL) are lymphocytes that are actually among and in contact with tumor cells (81). Non-infiltrating lymphocytes or "peritumoral lymphocytes" are not in contact with tumor cells and are not related to prognosis. The significance of TIL has been confirmed by the studies of Clemente and Mihm, in both primary and metastatic melanomas (86,87).

Ulceration

Ulceration is the strongest protective factor after thickness in the 2002 AJCC staging system, in which it is used as a stage modifier (79). However, ulceration does not enter some other models, especially in those in which mitotic rate is an attribute (81,82).

Vascular/Lymphatic Invasion

Invasion of lymphatics or of blood vessels in primary tumors is relatively uncommonly recognized. There has been lack of agreement as to the independent prognostic significance of this attribute (88–93), possibly partly because of its rarity which reduces the power of the studies to recognize its significance. Sagebiel has described "uncertain" vascular invasion, in which there is invasion of the wall of the vessels (or "mural invasion"), without tumor cells being present in the lumen (89). Both patterns of invasion appear to have prognostic significance.

Satellites, In-Transit Metastases, and Regional Lymph Node Metastases

As might be expected, evidence of spread of the tumor beyond the primary site is associated with reduced disease-free survival probability. Satellites are metastases that are present, by definition, within 5 cm of the primary tumor and may be present in a biopsy or in a re-excision specimen. In the AJCC staging system, the presence of satellites is indicative of a stage 4 lesion, although this is not based on extensive data (94). Nevertheless, a number of studies support the importance of satellites as a negative prognostic indicator (88,93,95).

PROGNOSTIC MODELS FOR MELANOMA

Attributes like those already described can be combined through statistical techniques to derive a model that can be used to estimate the likely survival for individual patients, based on the survival experience of a large group of patients. In the 2002 AJCC staging system for melanoma, the primary attribute used is thickness, stratified at 1-mm intervals and modified by the presence or absence of ulceration (79). The lowest risk group, AJCC stage 1, with a thickness < 1 mm, is also the single largest group of melanoma patients. The overall survival, though "low risk," is nevertheless a not inconsiderable 12% by 10 years, and this group therefore accounts for a substantial fraction of the mortality from melanoma. In a recent analysis, Gimotty et al. (23) have demonstrated that a prognostic tree utilizing the attributes of mitogenicity, tumorigenicity, and gender is more accurate than the AJCC model in this important stage 1 group. As demonstrated in Figure 2, the model separates the stage 1 group into four subgroups at minimum, slight, moderate, and high-risk disease. For example, men with a melanoma that has any mitoses have a 31% risk of metastasis by 10 years of follow-up. After validation in other populations, the proposed prognostic tree

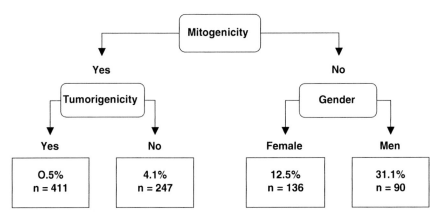

Figure 2 Tree analysis of the significance of mitogenicity and tumorigenicity in prognosis of melanoma. The numbers in the four "leaves" or cells of the tree at the bottom of the figure represent the percentage of patients who have experienced metastasis and the total number of patients in each cell. All patients were followed for at least 10 years or until the onset of the first metastasis.

will likely be useful in the design of clinical trials and clinical management for patients with "thin" melanomas.

MOLECULAR PATHOLOGY OF MELANOCYTIC TUMORS

The molecular pathways that drive and permit proliferation in melanocytic tumors are beginning to be understood. In a recent study of gene expression profiling using oligonucleotide microarrays, cluster analysis accurately separated nevi and primary melanomas, and two classes of metastatic melanomas. These gene expression signatures correlate well with previous understanding of diagnostic differences among melanomas and nevi, and provide the basis for beginning to develop a new molecular classification for melanoma, which may potentially correlate with prognosis and with therapy (96).

Molecular signaling pathways are important in many cancers and may provide therapeutic targets for a new generation of small molecule inhibitors of signaling. Activation of the "mitogenic activated protein (MAP) kinase" pathway has been demonstrated in most melanomas (97). This pathway can be activated by external mitogenic signals or by an autocrine loop, such as that involving basic fibroblast growth factor (bFGF). In 2002, it was discovered that about two-thirds of melanomas have a mutation of an oncogene that is a proximal member of the MAP kinase pathway, called BRAF (98). In melanomas that lack a mutation of BRAF, another oncogene from the same pathway, NRAS, tends to be mutated, and in a few melanomas, both genes are mutated (99). Thus, about two-thirds of melanomas have a mutation of one of the other of these proximal signaling members of the MAP kinase pathway (99). More recent studies have disclosed that these mutations are uncommon in melanomas on chronically sun-exposed skin, and on acral skin, in which other oncogenic mechanisms, such as activation of cyclin D1, occur. Interestingly, BRAF or NRAS mutations (which are typically mutually exclusive) have also been found in as many as 80% of benign nevi (100), associated with elevation of the inhibitory molecule p16 (101). This finding tends to confirm the tumor progression hypothesis that melanomas may arise in association with precursor nevi, and in a few cases the same mutations of oncogenes have been found in a melanoma and in its associated nevus, and in a VGP and its associated metastasis, providing further support for this idea (102,103). An inhibitor of BRAF has already been used in therapeutic trials, with some success when combined with a chemotherapeutic agent (104).

In parallel with the accumulation of mutated oncogenes, which are often also found to be amplified by CGH (105), there is a loss of suppressor genes in melanoma. Indeed, the first high-risk gene for melanoma that was detected in familial melanoma kindreds was the *p16* gene located on the short arm of chromosome 9 (106,107). One allele of this gene is mutated in about a third to one half of all families in which three or more melanomas have occurred (108). Loss of the other allele presumably gives a "selective growth advantage" to affected cells (109). Outside the hereditary melanoma situation, loss of p16 is documented in essentially all melanoma cell lines and in most primary tumors that have been studied, by a variety of mechanisms that include, in addition to inactivating mutations, deletion of the gene or loss of heterozygosity (110), methylation of the promoter (111), and mis-location of the protein from the nucleus to the cytoplasm (112). Thus, melanomagenesis appears to occur by a dual process of activation of oncogenes and loss of suppressor molecules.

The new molecular findings are beginning to provide novel therapeutic targets, which are beginning to make a difference to the appalling survival of patients with metastatic melanoma. In the future, one of the most important purposes of histopathology and molecular pathology will be the definition of pathways that are activated, or of suppresser genes that are inactivated, for the purpose of identifying therapeutic targets for selection of optimal therapeutic agents.

REFERENCES

1. Weinstock MA. Epidemiology of nonmelanoma skin cancer: clinical issues, definitions, and classification. J Invest Dermatol 1994; 102:4S–5S.
2. Petter G, Haustein UF. Squamous cell carcinoma of the skin—histopathological features and their significance for the clinical outcome. J Eur Acad Dermatol Venereol 1998; 11:37–44.
3. Chen GJ, Feldman SR, Williford PM, et al. Clinical diagnosis of actinic keratosis identifies an elderly population at high risk of developing skin cancer. Dermatol Surg 2005; 31:43–47.
4. Sexton M, Jones DB, Maloney ME. Histologic pattern analysis of basal cell carcinoma. Study of a series of 1039 consecutive neoplasms. J Am Acad Dermatol 1990; 23:1118–1126.
5. Yugueros P, Kane WJ, Goellner JR. Sweat gland carcinoma: a clinicopathologic analysis of an expanded series in a single institution. Plast Reconstr Surg 1998; 102:705–710.
6. Meyer T, Arndt R, Christophers E, Nindl I, Stockfleth E. Importance of human papillomaviruses for the development of skin cancer. Cancer Detect Prev 2001; 25:533–547.
7. Allen PJ, Bowne WB, Jaques DP, Brennan MF, Busam K, Coit DG. Merkel cell carcinoma: prognosis and treatment of patients from a single institution. J Clin Oncol 2005; 23:2300–2309.
8. Morgan MB, Swann M, Somach S, Eng W, Smoller B. Cutaneous angiosarcoma: a case series with prognostic correlation. J Am Acad Dermatol 2004; 50:867–874.
9. Pantanowitz L, Dezube BJ. Advances in the pathobiology and treatment of Kaposi sarcoma. Curr Opin Oncol 2004; 16:443–449.
10. Clark WH Jr. A classification of malignant melanoma in man correlated with histogenesis and biologic behavior. In: Montagna W, Hu F, eds. Advances in the Biology of the Skin. Vol. 8. New York: Pergamon Press, 1967:621–647.
11. Mihm MC Jr, Clark WH Jr, From L. The clinical diagnosis, classification and histogenetic concepts of the early stages of cutaneous malignant melanomas. N Engl J Med 1971; 284:1078–1082.

12. Elder DE, Guerry DIV, Epstein MN, et al. Invasive malignant melanomas lacking competence for metastasis. Am J Dermatopathol 1984; 6:55–62.
13. Foulds L. Neoplastic Development. London and New York: Academic press, 1969:41–86.
14. Alizadeh AA, Ross DT, Perou CM, Van de Rijn M. Towards a novel classification of human malignancies based on gene expression patterns. J Pathol 2005; 195: 41–52.
15. Friedman RJ, Rigel DS, Kopf AW. Early detection of malignant melanoma: the role of physician examination and self-examination of the skin. CA Cancer J Clin 1985; 35:130–151.
16. Wick MM, Sober AJ, Fitzpatrick TB, et al. Clinical characteristics of early cutaneous melanoma. Cancer 1980; 45:2684–2686.
17. Thomas L, Tranchand P, Berard F, Secchi T, Colin C, Moulin G. Semiological value of ABCDE criteria in the diagnosis of cutaneous pigmented tumors. Dermatology 1998, 197:11–17.
18. Gachon J, Beaulieu P, Sei JF, et al. First prospective study of the recognition process of melanoma in dermatological practice. Arch Dermatol 2005; 141:434–438.
19. Demierre MF, Chung C, Miller DR, Geller AC. Early detection of melanoma in the United States. Beware of the nodular subtype. Arch Dermatol 2005; 141: 745–750.
20. Clark WH Jr, Ainsworth AM, Bernardino EA, Yang CH Jr, Reed RJ. The developmental biology of primary human malignant melanomas. Semin Oncol 1975; 2:83–103.
21. Gimotty PA, Van Belle PA, Elder DE, et al. The biologic and prognostic significance of dermal Ki67 expression, mitoses and tumorigenicity in thin invasive cutaneous melanoma. J Clin Oncol 2005; 23:8048–8056.
22. Elder DE, Murphy GF. Benign melanocytic tumors (nevi). In: Elder DE, Murphy GF, eds. Melanocytic Tumors of the Skin. Washington, D.C.: Armed Forces Institute of Pathology, 1991:5–81.
23. Gimotty PA, Guerry D, Ming ME, et al. Thin primary cutaneous malignant melanoma: a prognostic tree for 10-year metastasis is more accurate than American joint committee on cancer staging. J Clin Oncol 2004; 22:3668–3676.
24. Guerry DIV, Synnestvedt M, Elder DE, Schultz D. Lessons from tumor progression: The invasive radial growth phase of melanoma is common, incapable of metastasis, and indolent. J Invest Dermatol 1993; 100:342S–345S.
25. Elder DE, Murphy GF. Melanocytic Tumors of the Skin. Washington, D.C.: Armed Forces Institute of Pathology, 1991.
26. Committee of Australian Pathologists. Moles and malignant melanoma: terminology and classification. Med J Aust 1967; 1:123–124.
27. Price NM, Rywlin AM, Ackerman AB. Histologic criteria for the diagnosis of superficial spreading melanoma: formulated on the basis of proven metastastic lesions. Cancer 1976; 38:2434–2441.
28. Elder DE, Green MH, Guerry DIV, Kraemer KH, Clark WH Jr. The dysplastic nevus syndrome: our definition. Am J Dermatopathol 1982; 4:455–460.
29. Bastian BC, Olshen AB, LeBoit PE, Pinkel D. Classifying melanocytic tumors based on DNA copy number changes. Am J Pathol 2003; 163:1765–1770.
30. Sagebiel RW. Unusual variants of melanoma: fact or fiction? Semin Oncol 1996; 23:703–708.

31. Whiteman DC, Watt P, Purdie DM, Hughes MC, Hayward NK, Green AC. Melanocytic nevi, solar keratoses, and divergent pathways to cutaneous melanoma. J Natl Cancer Inst 2003; 95:806–812.

32. Sauter ER, Yeo UC, Von Stemm A, et al. Cyclin d1 is a candidate oncogene in cutaneous melanoma. Cancer Res 2002; 62:3200–3206.

33. Bastian BC, Kashani-Sabet M, Hamm H, et al. Gene amplifications characterize acral melanoma and permit the detection of occult tumor cells in the surrounding skin. Cancer Res 2000; 60:1968–1973.

34. Elder DE, Goldman LI, Goldman SC, Greene MH, Clark WH Jr. Dysplastic nevus syndrome: a phenotypic association of sporadic cutaneous melanoma. Cancer 1980; 46:1787–1794.

35. Clemente C, Cochran A, Elder DE, et al. Histopathologic diagnosis of dysplastic nevi. Concordance among pathologists convened by the WHO melanoma programme. Hum Pathol 1991; 22:313–319.

36. Heenan PJ, Elder DE, Sobin LH. Histological classification of skin tumors. In: Heenan PJ, Elder DE, Sobin LH, eds. Histological Typing of Skin Tumors. Berlin, Heidelberg, New York: Springer, 1996:3–10.

37. Greene M, Clark WH Jr, Tucker MA, Kraemer KH, Elder DE, Fraser MC. High risk of malignant melanoma in melanoma-prone families with dysplastic nevi. Ann Intern Med 1985; 102:458–465.

38. Nordlund JJ, Kirkwood J, Forget BM, et al. Demographic study of clinically atypical (dysplastic) nevi in patients with melanoma and comparison subjects. Cancer Res 1985; 45:1855–1861.

39. Swerdlow AJ, English J, MacKie RM, et al. Benign melanocytic naevi as a risk factor for malignant melanoma. Br Med J (Clin Res Ed) 1986; 292:1555–1559.

40. Holly EA, Kelly JW, Shpall SN, Chiu SH. Number of melanocytic nevi as a major risk factor for malignant melanoma. J Am Acad Dermatol 1987; 17:459–468.

41. Roush GC, Nordlund JJ, Forget B, Gruber SB, Kirkwood JM. Independence of dysplastic nevi from total nevi in determining risk for nonfamilial melanoma. Prev Med 1988; 17:273–279.

42. Augustsson A, Stierner U, Rosdahl I, Suurküla M. Common and dysplastic naevi as risk factors for cutaneous malignant melanoma in a Swedish population. Acta Derm Venereol (Stockh) 1991; 71:518–524.

43. Halpern AC, Guerry DIV, Elder DE, et al. Dysplastic nevi as risk markers of sporadic (non-familial) melanoma: a case-control study. Arch Dermatol 1991; 127:995–999.

44. Tucker MA, Crutcher WA, Hartge P, Sagebiel RW. Familial and cutaneous features of dysplastic nevi: a case-control study. J Am Acad Dermatol 1993; 28:558–564.

45. Carey WP Jr, Thompson CJ, Synnestvedt M, et al. Dysplastic nevi as a melanoma risk factor in patients with familial melanoma. Cancer 1994; 74:3118–3125.

46. Kang S, Barnhill RL, Mihm MC Jr, Fitzpatrick TB, Sober AJ. Melanoma risk in individuals with clinically atypical nevi. Arch Dermatol 1994; 130:999–1001.

47. Tucker MA, Halpern A, Holly EA, et al. Clinically recognized dysplastic nevi. A central risk factor for cutaneous melanoma. JAMA 1997; 277:1439–1444.

48. Chaudru V, Chompret A, Bressac-de Paillerets B, Spatz A, Avril MF, Demenais F. Influence of genes, nevi, and sun sensitivity on melanoma risk in a family

sample unselected by family history and in melanoma-prone families. J Natl Cancer Inst 2004; 96:785–795.

49. Halpern AC, Guerry D, Elder DE, Trock B, Synnestvedt M. A cohort study of melanoma in patients with dysplastic nevi. J Invest Dermatol 1993; 100:346S–349S.
50. Arumi-Uria M, McNutt NS, Finnerty B. Grading of atypia in nevi: correlation with melanoma risk. Mod Pathol 2003; 16:764–771.
51. Busam KJ, Barnhill RL. Pagetoid Spitz nevus. Intraepidermal Spitz tumor with prominent pagetoid spread. Am J Surg Pathol 1995; 19:1061–1067.
52. Reed RJ, Ichinose H, Clark WH Jr, Mihm MC Jr. Common and uncommon melanocytic nevi and borderline melanomas. Semin Oncol 1975; 2:119–147.
53. Sagebiel RW, Chinn EK, Egbert BM. Pigmented spindle cell nevus. Clinical and histologic review of 90 cases. Am J Surg Pathol 1984; 8:645–653.
54. Barnhill RL, Barnhill MA, Berwick M, Mihm MC Jr. The histologic spectrum of pigmented spindle cell nevus: A review of 120 cases with emphasis on atypical variants. Hum Pathol 1991; 22:52–58.
55. Elder DE, Guerry D, Epstein MN, et al. Invasive malignant melanomas lacking competence for metastasis. Am J Dermatopathol 1984; 6(suppl 1):55–61.
56. Elder DE, Murphy GF. Malignant tumors (melanomas and related lesions). In: Elder DE, Murphy GF, eds. Melanocytic Tumors of the Skin. Washington, D.C.: Armed Forces Institute of Pathology, 1991:103–206.
57. Vollmer RT. Patient age in Spitz nevus and malignant melanoma: implication of Bayes rule for differential diagnosis. Am J Clin Pathol 2004; 121:872–877.
58. Vollmer RT. Use of Bayes rule and MIB-1 proliferation index to discriminate Spitz nevus from malignant melanoma. Am J Clin Pathol 2004; 122:499–505.
59. Paniago-Pereira C, Maize JC, Ackerman AB. Nevus of large spindle and/or epithelioid cells (Spitz's nevus). Arch Dermatol 1978; 114:1811–1823.
60. Weedon D, Little JH. The Spitz naevus. Aust N Z J Surg 1978; 48:21–22.
61. Spitz S. Melanomas of childhood. Am J Pathol 1948; 24:591–609.
62. Levene A. On the histological diagnosis and prognosis of malignant melanoma. J Clin Pathol 1980; 33:101–124.
63. Schmoeckel C, Castro CE, Braun-Falco O. Nevoid malignant melanoma. Arch Dermatol Res 1985; 277:362–369.
64. McNutt NS, Urmacher C, Hakimian J, Hoss DM, Lugo J. Nevoid malignant melanoma: morphologic patterns and immunohistochemical reactivity. J Cutan Pathol 1995; 22:502–517.
65. Zembowicz A, McCusker M, Chiarelli C, et al. Morphological analysis of nevoid melanoma: a study of 20 cases with a review of the literature. Am J Dermatopathol 2001; 23:167–175.
66. Tran TA, Carlson JA, Basaca PC, Mihm MC. Cellular blue nevus with atypia (atypical cellular blue nevus): a clinicopathologic study of nine cases. J Cutan Pathol 1998; 25:252–258.
67. Temple-Camp CR, Saxe N, King H. Benign and malignant cellular blue nevus. A clinicopathological study of 30 cases. Am J Dermatopathol 1988; 10:289–296.
68. Seab JA Jr, Graham JH, Helwig EB. Deep penetrating nevus. Am J Surg Pathol 1989; 13:39–44.
69. Cooper PH. Deep penetrating (plexiform spindle cell) nevus. A frequent participant in combined nevus. J Cutan Pathol 1992; 19:172–180.

70. Robson A, Morley-Quante M, Hempel H, McKee PH, Calonje E. Deep penetrating naevus: clinicopathological study of 31 cases with further delineation of histological features allowing distinction from other pigmented benign melanocytic lesions and melanoma. Histopathology 2003; 43:529–537.
71. Zembowicz A, Carney JA, Mihm MC. Pigmented epithelioid melanocytoma: a low-grade melanocytic tumor with metastatic potential indistinguishable from animal-type melanoma and epithelioid blue nevus. Am J Surg Pathol 2004; 28:31–40.
72. Elder DE, Xu X. The approach to the patient with a difficult melanocytic lesion. Pathology 2004; 36:428–434.
73. Xu X, Weber KS, Elenitsas R, Elder DE. Clinical and histological features of cellular nodules in congenital nevi. Am J Surg Pathol 2003; (in press).
74. Clark WH Jr, From L, Bernardino EA, Mihm MC Jr. The histogenesis and biologic behavior of primary human malignant melanomas of the skin. Cancer Res 1969; 29:705–727.
75. Clark WH. Tumour progression and the nature of cancer. Br J Cancer 1991; 64: 631–644.
76. Breslow A. Thickness, cross-sectional areas and depth of invasion in the prognosis of cutaneous melanoma. Ann Surg 1970; 172:902–908.
77. Breslow A. Tumor thickness, level of invasion and node dissection in stage I cutaneous melanoma. Ann Surg 1975; 182:572–575.
78. Breslow A, Macht SD. Optimal size of resection margin for thin cutaneous mela-noma. Surg Gynecol Obstet 1977; 145:691–692.
79. Balch CM, Soong SJ, Gershenwald JE, et al. Prognostic factors analysis of 17,600 melanoma patients: validation of the American joint committee on cancer melanoma staging system. J Clin Oncol 2001; 19:3622–3634.
80. Schmoeckel C, Braun-Falco O. Prognostic index in maligant melanoma. Arch Dermatol 1978; 114:871–873.
81. Clark WH Jr, Elder DE, Guerry DIV, et al. Model predicting survival in stage I mel-anoma based on tumor progression. JNCI 1989; 81:1893–1904.
82. Barnhill RL, Katzen J, Spatz A, Fine J, Berwick M. The importance of mitotic rate as a prognostic factor for localized cutaneous melanoma. J Cutan Pathol 2005; 32:268–273.
83. Kesmodel SB, Karakousis GC, Botbyl JD, et al. Mitotic rate as a predictor of sentinel lymph node positivity in patients with thin melanomas. Ann Surg Oncol 2005; 12:449–458.
84. Francken AB, Shaw HM, Thompson JF, et al. The prognostic importance of tumor mitotic rate confirmed in 1317 patients with primary cutaneous melanoma and long follow-up. Ann Surg Oncol 2004; 11:426–433.
85. Sondak VK, Taylor JM, Sabel MS, et al. Mitotic rate and younger age are predictors of sentinel lymph node positivity: lessons learned from the generation of a probabil-istic model. Ann Surg Oncol 2004; 11:247–258.
86. Clemente CG, Mihm MG, Bufalino R, Zurrida S, Collini P, Cascinelli N. Prognostic value of tumor infiltrating lymphocytes in the vertical growth phase of primary cutaneous melanoma. Cancer 1996; 77:1303–1310.
87. Mihm MC Jr, Clemente CG, Cascinelli N. Tumor infiltrating lymphocytes in lymph node melanoma metastases: A histopathologic prognostic indicator and an expression of local immune response. Lab Invest 1996; 74:43–47.

88. Nagore E, Oliver V, Botella-Estrada R, Moreno-Picot S, Insa A, Fortea JM. Prognostic factors in localized invasive cutaneous melanoma: high value of mitotic rate, vascular invasion and microscopic satellitosis. Melanoma Res 2005; 15:169–177.
89. Kashani-Sabet M, Sagebiel RW, Ferreira CM, Nosrati M, Miller JR III. Vascular involvement in the prognosis of primary cutaneous melanoma. Arch Dermatol 2001; 137:1169–1173.
90. Massi D, Borgognoni L, Franchi A, Martini L, Reali UM, Santucci M. Thick cutaneous malignant melanoma: a reappraisal of prognostic factors. Melanoma Res 2000; 10:153–164.
91. Niezabitowski A, Czajecki K, Rys J, et al. Prognostic evaluation of cutaneous malignant melanoma: a clinicopathologic and immunohistochemical study. J Surg Oncol 1999; 70:150–160.
92. Spatz A, Shaw HM, Crotty KA, Thompson JF, McCarthy SW. Analysis of histopathological factors associated with prolonged survival of 10 years or more for patients with thick melanomas (>5 mm). Histopathology 1998; 33:406–413.
93. Barnhill RL, Fine JA, Roush GC, Berwick M. Predicting five-year outcome for patients with cutaneous melanoma in a population-based study. Cancer 1996; 78:427–432.
94. Kim CJ, Reintgen DS, Balch CM. The new melanone staging system. Cancer Control 2002; 9:9–15.
95. León D, Daly JM, Synnestvedt M, Schultz DJ, Elder DE, Clark WH Jr. The prognostic implications of microscopic satellites in patients with clinical stage I melanoma. Arch Surg 1991; 126:1461–1468.
96. Haqq C, Nosrati M, Sudilovsky D, et al. The gene expression signatures of melanoma progression. Proc Natl Acad Sci USA 2005; 102:6092–6097.
97. Satyamoorthy K, Li G, Gerrero MR, et al. Constitutive mitogen-activated protein kinase activation in melanoma is mediated by both BRAF mutations and autocrine growth factor stimulation. Cancer Res 2003; 63:756–759.
98. Davies H, Bignell GR, Cox C, et al. Mutations of the BRAF gene in human cancer. Nature 2002; 417:949–954.
99. Kumar R, Angelini S, Hemminki K. Activating BRAF and N-Ras mutations in sporadic primary melanomas: an inverse association with allelic loss on chromosome 9. Oncogene 2003; 22:9217–9224.
100. Pollock PM, Harper UL, Hansen KS, et al. High frequency of BRAF mutations in nevi. Nat Genet 2003; 33:19–20.
101. Talve L, Sauroja I, Collan Y, Punnonen K, Ekfors T. Loss of expression of the $p16^{INK4}/CDKN2$ gene in cutaneous malignant melanoma correlates with tumor cell proliferation and invasive stage. Int J Cancer 1997; 74:255–259.
102. Omholt K, Platz A, Kanter L, Ringborg U, Hansson J. NRAS and BRAF mutations arise early during melanoma pathogenesis and are preserved throughout tumor progression. Clin Cancer Res 2003; 9:6483–6488.
103. Omholt K, Karsberg S, Platz A, Kanter L, Ringborg U, Hansson J. Screening of N-ras codon 61 mutations in paired primary and metastatic cutaneous melanomas: mutations occur early and persist throughout tumor progression. Clin Cancer Res 2002; 8:3468–3474.
104. Flaherty KT. New molecular targets in melanoma. Curr Opin Oncol 2004; 16:150–154.
105. Bastian BC. Understanding the progression of melanocytic neoplasia using genomic analysis: from fields to cancer. Oncogene 2003; 22:3081–3086.

106. Hussussian CJ, Struewing JP, Goldstein AM, et al. Germline p16 mutations in familial melanoma. Nat Genet 1994; 8:15–21.
107. Kamb A, Shattuck-Eidens D, Eeles R, et al. Analysis of the p16 gene (*CDKN2*) as a candidate for the chromosome 9p melanoma susceptibility locus. Nat Genet 1994; 8:22–26.
108. Newton Bishop JA. IL-15 The genetics of susceptibility to melanoma. Pigment Cell Res 2003; 16:578–579.
109. Nowell PC. The clonal evolution of tumor cell populations. Science 1976; 194:23.
110. Tran TP, Titus-Ernstoff L, Perry AE, Ernstoff MS, Newsham IF. Alteration of chromosome 9p21 and/or p16 in benign and dysplastic nevi suggests a role in early melanoma progression (United States). Cancer Causes Control 2002; 13:675–682.
111. Rocco JW, Sidransky D. p16(Mts-1/cdkn2/ink4a) in cancer progression. Exp Cell Res 2001; 264:42–55.
112. Ghiorzo P, Villaggio B, Sementa AR, et al. Expression and localization of mutant p16 proteins in melanocytic lesions from familial melanoma patients. Hum Pathol 2004; 35:25–33.

8

Epidemiology of Nonmelanocytic Skin Cancer

Richard P. Gallagher

Division of Dermatology and Cancer Control Research Program, British Columbia Cancer Agency, and Department of Health Care and Epidemiology, University of British Columbia, Vancouver, British Columbia, Canada

Tim K. Lee

Cancer Control Research Program, British Columbia Cancer Agency, Vancouver, and School of Computing Sciences, Simon Fraser University, Burnaby, British Columbia, Canada

Chris D. Bajdik

Cancer Control Research Program, British Columbia Cancer Agency, Vancouver, and Department of Health Care and Epidemiology, University of British Columbia, Vancouver, British Columbia, Canada

INTRODUCTION

Nonmelanocytic cancers of the skin are the most common malignancies worldwide and are particularly frequent in fair-skin populations. This review will describe the incidence in different populations, as well as discuss current knowledge concerning risk factors for the two most common types of the disease: basal cell carcinoma (BCC) and squamous cell carcinoma (SCC).

DESCRIPTIVE EPIDEMIOLOGY

Incidence

Cutaneous malignant melanoma is consistently recorded by cancer registries throughout the world and has been for at least 50 years, although there have been some concerns about underascertainment in more recent times (1–3). However, nonmelanocytic cancers are often not recorded by cancer registries. This is due to several reasons. First, these malignancies are rarely life-threatening. Secondly, these cancers are so numerous in fair-skin populations that their numbers amount to nearly 50% of the frequency of life-threatening cancers (4). Finally, it is likely that some proportion of these lesions are removed in physician offices, but do not go to pathological diagnosis, the main source of reports to cancer registries. Thus, rates from the few cancer registries that record these lesions should be regarded as minimal incidence estimates (5). Notwithstanding these concerns, incidence data from the few registry sources that collect it have proven very useful for assessing secular trends in incidence of BCC and SCC. This is especially true in jurisdictions with "socialized" medical plans, in which the entire population has access to uniform quality of diagnosis and treatment under a prepaid scheme. Because of the likelihood of registries missing cases, however, registry rates, as noted earlier, are likely to underestimate true incidence. For the same reason, registries are unlikely to be able to provide good prevalence estimates; in addition, many lesions may never be seen by practitioners and consequently remain unrecorded.

Perhaps the best way to accurately establish true incidence and prevalence rates of BCC and SCC in fair-skin population is through special periodic skin cancer surveys. Such surveys have been carried out at various times in the United States (6). Alternatively, enrollment of cohorts of adults from "normal" populations with longitudinal follow-up has also proven a practical way of estimating true incidence (7,8).

Secular Trends

Incidence rates of both BCC and SCC appear to have risen substantially in the white populations over the past 30 years. Registry data from North America indicate there was a annual increase in incidence of BCC of about 2% to 3% per year between 1960 and 2000 in the Canadian province of Manitoba and increases of similar magnitude in SCC (9). A similar pattern has been seen in British Columbia, Canada (10). Incidence rates in the United States also rose dramatically (11). The New Hampshire data showed an annual increase in BCC of 4% in both males and females from the period 1979–1980 to the period 1993–1994. Increases of 9% in males and 11% in females were seen for SCC. Even greater increases in incidence were seen for SCC in Rochester, Minnesota in the United States (12). In New Mexico, a high sunlight area in the United States, substantial increases in the incidence of both BCC and SCC have been seen over the period 1977–1999 (13).

In Australia, increases of greater magnitude (8% annually for BCC in both sexes; 6% and 7% for SCC in females and males, respectively) were seen over a 10-year period from 1978 to 1987 (14).

European countries have also experienced rising incidence rates for BCC and SCC. Nonmelanoma skin cancer (NMSC), and particularly BCC, increased in Finland during the time period 1956–1995, even though the overall rates were lower than those reported elsewhere in Europe (15). The Swiss canton of Vaud showed an increase in both types of skin cancer from 1976 to 1985 (16). However, more recently (1993–1998), trends in SCC incidence were reported to be leveling off, whereas BCC continued to rise (17). A similar trend in recent years was also reported for the canton of Neuchatel, with perhaps a decline in SCC (18).

Although, there is some evidence that melanoma incidence rates may be leveling in young men, and declining among young women (19), a recent paper suggests that both SCC and BCC may be actually increasing in U.S. women under the age of 40 (20). Caution is needed in interpreting the results of the U.S. paper, as the number of tumors per year on which the results were based is relatively small.

Geographic Variation

There is a substantial variation in the published rates of BCC and SCC in white populations; however, much of the variation in incidence is due to methods of data collection. Some data come from cancer registries and most are collected passively, whereas other data come from special surveys. As noted earlier, rates of BCC and SCC recorded in skin cancer surveys always exceed the rates reported by cancer registries. Skin pigmentation, a risk factor for SCC and BCC, also differs by geography and by population. In general, geographic differences in reported rates cannot be taken to be indicative of true underlying differences in SCC and BCC between different countries.

However, several special surveys conducted within countries with large susceptible (fair skin) populations can give some clues. In general, rates were found to be higher in U.S. whites, who reside in southern areas (with higher ambient UVB radiation levels) than in northern areas, in the special survey conducted in 1977–1978 (6). A similar trend with higher incidence rates closer to the equator is also seen in Australia (21). The information from both these countries was obtained through special surveys, in which data were collected in uniform ways over a short period of time with good quality control.

Gender and Anatomic Site Differences in Basal and Squamous Cell Carcinoma

Virtually, all data on incidence of BCC and SCC show overall rates to be higher in males than in females (6,7,9,10–18), although the male excess is more pronounced for SCC than BCC. Males have higher rates overall, prior to age 30–35, whereas BCC may be more common in females (20,22). A similar phenomenon is seen in cutaneous malignant melanoma—higher rates in females as young adults, with a male predominance after this age (23). Of concern, however, is the finding that rates of BCC in young women (<age 40) appear to be increasing at a faster rate than in men of the same age, particularly since 1990 (9,20). If this is real, and not due simply to females seeking care more consistently than males, and if the sex-specific incidence differences carry through to later life, the overall gender pattern in BCC may change dramatically in the next 20 years.

Both SCC and BCC occur predominantly on constantly sun-exposed sites such as the head and neck in both sexes (7,10,24). However, the rates of SCC on the face, head, and neck are substantially higher among males than among females (9,24). Rates of SCC on other anatomic sites (upper limbs, lower limbs, and trunk) are similar in males and females.

The relative differences in rates of BCC on the head and neck between males and females are much less pronounced than that seen in SCC. BCC also occurs with some frequency on the trunk (an intermittently sun-exposed site) in both males and females, although rates are higher in males. On the upper and lower limbs, BCC incidence rates are similar in females and males (9,24). There is some evidence that different histological subtypes of BCC may have slightly different site distributions and different mean ages at diagnosis, perhaps suggesting somewhat different etiologic relationships with sun exposure (25). Collection of individual susceptibility information and sunlight exposure history in a case-control manner would be of value in investigating this hypothesis.

ANALYTIC EPIDEMIOLOGY: HOST SUSCEPTIBILITY FACTORS

Pigmentation and Host Factors

Individuals with light skin and hair color are at elevated risk for both BCC and SCC (8,26–30) in countries with predominantly "fair" populations. The relationship also appears to hold for Mediterranean populations, where skin color tends to be darker overall (31,32). Light-colored eyes (blue or gray) appear to be better independent discriminators of risk in Mediterranean countries than in populations with fair skin, such as Australia and North America (31–33).

Cutaneous melanin density measured on a non-sun-exposed site (upper inner arm) by a skin-reflectance spectrometer set to read at 400 and 420 nm wavelength appears to be a stronger predictor of risk of both BCC and SCC than skin color, at least in males (34). More research using these newer tools may reveal more about the relationship between skin type and subsequent cancer than the simple skin tone comparisons done to date. Ethnic status may have an effect on risk of nonmelanocytic skin cancer, independent of skin color and other pigmentation factors (28), at least for BCC. This may be because measures of host susceptibility such as skin color are relatively crude, and when placed in a multivariate model cannot account for all the variations in risk that ethnic status carries, but it also may indicate that other (perhaps genetic) information is carried in "ethnic status," which deserves attention. Sun sensitivity is more pronounced in individuals at elevated risk of BCC and SCC (8,28–32,35), as is the presence of freckling (8,26–28).

Pigmented Lesions and Indicators of Solar Damage

Skin freckling appears to be a risk factor for both BCC and SCC in most studies in light skin populations (8,26–28,35). In Mediterranean populations, however, this appears not to be the case, at least for BCC (31,36). The presence of multiple melanocytic nevi is associated with increased risk for BCC in light skin populations (8,28) and perhaps Mediterranean populations also (31). There is little indication that melanocytic nevi are related to risk of SCC (28,35).

Presence of actinic keratoses, indicators of solar skin damage, and potential precursor lesions for SCC are, not surprisingly, more prevalent on those who develop SCC in light skin populations (8,28,35) and may also predict risk of BCC (28). In Mediterranean populations, actinic keratoses also appear to be risk factors for BCC (31,36). Of interest is a recent longitudinal study of individuals with a high prevalence of solar keratoses at enrollment, but no skin cancers. Examination of pigmentation variables, sun sensitivity, nevi, and other factors demonstrated that only increased age independently predicted occurrence of a BCC within five years of follow-up and only age and red hair color predicted occurrence of SCC (37). This suggests that the presence of solar keratoses is an important easily detected risk indicator for both nonmelanocytic skin cancers. This may have public health implications in the control and prevention of skin cancers.

Solar elastosis, an indicator of heavy solar exposure, is also an indicator of risk for SCC and BCC (8,28). Evidence for the value of solar lentigines, as an indicator of skin cancer risk, is mixed. When assessed on the arm (an intermittently exposed body site), one study appeared to indicate a modest elevated risk of BCC (36). However, when the same study assessed on the face (a constantly exposed site), they did not appear to predict risk. Kricker et al. (28) found them to be associated with neither BCC nor SCC.

Family History and Genetic Associations with Basal and Squamous Cell Carcinoma

Reported Family History of Basal and Squamous Cell Carcinoma

A number of investigations have shown an elevated risk of either BCC or SCC in subjects reporting a family history of skin cancer (31,38–40). Risk estimates for reported presence of a family history are variable; and questions used to elicit data sometimes fail to distinguish between history of nonmelanocytic skin cancer and cutaneous melanoma. In addition, most family history reports are not verified—thus the risk estimates must be treated with some caution.

Xeroderma Pigmentosum

Xeroderma pigmentosum (XP) is a rare genetic condition, which is transmitted in an autosomal recessive pattern, and affects from one in 25,000 to one in 40,000 newborns depending on ethnicity. The disease results in acute UV sensitivity, neurodegenerative changes, and premature aging. The defective gene is involved in repairing DNA damage that results from UV exposure. Those with XP must be carefully protected from solar UV radiation from birth because of their substantially increased risk of cutaneous melanoma, BCC, and SCC (41–44). Owing to its rarity, the condition contributes little to the population burden of nonmelanocytic skin cancer.

Basal Cell Nevus Syndrome

Basal cell nevus syndrome is a mutation in chromosome 9q22.3, transmitted as an autosomal dominant disorder, and characterized by multiple BCCs, skeletal abnormalities, palmoplantar pits, and epidermoid cysts (45,46). The condition is uncommon (one in 60,000) and does not account for a significant proportion of BCCs. However, investigation has indicated that loss of heterozygosity at 9q22.3 is also present in sporadic BCCs, suggesting that the "patched" gene, when intact, functions as a tumor suppressor (47).

Other Genetic Predictors of Risk

There are several genes for which a germline variation affects risk of nonmelanocytic skin cancer. The simplest form of variation is a single nucleotide polymorphism (SNP).

The DNA repair gene XRCC1 encodes a protein involved in the DNA repair pathway, specifically with the repair of single-strand DNA breaks, including those caused by ionizing and nonionizing (UV) radiation. A large case-control study in the U.S.A. found that certain SNPs in XRCC1 are associated with a reduced risk of both SCC and BCC and that the effect of sunburn on SCC risk may be mediated by a specific XRCC1 genotype (48).

The melanocortin receptor gene (MC1R) helps determine skin and hair color. Two SNPs are associated with an increased risk of both SCC and BCC, whereas other SNPs appear to be associated with phenotypic traits (light skin and red hair color) that are related to NMSC risk (49,50). Recent evidence from Tasmania confirmed that MC1R is associated with both SCC and BCC, but in the presence of information on skin color and sun sensitivity, MC1R genotype did not appear to improve prediction of disease risk (51).

The glutathione-S-transferase (GST) family of genes help detoxify mutagenic compounds induced by UV exposure. A study of renal transplant patients in the U.K. found an association between GSTP1 and SCC risk (52). A more recent study of renal transplant patients in Australia found that specific GSTM1 and GSTM3 were also associated with SCC risk; and GSTT1 and GSTP1 interacted with the immunosuppressive drug prednisolone to affect both SCC and BCC risks (53).

ANALYTIC EPIDEMIOLOGY: UV RADIATION EXPOSURE

Solar UV Exposure

Residence History and Ambient Solar Exposure

Several lines of evidence from epidemiological studies suggest that ambient solar UV is a risk factor for BCC and SCC, the most basic coming from studies of latitude and incidence. Scotto and Fears (6) in their 1977–1978 survey of nonmelanocytic skin cancer found that incidence rates were directly correlated with the indices of solar UVB. The latitude gradient was somewhat stronger for SCC than for BCC, suggesting some differences in the relationship of the two types to sun exposure. Similar results were later seen with distance to the equator in Australian studies (21).

Studies of female migrants within the U.S.A. who have moved to a state with high sunlight from a state with low sunlight showed a reduced risk of SCC compared with individuals who have lived their lives in high sunlight states (35,54), but the same effect is not seen for BCC, at least among male migrants (55). Migrants to Australia who arrived after age nine showed a much lower risk of BCC (28) and SCC (35).

Exposure Implied from Anatomic Site of the Tumor

The U.S. skin cancer survey (6) showed a predominance of SCCs on constantly sun-exposed sites. BCCs demonstrated a pattern similar to SCC, but the differences between constantly and intermittently exposed sites were less pronounced than those seen for SCC. Similarly, Armstrong et al. (56) showed that the "density" (incidence per unit surface area) of both SCC and BCC was highest on usually sun-exposed sites, intermediate on occasionally sun-exposed sites, and lowest on rarely sun-exposed sites. Again, the density gradient was more pronounced for SCC than for BCC, among both males and females.

Recalled Sun Exposure History

Early studies of the relationship between sun exposure and BCC or SCC (6) suggested a linear relationship between solar UV exposure and risk. However, when analytic studies were conducted with adequate control for pigmentation and host susceptibility factors, the results suggested that the patterns of solar UV exposure were different for BCC and SCC.

Basal cell carcinoma: The Australian case-control data (57) showed an increasing risk of BCC with intermittent or recreational sun exposure, between ages 15 and 19. Little evidence of association was seen with recreational exposure patterns at later ages. Data from a Canadian study conducted in the province of Alberta showed a similar association with early life recreational exposure (age 0–19), but no relationship with lifetime mean annual recreational exposure (26). Neither the Australian nor the Canadian study showed an association with occupational sun exposure. A study conducted in a Southern European population (58) demonstrated a relationship between sun exposure during beach holidays taken in childhood and a similar association with lifetime holiday exposure (again largely beach exposure). Several Italian studies also showed an increased risk of BCC with beach sun exposure before age 20 (31,36) with no increase in risk seen for recreational exposure after age 20 or with occupational sun exposure.

In the Canadian and Australian studies, risk was largely confined to those who had difficulty tanning, whereas in the European study, risk among poor tanners appeared to plateau after relatively little holiday exposure but a linear response was seen in good tanners with increasing holiday sun.

Squamous cell carcinoma: Patterns of recalled sun exposure in subjects who develop SCC differ from those seen for individuals with BCC. English et al. (59), in Australia, found a relationship between risk of SCC and total sun exposure to the site at which the tumor developed, although the risk appeared to drop off slightly in those with the highest exposure. Gallagher et al. (27), in Canada, showed a similar increasing risk of SCC with occupational sun exposure, particularly in 10 years prior to diagnosis. The Southern European study (58) showed an increased risk of SCC with lifetime occupational sun exposure. None of the studies demonstrated a significant relationship between SCC and recreational sun exposure or activities.

In summary, the recalled pattern of sun exposure that predisposes to BCC appears to be similar to that seen in cutaneous melanoma. There is an increased risk with intermittent solar exposure, particularly that accrued early in life, but no increase in risk with chronic occupational exposure or with cumulative exposure (recreational plus occupational). SCC, on the contrary, appears to be related to constant occupational or cumulative exposure, with little or no increase resulting from the intermittent exposure accrued during outdoor recreation. A recent detailed review of solar exposure and the three major types of skin cancer suggest that pattern and amount of solar exposure operate independently. For cutaneous melanoma and BCC, risk increases monotonically with increasing intermittency of exposure if the amount is held constant and also increases monotonically with the amount of exposure, if degree of intermittency is held constant (60). SCC is dependent on the cumulative amount of sun exposure, but not on the degree of intermittency of that exposure.

Sunburn as an Indicator of Solar Exposure

Episodes of sunburn may be viewed as indicators of high solar exposure and provide an indication of the time of life when the heaviest sun exposure (particularly recreational exposure) took place. Several systematic reviews of sun exposure and cutaneous melanoma have shown the relationship with recalled episodes of sunburn to be at least as strong as that with recalled recreational sun exposure (61,62). Risk of BCC increases with episodes of sunburn at any age (30,55,57) and when restricted to those occurring in early life in most (26,29,30,31), but not all (36) studies.

Relationship of lifetime sunburn history to SCC is inconsistent. The study of Grodstein et al. (54) found an association with lifetime sunburn index and that of Gallagher et al. (27) with burns in the decade prior to diagnosis; but other studies have not found an association with recent or lifetime sunburns (29). An association with severe or "blistering" sunburn was found in the Australian study of English et al. (59), but none with overall sunburn history. An association with severe childhood sunburn (causing pain for two or more days) was seen in the Canadian study (27), but no association with overall sunburn history as a child was detected. The European study also showed no association between childhood or lifetime sunburn history and SCC (29).

In summary, a positive association between childhood sunburn history and BCC seen in studies from various parts of the world is fairly consistent and mirrors the importance of reported childhood sun exposure in accounting for risk. Lifetime sunburn history may be less important. In SCC, there is little evidence that lifetime or childhood sunburn history is important in accounting for risk of SCC.

Artificial UV Exposure

There are relatively few studies of nonmelanocytic skin cancer and artificial UV exposure. A recent American study demonstrated a fairly strong association between use of tanning lamps and SCC, with more than a doubling of risk of this disease (63). A more modest elevated risk was seen for BCC. One of the earlier studies also showed a substantially increased risk of SCC with use of sunlamps (64); however, this must be treated with caution due to wide confidence intervals around the point estimate of risk. Two other studies did not demonstrate an increased risk of either SCC or BCC with use of sunlamps (30,65). Power to detect associations was limited in the negative studies because of low exposure prevalence.

Medical use of artificial UV, in the form of either psoralen + UVA, or use of UVB to treat severe psoriasis increases risk of both BCC and SCC (66,67), and the increased risk appears to persist even 15 years after discontinuing treatment, at least for psoralen + UVA (68).

OTHER FACTORS

Although at least 85% of BCCs and SCCs are thought to be caused by UVR exposure (69), a number of other factors have been found to be associated with risk of nonmelanocytic skin cancer. For the most part, these exposures separately account for very small proportions of these cancers.

Physical and Chemical Exposures

Exposure to ionizing radiation appears to increase risk of nonmelanocytic skin cancer (70–73). Although this association is seen relatively consistently, the exposure itself is relatively rare.

Exposure to arsenic increases risk of BCC (74), and both BCC and SCC (75), although risks in the U.S. study appear to be modest. A variety of occupational exposures may also increase risk of nonmelanocytic skin cancer; however, the population attributable risk from each of the exposures is likely to be small.

Immune Compromise

Renal transplant recipients are known to be at increased risk of nonmelanocytic skin cancer (76–78). Persons with HIV/AIDS are also at a substantially elevated risk and the advent of the HAART therapy may actually increase this risk further by virtue of increasing life-expectancy and consequent time-at-risk (79). Individuals previously diagnosed with non-Hodgkin lymphoma (NHL) may be at elevated risk of subsequent SCC and those previously diagnosed with SCC are at increased risk of subsequent NHL (80). In addition, a two-fold risk of NHL has been seen in a cohort of 11,878 BCC patients (81). These findings indicate that immune compromise in any form can increase risk of nonmelanocytic skin cancer.

SUMMARY

BCC and SCC of the skin together constitute the most common form of cancer in countries with the Caucasian populations. Although they rarely become life-threatening, treatment can result in disfigurement and substantial morbidity. Costs for treatment will become a major burden on healthcare systems in Western countries, as life expectancy continues to rise in the 21st century. It is well known that the principal causes of these tumors are phenotypic susceptibility factors and exposure to solar UV radiation. Efforts to stem the rising incidence rates by simply advising people to avoid UV exposure by reducing outdoor activities may have unanticipated adverse consequences such as increased obesity because of the lack of physical activity and vitamin D deficiency in certain groups.

In the near future, more research will be needed to try to estimate the reduction in UV exposure necessary to reduce risk of skin cancer without incurring other health problems. Skin cancer prevention programs also need to be constantly evaluated, and public health messages examined in light of the latest scientific evidence, in order to ensure that they are having only positive effects on human health.

REFERENCES

1. Karagas MR, Thomas DB, Roth GJ, et al. The effects of changes in health care delivery on the reported incidence of cutaneous melanoma in Washington State. Am J Epidemiol 1991; 133:58–62.
2. Koh HJ, Clapp RW, Barnett JM, et al. Systematic underreporting of cutaneous malignant melanoma in Massachusets. J Am Acad Dermatol 1991; 24:545–550.
3. Melia J, Frost T, Graham-Brown R, et al. Problems with registration of cutaneous malignant melanoma in England. Br J Cancer 1995; 72:224–228.
4. National Cancer Institute of Canada. Canadian Cancer Statistics, Toronto, Canada April 2005, p. 24.
5. Gallagher RP, Lee TK. Assessing incidence rates and secular trends in nonmelanocytic skin cancer: which method is best? J Cutan Med Surg 1998; 3:35–39.
6. Scotto J, Fears TR. Incidence of non-melanoma skin cancer in the United States. National Institutes of Health Publication 83-2433, Washington D.C.: U.S. Dept of Health and Human Services, 1983.
7. Kricker A, English DR, Heenan PJ, Randell PL, et al. Skin cancer in Geraldton, Western Australia: a survey of incidence and prevalence. Med J Aust 1990; 152:399–407.
8. Green A, Battistutta D, Hart V, et al. and the Nambour Study Group. Skin cancer in a subtropical Australian population: incidence and lack of association with occupation. Am J Epidemiol 1996; 144:1034–1040.
9. Demers AA, Nugent Z, Mihalcioiu C, et al. Trends of nonmelanoma skin cancer from 1960–2000 in a Canadian population. J Am Acad Dermatol 2005; 53:320–327.
10. Gallagher RP, Ma B, McLean DI, et al. Trends in basal cell carcinoma, squamous cell carcinoma, and melanoma of the skin from 1973–1987. J Am Acad Dermatol 1990; 23:413–421.
11. Karagas MR, Greenberg ER, Spencer SK, et al. for the New Hampshire Skin Cancer Study Group. Increase in incidence rates of basal cell and squamous cell skin cancer in New Hampshire, U.S.A. Int J Cancer 1999; 81:555–559.
12. Gray DT, Suman VJ, Su WP, et al. Trends in the population-based incidence of squamous cell carcinoma of the skin first diagnosed between 1984 and 1992. Arch Dermatol 1997; 133:735–740.
13. Athas WF, Hunt WC, Key CR. Changes in nonmelanoma skin cancer incidence between 1977–1978 and 1998–1999 in Northcentral New Mexico. CEPB 2003; 12:1105–1108.
14. Kaldor J, Shugg D, Young B, et al. Non-melanoma skin cancer: ten years of cancer-registry-based surveillance. Int J Cancer 1991; 53:886–891.
15. Hannuksela-Svahn A, Pukkala E, Karvonnen K. Basal cell skin cancer and other non-melanoma skin cancers in Finland 1956–1995. Arch Dermatol 1999; 135:781–786.
16. Levi F, LaVecchia C, Te V-C, Mezzanotte G. Descriptive epidemiology of skin cancer in the Swiss Canton of Vaud. Int J Cancer 1998; 42:811–816.
17. Levi F, Te V-C, Randimbison L, Erler G, LaVecchia C. Trends in skin cancer in Vaud: an update, 1976–1998. Eur J Cancer Prev 2001; 10:371–373.
18. Levi F, Erler G, Te V-C, et al. Trends in skin cancer incidence in Neuchatel, 1976–1998. Tumori 2001; 87:288–289.
19. Marrett LD, Nguyen HL, Armstrong BK. Trends in incidence of cutaneous malignant melanoma in New South Wales, 1983–1996. Int J Cancer 2001; 92:457–462.

20. Christensen LJ, Borrowman TA, Vachon CM, et al. Incidence of basal cell and squamous cell carcinoma in a population younger than 40 years. JAMA 2005; 294:681–690.
21. Giles GG, Marks R, Foley P. Incidence of non-melanocytic skin cancer treated in Australia. BMJ 1988; 296:13–17.
22. Cox NH. Basal cell carcinoma in young adults. Br J Dermatol 1992; 127:26–29.
23. Parkin DM, Whelan SL, Ferlay J, et al. Cancer Incidence in 5 Continents, Vol. VII. Lyon: IARC Press, International Agency for Research on Cancer, 1997.
24. Osterlind A, Hou-Jensen K, Jensen OM. Incidence of cutaneous malignant melanoma in Denmark, 1978–1982. Anatomic site distribution, histologic types, and comparison with non-melanoma skin cancer. Br J Cancer 1988; 58:385–391.
25. McCormack CJ, Kelly JW, Dorevitch AP. Differences in age and body site distribution of the histological subtypes of basal cell carcinoma; a possible indicator of differing causes. Arch Dermatol 1997; 133:593–596.
26. Gallagher RP, Hill GB, Bajdik CD, et al. Sunlight exposure, pigmentary factors and risk of nonmelanocytic skin cancer I. Basal cell carcinoma. Arch Dermatol 1995; 101:157–163.
27. Gallagher RP, Hill GB, Bajdik CD, et al. Sunlight exposure, pigmentation factors and risk of nonmelanocytic skin cancer II. Squamous cell carcinoma. Arch Dermatol 1995; 131:164–169.
28. Kricker A, Armstrong BK, English DR, et al. Pigmentary and cutaneous risk factors for non-melanocytic skin cancer—a case-control study. Int J Cancer 1991; 48:650–662.
29. Zanetti R, Rosso S, Martinez C, et al. The multicentre south European study "Helios" I: skin characteristics and sunburns in basal cell and squamous cell carcinoma of the skin. Br J Cancer 1996; 73:1440–1446.
30. Rosso S, Joris F, Zanetti R. Risk of basal and squamous cell carcinomas of the skin in Sion, Switzerland: a case-control study. Tumori 1999; 85:435–442.
31. Naldi L, DiLandro A, D'Avenzo B, et al. Host-related and environmental risk factors for cutaneous basal cell carcinoma; evidence from an Italian case-control study. J Am Acad Dermatol 2000; 42:446–452.
32. Khwsky FE, Bedwani R, D'Avanzo B, et al. Risk factors for non-melanonomatous skin cancer in Alexandria Egypt. Int J Cancer 1994; 56:375–378.
33. Suarez-Varela MM, Gonzalez AL, Caraco EF. Non-melanoma skin cancer: a case–control study on risk factors and protective measures. J Environ Pathol Toxicol Oncology 1996; 15:255–261.
34. Dwyer T, Blizzard L, Ashbolt R, et al. Cutaneous melanin density of Caucasians measured by spectrophotometry, and risk of malignant melanoma, basal cell carcinoma, and squamous cell carcinoma of the skin. Am J Epidemiol 2002; 155:614–621.
35. English DR, Armstrong BK, Kricker A, et al. Demographic characteristics, pigmentary and cutaneous risk factors for squamous cell carcinoma of the skin: a case-control study. Int J Cancer 1998; 76:628–634.
36. Corona R, Dogliotti W, D'Errico M, et al. Risk factors for basal cell carcinoma in a Mediterranean population—role of recreational sun exposure early in life. Arch Dermatol 2001; 137:1162–1168.
37. Foote JA, Harris RB, Giuliano AR, et al. Predictors for cutaneous basal and squamous cell carcinoma among actinically damaged adults. Int J Cancer 2001; 95:7–11.
38. Gafa L, Filippazzo MG, Tumino R, et al. Risk factors of nonmelanoma skin cancer in Ragusa Sicily: a case-control study. CCC 1991; 2:395–399.

39. Hogan DJ, To T, Gran L, et al. Risk factors for basal cell carcinoma. Int J Dermatol 1989; 28:591–594.
40. Herity B, O'Loughlin G, Moriarty MJ, Conroy R. Risk factors for non-melanoma skin cancer. Irish Med J 1989; 82:151–152.
41. Kraemer KH, Lee MM, Scotto J. Xeroderma pigmentosum. Cutaneous, ocular, and neurologic abnormalities in 830 published cases. Arch Dermatol 1987; 123:241–250.
42. Han J, Colditz GA, Liu JS, Hunter DJ. Genetic variation in XPD, sun exposure, and the risk of skin cancer. Cancer Epidemiol Biomarkers Prev 2005; 14:1539–1544.
43. Dybdahl M, Vogel U, Frentz G, et al. Polymorphisms in the DNA repair gene *XPD*: correlations with risk and age at onset of basal cell carcinoma. Cancer Epidemiol Biomarkers Prev 1999; 8:77–81.
44. Vogel U, Hedayati M, Dybdahl M, et al. Polymorphisms of the DNA repair gene *XPD*: correlations with the risk of basal cell carcinoma revisited. Carcinogenesis 2001; 22:899–904.
45. Compton JG, Goldstein AM, Turner M, et al. Fine mapping of the locus for nevoid basal cell carcinoma syndrome on chromosome 9q. Arch Dermatol 1994; 103:178–181.
46. Gorlin RJ, Goltz RW. Multiple nevoid basal cell epithelioma, jaw cysts, and bifid rib: a syndrome. N Engl J Med 1960; 262:908–912.
47. Gailani MR, Bale AE. Developmental genes and cancer: role of patched in basal cell carcinoma of the skin. J Natl Cancer Inst 1997; 89:1103–1109.
48. Nelson HH, Kelsey KT, Mott LA, Karagas MR. The XRCC1 Arg399Gln polymorphism, sunburn and non-melanoma skin cancer; evidence of a gene-environment interaction. Cancer Res 2002; 62:152–155.
49. Box NF, Duffy DL, Irving RE, et al. Melanocortin-1 receptor genotype is a risk factor for both basal and squamous cell carcinoma. J Invest Dermatol 2001; 116:224–229.
50. Bastiaens MT, Huurne AC, Kielich C, et al. Melanocortin-1 receptor gene variants determine the risk of nonmelanoma skin cancer independently of fair skin and red hair. Am J Hum Genet 2001; 68:884–894.
51. Dwyer T, Stankovich JM, Blizzard L, et al. Does the addition of information on genotype improve prediction of the risk of melanoma and nonmelanoma skin cancer beyond that obtained from skin phenotype? Am J Epidemiol 2004; 159:826–833.
52. Marshall SE, Bordea C, Haldar NA, et al. Glutathione S-transferase polymorphisms and skin cancer after renal transplantation. Kidney Int 2000; 58:2186–2193.
53. Fryer AA, Ramsay HM, Lovatt TJ, et al. Polymorphisms in glutathione S-transferases and non-melanoma skin cancer risk in Australian renal transplant recipients. Carcinogenesis 2005; 26:185–191.
54. Grodstein F, Speizer FE, Hunter DJ. A prospective study of incident squamous cell carcinoma of the skin in the Nurses' Health Study. J Natl Cancer Inst 1995; 87:1061–1066.
55. van Dam RM, Huang Z, Rimm E, et al. Risk factors for basal cell carcinoma of the skin in men: results from the Health Professional Follow-up study. Am J Epidemiol 1999; 150:459–468.
56. Armstrong BK, Kricker A, English DR. Sun exposure and skin cancer. Aust J Dermatol 1997; 38:s1–s6.
57. Kricker A, Armstrong BK, English DR, Heenan PJ. Does intermittent sun exposure cause basal cell carcinoma? A case-control study in Western Australia. Int J Cancer 1995; 60:489–494.

58. Rosso S, Zanetti R, Martinez C, et al. The multicentre south European study "Helios" II: different sun exposure patterns in the etiology of basal cell and squamous cell carcinomas of the skin. Br J Cancer 1996; 73:1447–1453.

59. English DR, Armstrong BK, Kricker A, et al. Case-control study of sun exposure and squamous cell carcinoma of the skin. Int J Cancer 1998; 77:347–353.

60. Armstrong BK. How sun exposure causes skin cancer: an epidemiological perspective. In: Hill D, Elwood JM, English DR, eds. Prevention of Skin Cancer. Dordrecht: Kluwer Academic Publishers, 2004:89–116.

61. Gandini A, Sera F, Cattaruzza MS, et al. Meta-analysis of risk factors for cutaneous melanoma: II sun exposure. Eur J Cancer 2004; 41:45–60.

62. Elwood JM, Jopson J. Melanoma and sun exposure: an overview of published studies. Int J Cancer 1997; 73:198–203.

63. Karagas MR, Stannard VA, Mott LA, et al. Use of tanning devices and risk of basal cell and squamous cell carcinoma. J Natl Cancer Inst 2002; 94:224–226.

64. Aubrey F, MacGibbon B. Risk of squamous cell carcinoma of the skin; a case-control study in the Montreal area. Cancer 1985; 55:907–911.

65. Bajdik CD, Gallagher RP, Astrakianakis G, et al. Non-solar ultraviolet radiation and risk of basal and squamous cell skin cancer. Br J Cancer 1996; 73:1612–1614.

66. Stern RS, Laird N for the Photochemotherapy Follow-up Study. The carcinogenic risk of treatments for severe psoriasis. Cancer 1994; 73:2759–2764.

67. Lim JL, Stern RS. High levels of ultraviolet B exposure increase the risk of non-melanoma skin cancer in psoralen and ultraviolet A treated patients. J Invest Dermatol 2005; 24:505–513.

68. Nijsten TE, Stern RS. The increased risk of skin cancer is persistent after discontinuation of psoralen + UVA: a cohort study. J Invest Dermatol 2003; 12:252–258.

69. Armstrong BK, Kricker A. Skin cancer. Dermatol Clin 1995; 13:583–594.

70. Ron E, Modan B, Preston D, et al. Radiation-induced skin carcinomas of the head and neck. Radiat Res 1991; 125:318–325.

71. Lichter MD, Karagas MR, Mott LA, et al. Therapeutic ionizing radiation and the incidence of basal cell carcinoma and squamous cell carcinoma. The New Hampshire Skin Cancer Study Group. Arch Dermatol 2000; 136:1007–1011.

72. Sadamori N, Mine M, Honda T. Incidence of skin cancer among Nagasaki atomic bomb survivors. J Radiat Res 1991; 2(suppl):217–225.

73. Karagas MR, McDonald JA, Greenberg ER, et al. Risk of basal cell and squamous cell skin cancers after ionizing radiation therapy. For the Skin Cancer Prevention Study Group. J Natl Cancer Inst 1996; 88:1848–1853.

74. Boonchai W, Green A, Ng J, et al. Basal cell carcinoma in chronic arsenicism occurring in Queensland, Australia after ingenstion of an asthma medication. J Am Acad Dermatol 2000; 43:664–669.

75. Karagas MR, Stukel TA, Morris JS, et al. Skin cancer in relation to toenail arsenic concentrations in a US population-based case-control study. Am J Epidemiol 2001; 153:559–565.

76. Hartevelt MM, Bouwes-Bavinck JN, Kootte AMM, et al. Incidence of skin cancer after renal transplantation in the Netherlands. Transplantation 1990; 49:506–509.

77. Fuente MJ, Sabat M, Roca J, et al. A prospective study of the incidence of skin cancer and its risk factors in a Spanish Mediterranean population of kidney transplant recipients. Br J Dermatol 2003; 149:1221–1226.

78. Bordea C, Wojnarowska F, Millard PR, et al. Skin cancers in renal-transplant recipients occur more frequently than previously recognized in a temperate climate. Transplantation 2004; 77:574–579.
79. Adami J, Frisch M, Yuen J, et al. Evidence of an association between non-Hodgkins lymphoma and skin cancer. BMJ 1995; 310:1491–1495.
80. Levi F, La Vecchia C, Van-Cong T, et al. Incidence of invasive cancers following basal cell carcinoma. Int J Cancer 1998; 147:722–726.
81. Clifford GM, Polesel J, Rickenbach M, et al. Cancer risk in the Swiss HIV cohort study: associations with immunodeficiency, smoking, and highly active antiretroviral therapy. J Natl Cancer Inst 2005; 97:425–432.

9

Epidemiology of Cutaneous Malignant Melanoma

Johan Moan

Department of Radiation Biology, Institute for Cancer Research, Montebello and Department of Physics, University of Oslo, Oslo, Norway

Alina Carmen Porojnicu

Department of Radiation Biology, Institute for Cancer Research, Montebello, Oslo, Norway and Department of Biophysics and Cell Biotechnology, Carol Davila University of Medicine and Pharmacy, Bucharest, Romania

Arne Dahlback

Department of Physics, University of Oslo, Oslo, Norway

INTRODUCTION

Ultraviolet radiation (UVR) from the sun is by far the most important risk factor for nonmelanoma skin cancer, notably for squamous cell carcinoma (SCC) (1,2). Also for basal cell carcinoma (BCC), practically all investigations equivocally indicate a relationship (1,2). However, in the case of the most dangerous form of skin cancer, cutaneous malignant melanoma (CMM), the relationship is less clear and has been debated for decades (1–7). Recently, the confusion is increasing because numerous reports claim that solar radiation protects against several forms of cancer, even CMM, or at least improves their prognosis, through its production of vitamin D_3 in skin (8,9).

Our own research, mainly based on epidemiological data from Scandinavia, clearly points to a relationship, although the dose–response curve for CMM is different from that of SCC and BCC (2). Discrepancies may arise from the following two facts, in addition to UV induction of vitamin D_3: Intermittent and not accumulated sun exposure may be melanomagenic, while prolonged and moderate UV exposure may afford protection through skin thickening and melanin accumulation in the upper, dead layers of the epidermis.

After briefly reviewing the arguments in the debate, we will shed light on them and try to arrive at a conclusion in view of recent epidemiological observations. We will also consider what might be a wise message to bring to the public, one that minimizes melanoma risk and maximizes the overall vitamin D_3 status.

ARGUMENTS AGAINST AND FOR A RELATIONSHIP BETWEEN ULTRAVIOLET RADIATION AND CUTANEOUS MALIGNANT MELANOMA

The main arguments against a relationship are as follows (10–14):

- In the surroundings of many CMMs, there is little solar elastosis. Solar elastosis is related to the accumulated UV exposure.
- Epidemiological case control studies give conflicting results; some show a dependency of CMMs on UV exposure, while some even show protection.
- The localization pattern of CMMs on different parts of the body is widely different from that of SCCs. In some cases, the density of CMMs is smaller on the face than on body sites normally shielded from solar radiation, like the back.
- CMM appears to be more frequent among people in "white collar" occupations than among people in "blue collar" occupations. CMMs are relatively uncommon among farmers and fishermen.
- While BCCs and SCCs are common among albino Africans, CMMs are not.
- The incidence of CMM does not generally increase with decreasing latitude.
- The use of sunscreens is, in some investigations, correlated with increased CMM incidence rates.

The main arguments for a relationship are more numerous (2,5,10–20).

- Several recent investigations, comparing people with similar skin type, show increasing CMM incidence (or death) rates with decreasing latitude.
- CMM is more common in people with a light skin color than in people with dark skin color. Melanin absorbs UVR.
- Migration to more sunny countries increases the risk of getting CMMs.
- UVR induces pigmented nevi. CMMs sometimes arise in borders of such nevi.
- The CMM density on different body sites appears to correlate to some extent with intermittent sun exposure.

- Episodes of sunburn, notably in childhood, appear to increase the CMM risk.
- CMM patients often have low minimum erythema doses and impaired DNA repair capacity.
- Lentigo maligna melanomas (Hutchinson's melanotic freckles) are clearly related to sun exposure.
- Persons with xeroderma pigmentosum have at least a 1000 times larger risk of getting CMM than other persons.
- Some CMMs contain cells with UV fingerprint mutations.
- CMM-like tumors can be induced in some animals by UVR. Examples are *Xiphophorus* (a fish), *Monodelphis domestica* (an opossum), angora goats, Sinclair swine, and white horses.
- Patients with CMM often also have BCC.
- Psoralen + UV-A treatment of psoriasis patients seems to increase their CMM risk.
- Some investigations indicate that sunbeds users have an increased risk of CMM.

MATERIALS AND METHODS

New data presented in this work are mainly extracted from the population based Norwegian Cancer Registry. Norway is divided into 19 regions according to

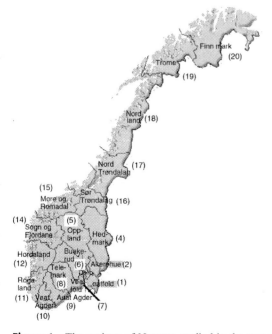

Figure 1 The regions of Norway studied in the present work.

latitude and UV exposure (Fig. 1). Whenever rates (R) are given, they are age adjusted to the European standard population. The two largest cities, Oslo and Bergen, are excluded from the study, to reduce the errors that may arise from different sun-exposure habits of urban and rural populations, although this does not seem to be of major importance for skin cancer incidence in Norway (2).

The global solar UV irradiance (i.e., direct + diffuse radiation on a horizontal surface) was calculated with a radiative transfer model (21,22). The daily total ozone column amounts measured by the TOMS instruments aboard the Nimbus-7 and Earth Probe satellites were used as input to the model. The daily cloud cover for each site used in the calculations was derived from measured reflectivities from an ozone-insensitive channel in the same satellite instruments. Notably, the coastal regions (Regions 11–15, Fig. 1) are cloudier than the inland areas (Regions 1,2,4–6,8, Fig. 1). The effect of snow cover at different regions in Norway was estimated by comparing the calculations with UV measurements from the Norwegian UV monitoring network. The calculated annual UV exposures in this chapter are based on available satellite measurements in the period 1980–2000.

The fluences of carcinogenic UVR from the sun were determined under the assumption that the action spectrum of CMM is similar to the CIE reference spectrum for human erythema (2). For considerations of north–south gradients of UV in Norway, similar results, although with slightly different slopes of the incidence curves, would have been obtained if the fish melanoma spectrum (2) had been used.

Average annual fluences are given, although the summer values (May–August) are dominant with respect to UVR. Average summer temperatures may be relevant for CMM induction and are shown as given by The Norwegian Meteorological Institute (Fig. 8).

TIME TRENDS

For the period 1980–2001, there is no significant increasing trend of the UV fluence in south Norway (Fig. 2). Thus, in agreement with earlier findings (2), if ozone depletion has occurred over these latitudes, it is not large enough to influence the UV fluence significantly. Variations in cloud cover in the summer months play a much larger role (15). The most abrupt change took place from 1997 to 1998 (Fig. 2). In fact, the fluence was 20% lower in 1998 than in 1997. For persons older than 50 years, there is no significant change of CMM incidence that can be related to this UV change. For younger women (0 to 49 years), there is a tendency of a decrease of CMM incidence from 1997 to 1998 and the following years. This may indicate a short latency time, for the last step of CMM carcinogenesis, although the observed changes are hardly significant. It has been shown that high fluences of UV during a summer increase the number and size of nevi (23).

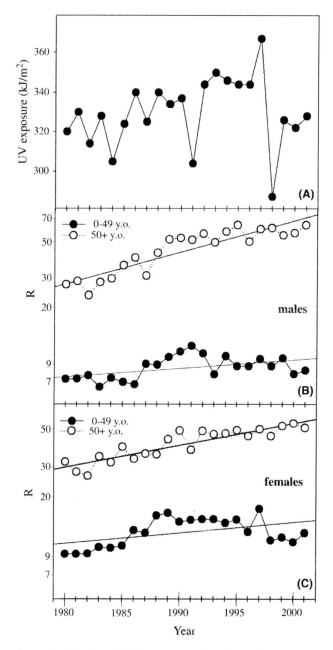

Figure 2 (**A**) Annual UV exposures from the sun in southern Norway. (**B, C**) Annual age-adjusted incidence rates for cutaneous malignant melanoma in southern Norway for men and women aged 0 to 49 years and 50+ years.

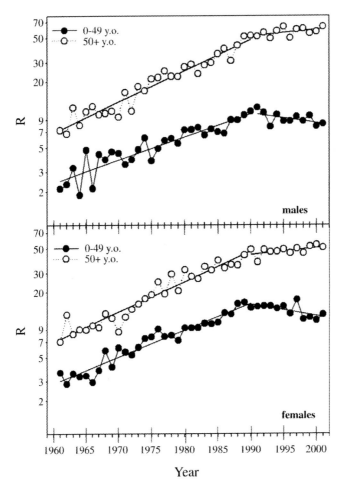

Figure 3 Annual age adjusted incidence rates as described in Figure 2, for the period 1960–2001.

For CMM, incidence data are available for a longer period (Fig. 3). Two conclusions can be drawn from these data. First, the increasing trend of the incidence rates stopped at about 1990. For the younger generation, there is even a decrease after that time. Second, for the period 1961–1990, the doubling time is longest for the younger generation (15 years for males, 14 years for females versus 11 years for older generation, for which the incidence rates are roughly similar for males and females). As can be seen from Figure 4, the ratio of the incidence rates of old (50+) to young (0 to 49) males are increasing with time, from ~2.5 in 1960 to ~6.5 in 2001 in the southern part of the country. A similar trend is found for the northern counties, although the data are more

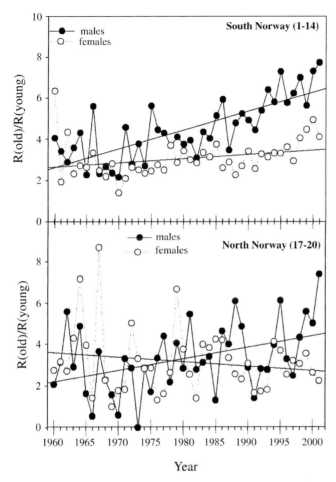

Figure 4 Similar data as shown in Figure 3, but given for south and north Norway separately. The numbers of the regions correspond to Figure 1.

scattered due to fewer annual incidences. Surprisingly, no similar trend is found for females.

From these data (Figs. 2–4), we conclude that after 1990 there has been a slight decreasing trend of the incidence rates of CMM in Norway for young people. Similar trends have been found for a number of other countries, and may indicate that the public campaigns for awareness of the carcinogenic effects of sun exposure have been successful (24). It should be remembered that the use of sunbeds has increased over the last decades. Thus, for the population as a whole, sunbeds do not yet constitute a major threat. This is not surprising, because even now relatively few persons use sunbeds or other kinds of sunbeds regularly. No conclusion concerning frequent users can be drawn from the present data.

DEPENDENCY ON LIVING STANDARD

As shown in Figure 5, the incidence rates of CMM in European countries appear to increase with increasing GDP/capita (25). GDP/capita is defined as the total gross domestic product of a country divided by its number of people, and provides a rough estimate of the living standard. This dependency is in agreement with several earlier investigations, as well as with the common view that CMM is particularly common among rich, indoor workers, and more rare among "blue collar" workers like fishermen and farmers (26,27). Such data lay credibility to the "intermittent exposure" hypothesis, which says that intermittent, high-intensity exposures, as one would get in weekends and holidays in sunny areas, are particularly dangerous with respect to CMM.

When comparing incidence rates in different countries or regions, one should be aware that significant differences might arise due to different skin types. In southern Europe (Greece, Portugal, Spain, Italy) darker skin types are certainly more frequent than in the northern countries. Thus, when Australia and New Zealand on one hand and Scandinavia on the other are compared, GDPs/capita are generally lower in the former countries (27 and 19 USD for Australia and New Zealand, respectively, versus 36 USD for Norway) (Fig. 5), skin types are presumably similar, while CMM incidence rates are factors between 2 and 3.7 larger.

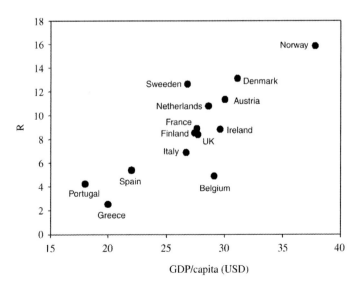

Figure 5 Cutaneous malignant melanoma incidence rates, both sexes combined, for different European countries as a function of their GDP/capita. *Abbreviation*: GDP, gross domestic product.

LATITUDE GRADIENTS

As shown in Figure 6, the incidence rates, as well as the death rates, in the major European countries decrease with increasing UV exposure. The ratios of the death rates to the incidence rates are roughly constant. The decrease of the rates with increasing latitude is certainly related to differences in skin types. Thus, when populations with fair skin are considered, there is, as earlier shown (2), a positive dose gradient (Fig. 7). The gradient of the incidence rates in Norway (Fig. 8) is larger than that for other populations. This is in agreement with earlier findings (15) and may be related to differences in sun-exposure patterns in different counties (Fig. 8). There is a significant increase, both of the death rates and of incidence rates from north to south in Norway (Fig. 8).

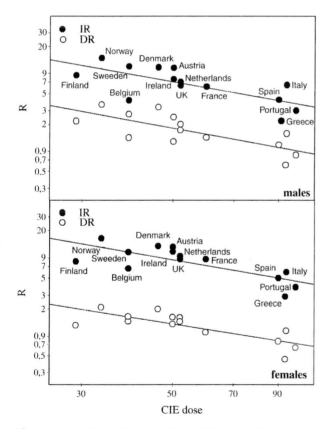

Figure 6 Incidence (●) and death (○) rates of cutaneous malignant melanoma in Europe as a function of the UV exposure from the sun, adjusted according to the CIE reference spectrum for erythema (2). The CMM incidence rates were obtained from IARC publications: *Cancer Incidence in Five Continents* (Vol. VII and Vol. VIII) and *Trends in Cancer Incidence and Mortality*. CMM death rates were obtained from WHO mortality database (75).

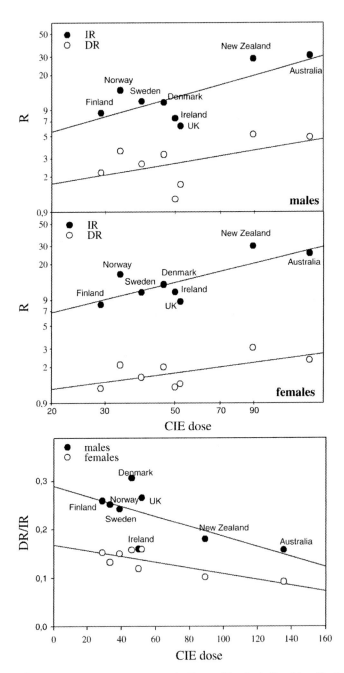

Figure 7 Similar data as shown in Figure 6 but including New Zealand and Australia and excluding south Europe where the populations have a darker skin and hair color. Data were extracted from the same source as mentioned in Figure 6.

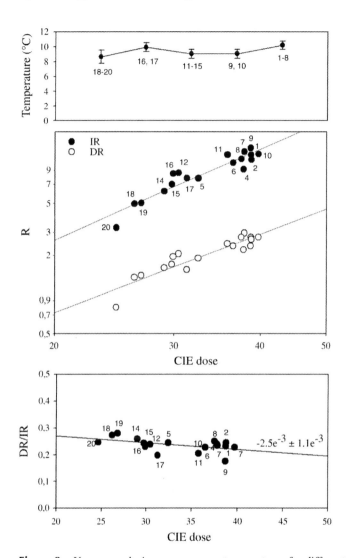

Figure 8 *Upper panel*: Average summer temperatures for different regions of Norway (1961–1990). *Middle panel*: Incidence and death rates of cutaneous malignant melanoma (1957–2001) in different counties of Norway (Fig. 1). *Lower panel*: The ratio of the death rates to the incidence rates for the same counties.

The slope for the death rate is smaller than that for the incidence rates, as also shown by the ratios of the death to the incidence rates in the lower panels of Figures 7 and 8. This may be due to higher awareness of the carcinogenic effects of the sun in populations living in high-exposure regions, resulting in earlier detection of CMMs. More likely, however, is that solar radiation has a dual effect on death rates of CMM. On one hand CMMs are induced by UVR and, on the other hand, UVR seems to improve the prognosis of CMMs (8). Such an improvement may be related to the fact that vitamin D_3 is produced in human skin by UVR (28). The level of calcidiol (25 hydroxy vitamin D_3) in most populations is higher in the summer than in the winter. We have earlier shown that this may give better prognosis for colon cancer, breast cancer, prostate cancer, and Hodgkin's lymphoma, diagnosed in seasons of high serum concentrations of calcidiol than in seasons of low concentrations of calcidiol (29–31). Temperature differences may play a role both for the carcinogenic process and for the exposure pattern. However, this probably plays an insignificant role for the Norwegian data, because the summer temperature differences are small from region to region (Fig. 8, upper panel).

Ratios of death rates to incidence rates should be interpreted with care, because there is a delay between incidence and death. However, for populations with exponential time trends in incidence increase, that is, constant doubling time (Fig. 3, 1960–1990), ratios may give useful information.

Figure 9 shows that in Norway slightly more CMM cases are diagnosed in the summer than in the winter, as recently found for Europe as a whole (32). The high number of diagnosed cases in June and the low number in July and December are probably related to vacations. For persons older than 30 years this does not have any significant influence on the prognosis, which is similar for all seasons (Fig. 9, lower panel). It is well known that the induction of vitamin D_3 in the skin is much more potent for younger than for older persons (33). In agreement with this, the prognosis, as measured at 18 and 36 months, is better and the death rates are lower for cases diagnosed in the summer than in the winter (Fig. 9, middle panel). However, the effect is only manifested as a delay in progression, because the overall survival is constant through the year.

Thus, the data shown in Figures 8 and 9 constitute an indication, although a weak one, that solar radiation, through its production of vitamin D_3 improves the prognosis of CMM, as already suggested by others (8).

INTERMITTENT EXPOSURE HYPOTHESIS

A number of epidemiological observations indicate that intermittent, rather than constant and occupational, sun exposures, are melanomagenic (10–20). A number of case-control studies are summarized in Figure 10 [for references, see (4,10–20,34,35)]. No time trend can be seen. Occupational sun exposure hardly increases the odds ratio for CMM incidence. On the average, this ratio is 1.3 ± 0.2. On the other hand, intermittent exposures give increased odds ratios (2.3 ± 0.2 in this studies). Note that Figure 10 is given with exponential ordinates, while the average odds ratios are calculated on a linear basis.

The distribution of CMMs on different body localizations also lays support to the intermittent exposure hypothesis. For younger generations, the density of diagnosed CMMs (i.e., the relative number of CMMs arising per cm^2 of skin) is higher on the trunk (men) and on the lower legs (women) than on the face which

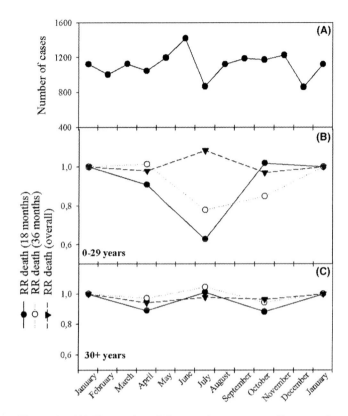

Figure 9 (A) The number of diagnosed cutaneous malignant melanoma cases per month in Norway for the period 1960–1993. (**B** and **C**) The relative death rates of CMM, as determined 18 months, 36 months, and 156 months (overall) after diagnosis in the four seasons of the year, for the age groups 0–29 years and 30+ years.

certainly gets the largest accumulated exposure (2,8). For the older generation, which most likely had lower intermittent exposures on non-facial body localizations, the density is always largest for the face. Thus, CMMs on the face and neck are predominantly a disease of accumulated exposure and age (Fig. 11), while CMMs on the trunk is a disease of middle-aged persons and follows an intermittent exposure relationship. The habit of sun exposure of the breasts is a relatively new one for women. In agreement with this, hardly any CMMs arose on female breasts prior to 1973. Later, however, it has become more common. The peak of the age-distribution curve is at about 40 years of age, while that for face and neck is at 70–80 (Fig. 11). The ratio of the increased rate of diagnosed cases from the period 1954–1976 to the period 1977–1998 (Fig. 12) is a factor of 3 for face and neck, a factor of 4–5 for trunk and legs, and a factor of 19 for the breasts. Still, the density is smaller by a factor of ~7 for the

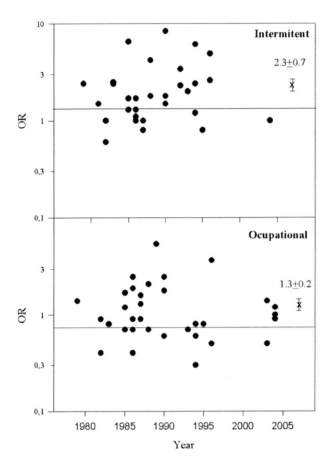

Figure 10   Odds ratios for cutaneous malignant melanoma persons with high intermittent (*upper panel*) and occupational (*lower panel*) lifetime doses of solar radiation. The data are taken from a number of published case-control investigations. For references, see the text.

breasts than for the rest of the female trunk (2). The constitution of the skin is hardly different on the breast and on the rest of the trunk, so the only difference is the dose of intermittent sun exposure.

OTHER FACTORS RELEVANT FOR CUTANEOUS MALIGNANT MELANOMA

Genetic Factors (3,8,10,36–42)

A number of inherited properties are related to the risk of getting CMM, the most important one being skin pigmentation. Generally, dark skin has a protective effect against all forms of skin cancer caused by absorption of UVR by

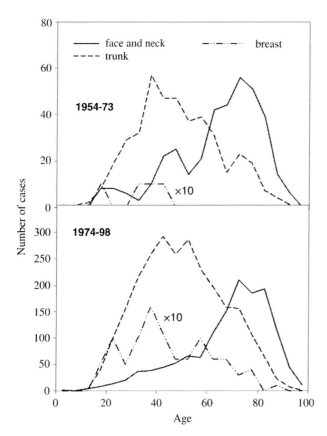

Figure 11 Cutaneous malignant melanoma in women in Norway. The number of diagnosed cases for the period 1954–1973 (*upper panel*) and 1974–1998 (*lower panel*).

melanin. Thus, the DNA in living and proliferating basal cells and melanocytes is shielded. However, the protective role of melanin seems to be smaller for CMM than for BCC and SCC. For the latter two skin cancer types, the incidence rates are between 20 and 70 times larger among Caucasians than among black Africans living at the same latitudes (41,43), while those for CMM are 10 to 20 times larger (43). Furthermore, albinism is a risk factor for BCC and SCC, but evidently not to the same degree for CMM (14). We have proposed that pheomelanin in melanocytes may be a chromophore for CMM, because free radicals are formed from this kind of melanin under UV exposure and such radicals can reach the nucleus of melanocytes (44). Melanin present in the upper, dead skin layers, however, may be protective, because radicals formed there can presumably not reach the melanocytes. Such a hypothesis would also explain the relatively low CMM risk among out-door workers who have a permanent tan and be in

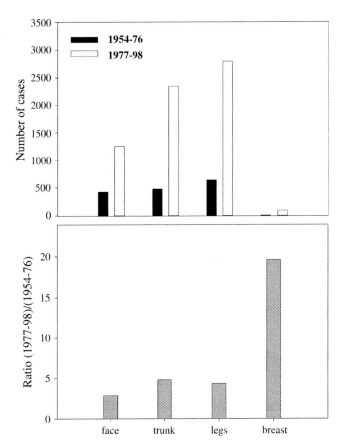

Figure 12 The number of diagnosed cases of cutaneous malignant melanoma in women in Norway for the given time periods (*upper panel*). The ratios of the numbers for 1977–1998 to those for 1954–1976 (*lower panel*).

agreement with the dose–response relationship proposed, namely that CMM incidence seems to increase with the dose up to a certain limit, above which it decreases (5).

Convincing proofs for the involvement of genetic factors in combination with UV induce DNA damage are that CMM rates are high among patients with xeroderma pigmentosum and ataxia telangiectazia (inherited deficiencies in DNA repair).

Other factors that increase the risk of getting CMMs are pigmented nevi, red hair color, blue eye color, freckles, and low minimal erythema doses. Inherited or acquired immunological deficiencies may also play a role because immunosuppression increases the risk of CMM and also because there seems to be a correlation of CMM risk and the risk to get non-Hodgkin's lymphoma (45–47).

Diet, Alcohol Consumption, Smoking, and Cutaneous Malignant Melanoma (48)

Diets rich in vitamin D and carotenoids and low alcohol consumption seem to be associated with reduced CMM risk (48). This role of vitamin D is in agreement with our findings (Fig. 9) and with those of Berwich et al. (8) showing that the prognosis of CMMs originating in skin with signs of sun damage have a better prognosis than those in less sun-damaged skin. Furthermore, the facts that increasing total UV exposure does not seem to increase the CMM risk (Fig. 10) and that sun exposure in childhood is a protective factor for CMM (49) are in agreement with this. Also, in-vitro experiments indicate a protective role of vitamin D_3. The UV absorbing, radical scavenging, and antioxidant properties of carotenoids make them likely candidates for protectors. Smoking has been reported to be a risk factor for SCC but not for CMM (50).

Sunbeds

Sunbed use has increased rapidly during the last two decades. In spite of this, the incidence rate of CMM after 1990 (Fig. 3) has decreased for younger persons, that is, for those who use sunbeds most frequently. From this we can conclude that sunbeds do not play a significant role for the population as a whole. This is in agreement with the early investigations, which show insignificant or no association between sunbed use and CMM (6,51–53). Later reviews of case-control studies between 1988 and 2003 come to the conclusion that there is still no conclusive evidence on the influence of tanning devices and CMM occurrence, or that severe methodological limitations have to be overcome before reliable conclusions can be drawn (54,55). While some of the cited studies show a possible association, others suggest either no or even a slight protective role of sunbeds. In a recent study from the United Kingdom, it was found that the risk of CMM did not increase with increasing number of hours or years of sunbed exposure (56). The fact that the spectra of modern sunbeds are more weighted in the UV-A region, where DNA absorbs minimally (hence the term "UV-A-sunbeds"), is probably of no major concern, because we and others have shown that even in such beds the small percentage of UV-B they emit gives the strongest biological effect, both with respect to tanning and erythema (57,58).

Little attention has so far been paid to the facts that sunbeds generally emits a much smaller fraction of visible light than that present in solar radiation and that visible light contributes to photorepair of UV-induced DNA damage.

On a personal basis, misuse or exaggerated use of sunbeds may certainly increase the CMM risk. However, in evaluations of the health effects of sunbeds, one should not forget the fact that use of sunbeds improves the bone mass density through substantial production of vitamin D_3 [(59,60) and unpublished data from our laboratory]. The protecting and/or delaying effects of vitamin D_3 metabolites are relevant for several major cancer forms, like prostate cancer, breast cancer, colon cancer, lymphomas, and even CMMs (8,9,29,30,61,62).

Thus, one should not completely overlook the possibility that moderate sunbeds use may be beneficial for certain groups, notably for elderly people. It has been proposed that increased UV exposure may prolong more lives than it shortens (63).

Sunscreens

The effect of sunscreens on the incidence of CMM is even more controversial and debated than the effect of sunbeds. Several reviews have been published (64–66). Surprisingly, many investigations indicate a higher CMM rate among sunscreen users than among non-users. In most cases, no significant effects are found. A serious confounding factor in such investigations is that sunscreen use may tempt people to spend more time in the sun. Some authors have suggested that certain sunscreens may be risk factors for CMM (67). Sunscreen ingredients may act as mutagens during sun exposure (68). This is not surprising, because they are small, aromatic molecules, which are often strong photosensitizers and free radical generators. Furthermore, it is likely that they can penetrate the skin, reach the circulation, and act systemically. Animal experiments indicate that some common sunscreens provide protection against sunburn, but not against CMM (69). After the introduction of sunscreens in the 1960s and their rapidly increasing use in the following decades, there has been a striking increase in the incidence rates of CMM in most countries. It should be kept in mind that sunscreens strongly suppress vitamin D_3 production (70,71), and may, therefore, potentially promote progression of cancers. A controversial statement is that sunscreen use may cause more cancer deaths than it prevents (72).

In view of this, one should probably not encourage people to use more sunscreens but rather to reduce their UV exposure. Exaggerated exposure may even decrease the vitamin D_3 level under certain conditions, because both provitamin D_3 and vitamin D_3 itself stay for some time in the skin, and both are sensitive to UVR (73).

Temperature

Carcinogenesis, like most other biological processes, is faster when the temperature increases, and it has been suggested that the north–south gradient in CMM incidence rates (see "Dependency on living standard" already discussed) is related to temperature gradients rather than to UV gradients (14). Our data, as shown in Fig. 8, do not support this view.

CONCLUSIONS

In view of the new data presented here, as well as of a number of cited investigations and earlier data from Norway (74), solar radiation seems to be a major cause of CMM in Europe. Sunbeds may possibly cause CMM in individuals using them frequently and exposing themselves to large doses, but for the population as a whole they play no major role. The action of sunscreens with UV-A and UV-B absorbers is controversial. Thus, a safe way to avoid CMM would be to limit the sun exposure rather than to apply sunscreens and stay longer in the sun. Solar radiation and sunbeds give substantial contributions to the vitamin D_3 status, and because this vitamin reduces the mortality of a number of internal cancers, possibly also of CMM, and is beneficial in relation to several other diseases with increasing incidence rates, one should not advise people to stay completely out of the sun and totally avoid sunbeds, but rather get moderate UV exposures regularly.

ACKNOWLEDGMENTS

The authors want to thank Frøydis Langmark, Steinar Hansen, and Trude Eid Robsahm at the Norwegian Cancer Registry who helped with the epidemiological data and gave valuable comments to the manuscript but who are not responsible for the interpretations or for the conclusions. The TOMS data were provided by NASA/GSFC.

REFERENCES

1. Armstrong BK, Kricker A, English DR. Sun exposure and skin cancer. Australas J Dermatol 1997; 38(suppl 1):S1–S6.
2. Moan J, Dahlback A. Ultraviolet radiation and skin cancer: epidemiological data from Scandinavia. 1993; 10:255–293.
3. Armstrong BK, Kricker A. The epidemiology of UV induced skin cancer. J Photochem Photobiol B 2001; 63(1–3):8–18.
4. Elwood JM. Melanoma and sun exposure: contrasts between intermittent and chronic exposure. World J Surg 1992; 16(2):157–165.
5. Holman CD, Armstrong BK, Heenan PJ. Relationship of cutaneous malignant melanoma to individual sunlight-exposure habits. J Natl Cancer Inst 1986; 76(3):403–414.
6. Osterlind A, Tucker MA, Stone BJ, et al. The Danish case-control study of cutaneous malignant melanoma. II. Importance of UV-light exposure. Int J Cancer 1988; 42(3):319–324.
7. Teppo L, Pakkanen M, Hakulinsen T. Sunlight as a risk factor of malignant melanoma of the skin. Cancer 1978; 41(5):2018–2027.
8. Berwick M, Armstrong BK, Ben Porat L, et al. Sun exposure and mortality from melanoma. J Natl Cancer Inst 2005; 97(3):195–199.
9. Hughes AM, Armstrong BK, Vajdic CM, et al. Sun exposure may protect against non-Hodgkin lymphoma: a case-control study. Int J Cancer 2004; 112(5):865–871.
10. Weinstock MA. Ultraviolet radiation and skin cancer: epidemiological data from the United States and Canada. 1993; 295–344.
11. Rockley PF, Trieff N, Wagner RF Jr, et al. Nonsunlight risk factors for malignant melanoma. Part I: Chemical agents, physical conditions, and occupation. Int J Dermatol 1994; 33(6):398–406.
12. Rampen FH, Fleuren E. Melanoma of the skin is not caused by ultraviolet radiation but by a chemical xenobiotic. Med Hypotheses 1987; 22(4):341–346.

13. Koh HK, Kligler BE, Lew RA. Sunlight and cutaneous malignant melanoma: evidence for and against causation. Photochem Photobiol 1990; 51(6):765–779.
14. Christophers AJ. Melanoma is not caused by sunlight. Mutat Res 1998; 422(1):113–117.
15. Moan J, Dahlback A. Predictions of health consequences of a changing UV-fluence. 1995; 87–100.
16. Magnus K. Habits of sun exposure and risk of malignant melanoma: an analysis of incidence rates in Norway 1955–1977 by cohort, sex, age, and primary tumor site. Cancer 1981; 48(10):2329–2335.
17. Maestro R, Boiocchi M. Sunlight and melanoma: an answer from MTS1 (p16). Science 1995; 267(5194):15–16.
18. Green A, Williams G. Ultraviolet radiation and skin cancer: epidemiological data from Australia. 1993; 233–254.
19. Elwood JM, Whitehead SM, Gallagher RP. Epidemiology of human malignant skin tumours with special reference to natural and artificial ultraviolet radiation exposure. 1989; 55–84.
20. Beitner H, Ringborg U, Wennersten G, et al. Further evidence for increased light sensitivity in patients with malignant melanoma. Br J Dermatol 1981; 104(3):289–294.
21. Dahlback A, Stamnes K. A new spherical model for computing the radiation field available for photolysis and heating rate at twilight. Planet Space Sci 1991; 39:671–683.
22. Stamnes K, Tsay SC, Wiscombe W, et al. Numerically stable algorithm for discrete-ordinate-method for radiative transfer in multiple scattering and emitting layered media. Appl Opt 1988; 27:2502–2509.
23. Harrison SL, MacLennan R, Speare R, et al. Sun exposure and melanocytic naevi in young Australian children. Lancet 1994; 344(8936):1529–1532.
24. La Vecchia C, Lucchini F, Negri E, et al. Recent declines in worldwide mortality from cutaneous melanoma in youth and middle age. Int J Cancer 1999; 81(1):62–66.
25. http://www.cia.gov/cia/publications/factbook/rankorder/2004rank.html (accessed April 2005).
26. Lee PY, Silverman MK, Rigel, DS, et al. Level of education and the risk of malignant melanoma. J Am Acad Dermatol 1992; 26(1):59–63.
27. Social inequalities and cancer. IARC Sci Publ 1997; 138:1–15.
28. Holick MF. Vitamin D: A millennium perspective. J Cell Biochem 2003; 88(2):296–307.
29. Robsahm TE, Tretli S, Dahlback A, et al. Vitamin D3 from sunlight may improve the prognosis of breast-, colon- and prostate cancer (Norway). Cancer Causes Control 2004; 15(2):149–158.
30. Moan J, Porojnicu AC, Robsahm TE, et al. Solar radiation, vitamin D and survival rate of colon cancer in Norway. J Photochem Photobiol B 2005; 78(3):189–193.
31. Porojnicu AC, Robsahm TE, Hansen Ree A, et al. Season of diagnosis is a strong prognostic factor in Hodgkin lymphoma. A possible role of sun-induced vitamin D. Br J Cancer 2005; submitted.
32. Boniol M, De Vries E, Coebergh JW, et al. Seasonal variation in the occurrence of cutaneous melanoma in Europe: influence of latitude. An analysis using the EUROCARE group of registries. Eur J Cancer 2005; 41(1):126–132.

33. Holick MF, Matsuoka LY, Wortsman J. Age, vitamin D, and solar ultraviolet. Lancet 1989; 2(8671):1104–1105.
34. Elwood JM, Jopson J. Melanoma and sun exposure: an overview of published studies. Int J Cancer 1997; 73(2):198–203.
35. Nelemans PJ, Rampen FH, Ruiter DJ, et al. An addition to the controversy on sunlight exposure and melanoma risk: a meta-analytical approach. J Clin Epidemiol 1995; 48(11):1331–1342.
36. Rivers JK. Is there more than one road to melanoma? Lancet 2004; 363(9410): 728–730.
37. Kraehn GM, Schartl M, Peter RU. Human malignant melanoma. A genetic disease? Cancer 1995; 75(6):1228–1237.
38. Ichii-Jones F, Lear JT, Heagerty AH, et al. Susceptibility to melanoma: influence of skin type and polymorphism in the melanocyte stimulating hormone receptor gene. J Invest Dermatol 1998; 111(2):218–221.
39. Rees JL, Healy E. Melanocortin receptors, red hair, and skin cancer. J Investig Dermatol Symp Proc 1997; 2(1):94–98.
40. Graham S, Marshall J, Haughey B, et al. An inquiry into the epidemiology of melanoma. Am J Epidemiol 1985; 122(4):606–619.
41. Armstrong BK, Kricker A. Skin cancer. Dermatol Clin 1995; 13(3):583–594.
42. Desmond RA, Soong SJ. Epidemiology of malignant melanoma. Surg Clin North Am 2003; 83(1):1–29.
43. Halder RM, Bridgeman-Shah S. Skin cancer in African Americans. Cancer 1995; 75(suppl 2):667–673.
44. Moan J, Dahlback A, Setlow RB. Epidemiological support for an hypothesis for melanoma induction indicating a role for UVA radiation. Photochem Photobiol 1999; 70(2):243–247.
45. McKenna DB, Doherty VR, McLaren KM, et al. Malignant melanoma and lympho-proliferative malignancy: is there a shared aetiology? Br J Dermatol 2000; 143(1):171–173.
46. Hemminki K, Jiang Y, Steineck G. Skin cancer and non-Hodgkin's lymphoma as second malignancies. markers of impaired immune function? Eur J Cancer 2003; 39(2):223–229.
47. Goggins WB, Finkelstein DM, Tsao H. Evidence for an association between cutaneous melanoma and non-Hodgkin lymphoma. Cancer 2001; 91(4):874–880.
48. Millen AE, Tucker MA, Hartge P, et al. Diet and melanoma in a case-control study. Cancer Epidemiol Biomarkers Prev 2004, 13(6):1042–1051.
49. Kaskel P, Sander S, Kron M, et al. Outdoor activities in childhood: a protective factor for cutaneous melanoma? Results of a case-control study in 271 matched pairs. Br J Dermatol 2001; 145(4):602–609.
50. De Hertog SA, Wensveen CA, Bastiaens MT, et al. Relation between smoking and skin cancer. J Clin Oncol 2001; 19(1):231–238.
51. Gallagher RP, Elwood JM, Hill GB. Risk factors for cutaneous malignant melanoma: the Western Canada Melanoma Study. Recent Results Cancer Res 1986; 102:38–55.
52. Holman CD, Armstrong BK, Heenan PJ, et al. The causes of malignant melanoma: results from the West Australian Lions Melanoma Research Project. Recent Results Cancer Res 1986; 102:18–37.

53. Garbe C, Weiss J, Kruger S, et al. The German melanoma registry and environmental risk factors implied. Recent Results Cancer Res 1993; 128:69–89.
54. Autier P. Issues about sunbeds. In: Hill DJ, Elwood JM, English DR, eds. Prevention of Skin Cancer. Dordrecht: Kluwer Academic Publishers, 2004:157–176.
55. Swerdlow AJ, Weinstock MA. Do tanning lamps cause melanoma? An epidemiologic assessment. J Am Acad Dermatol 1998; 38(1):89–98.
56. Bataille V, Winnett A, Sasieni P, et al. Exposure to the sun and sunbeds and the risk of cutaneous melanoma in the UK: a case-control study. Eur J Cancer 2004; 40(3):429–435.
57. Woollons A, Kipp C, Young AR, et al. The 0.8% ultraviolet B content of an ultraviolet A sunlamp induces 75% of cyclobutane pyrimidine dimers in human keratinocytes in vitro. Br J Dermatol 1999; 140(6):1023–1030.
58. Moan J, Johnsen B. What kind of radiation is efficient in sunbeds, UVA or UVB? J Photochem Photobiol B 1994; 22(1):77–79.
59. Studzinski GP, Moore DC. Sunlight—can it prevent as well as cause cancer? Cancer Res 1995; 55(18):4014–4022.
60. Tangpricha V, Turner A, Spina C, et al. Tanning is associated with optimal vitamin D status (serum 25-hydroxyvitamin D concentration) and higher bone mineral density. Am J Clin Nutr 2004; 80(6):1645–1649.
61. Grant WB. An ecologic study of dietary and solar ultraviolet-B links to breast carcinoma mortality rates. Cancer 2002; 94(1):272–281.
62. Grant WB. Geographic variation of prostate cancer mortality rates in the United States: Implications for prostate cancer risk related to vitamin D. Int J Cancer 2004; 111(3):470–471.
63. Grant WB. An estimate of premature cancer mortality in the U.S. due to inadequate doses of solar ultraviolet-B radiation. Cancer 2002; 94(6):1867–1875.
64. Dennis LK, Beane Freeman LE, VanBeek MJ. Sunscreen use and the risk for melanoma: a quantitative review. Ann Intern Med 2003; 139(12):966–978.
65. Huncharek M, Kupelnick B. Use of topical sunscreens and the risk of malignant melanoma: a meta-analysis of 9067 patients from 11 case-control studies. Am J Public Health 2002; 92(7):1173–1177.
66. Autier P, Dore JF, Schifflers E, et al. Melanoma and use of sunscreens: an Eortc case-control study in Germany, Belgium and France. The EORTC Melanoma Cooperative Group. Int J Cancer 1995; 61(6):749–755.
67. Westerdahl J, Olsson H, Masback A, et al. Is the use of sunscreens a risk factor for malignant melanoma? Melanoma Res 1995; 5(1):59–65.
68. Knowland J, McKenzie EA, McHugh PJ, et al. Sunlight-induced mutagenicity of a common sunscreen ingredient. FEBS Lett 1993; 324(3):309–313.
69. Wolf P, Donawho CK, Kripke ML. Effect of sunscreens on UV radiation-induced enhancement of melanoma growth in mice. J Natl Cancer Inst 1994; 86(2):99–105.
70. Matsuoka LY, Ide L, Wortsman J, et al. Sunscreens suppress cutaneous vitamin D3 synthesis. J Clin Endocrinol Metab 1987; 64(6):1165–1168.
71. Matsuoka LY, Wortsman J, Hanifan N, et al. Chronic sunscreen use decreases circulating concentrations of 25-hydroxyvitamin D. A preliminary study. Arch Dermatol 1988, 124 (12), 1802–1804.
72. Ainsleigh HG. Beneficial effects of sun exposure on cancer mortality. Prev Med 1993; 22(1):132–140.

73. Webb AR, DeCosta BR, Holick MF. Sunlight regulates the cutaneous production of vitamin D3 by causing its photodegradation. J Clin Endocrinol Metab 1989; 68(5):882–887.
74. Magnus K. The Nordic profile of skin cancer incidence. A comparative epidemiological study of the three main types of skin cancer. Int J Cancer 1991; 47(1):12–19.
75. http://www-depdb.iarc.fr/who/menu.htm.

10

Descriptive Epidemiology of Skin Cancer Incidence and Mortality

Mathieu Boniol
International Agency for Research on Cancer, Lyon, France

Jean-François Doré
International Agency for Research on Cancer and INSERM Unit 590, Centre Léon Bérard, Lyon, France

Philippe Autier, Michel Smans, and Peter Boyle
International Agency for Research on Cancer, Lyon, France

INTRODUCTION

Cancer of the skin is a very common form of neoplasm. These cancers are commonly divided between cutaneous melanoma and nonmelanoma skin cancer. Cutaneous melanoma has shown a rapid increase of incidence in last decades, and because of its poor prognosis, this neoplasm has received a great deal of interests in epidemiological studies. In marked contrasts, and despite the important prevalence of this disease in the population, few reliable epidemiological data exists about nonmelanoma skin cancers.

CUTANEOUS MELANOMA

Even if cutaneous melanoma has been the subject of a great deal of interest in cancer research in recent years, it is not a disease of modern times. The oldest case of melanoma described in the literature was found on a mummy of an Inca adept of solar cult, 2400 years ago (1). This disease also attracted the eye of the painter Goya in 1800 on the famous painting of *Doña Maria Josefa*. But the first medical description of cutaneous melanoma is attributed to René Laennec in 1804 (2) under the term melanose. In 1838, Carswell invented the term melanoma for this disease (3).

Melanoma was assimilated and further considered as a cancer in 1857, when Norris published the description of eight melanoma patients (4).

INCIDENCE OF CUTANEOUS MELANOMA WORLDWIDE

Geographical Variations

First and foremost, melanoma is a disease of white populations. A recent analysis in the United States showed that melanoma incidence is 17 times higher in white males than in black males, and 29 times higher for white females than for black females (5). The incidence of cutaneous melanoma is also lower among other ethnic groups compared with whites (Table 1). In the United States in 2003, the individual lifetime risk of incidence of cutaneous melanoma was 1.87% for whites and 0.077% for blacks. But this white/black dichotomy is not sufficient to summarize populations at risk, as cutaneous melanoma appears to be a disease more specifically of Caucasian populations. Hispanic, Asian, and Indian populations have very low rates of cutaneous melanoma.

In 2002, 82% of melanoma cases occurred in developed countries and the IARC estimated that there were 8.3/100,000 new melanoma case among men and 7.5/100,000 in women in developed countries, and only 0.7/100,000 for men and women in less developed countries (6). Among Caucasian populations, the highest incidence rates are found in Australia and New Zealand (Table 2).

Melanoma incidence varies greatly by latitude of residence. Even in Australia where the incidence is the highest, there is a south to north gradient of incidence: the incidence steadily increases for latitudes closer to the equator

Table 1 Incidence of Cutaneous Melanoma, Age-Standardized on U.S. Population, in Surveillance Epidemiology and End Result Registry Between 1997 and 2000 by Sex and Race

Ethnicity	Males		Females	
	Incidence[a]	CI 95%	Incidence	CI 95%
All ethnicity	21.41	21.09–21.74	13.83	13.59–14.06
Whites	25.36	24.96–25.76	16.82	16.53–17.12
Blacks	1.48	1.16–1.87	0.73	0.57–0.93
American Indians or Alaska natives	2.46	1.36–4.35	1.50	0.80–2.69
Asians	1.68	1.40–2.01	1.51	1.28–1.78
Hispanics	4.41	3.91–4.98	4.46	4.06–4.90

[a]Incidence per 100,000 person-years age standardized on U.S. population in 2000 estimated by the National Census Bureau, SEER cancer statistics 2003.

Table 2 Incidence in 2002 in Different Regions of the World Including an Important Minority or More Caucasian Populations

Regions	Males	Females
Australia and New Zealand	37.8	29.4
North America	16.4	11.7
Northern Europe	8.4	10.0
Western Europe	7.3	10.3
Southern Europe	6.0	5.5
South Africa	5.4	4.1
Eastern Europe	3.3	3.8
South America	2.4	2.3

Note: Incidence rates age-standardized on the world population expressed as number of annual new cases per 100,000 person-years.
Source: From Ref. 6.

(7). This gradient was also described in other parts of the world such as U.S. (8), or Sweden (9) and Norway (10). However, Europe presents a particular geographical pattern of incidence, Nordic countries present the greatest melanoma incidence. But this reverse trend is only observed for western Europe, whereas in central Europe there is the classical north to south gradient of latitude (11). This western Europe trend was sometimes attributed to the distribution of skin sensitivity, with more sensitive population living in Nordic countries. But as there is no difference in distribution of population between central Europe and western Europe, this hypothesis is no longer valid. Difference in sun exposure habits could explain this unique inverse trend in incidence. In western Europe, Nordic populations have important skin sensitivity and they seek sun tanning and intermittent sun exposures mostly by travelling to the south of Europe for holidays, whereas these opportunities for solar exposure were only recently available for resident of central European countries.

Seasonal Variation of Incidence of Cutaneous Melanoma

Melanoma incidence presents an intriguing seasonal variation in incidence with a summer peak, and this has been demonstrated in both hemispheres.

The first study describing this phenomenon was conducted in the U.S. in 1980 (12). The author evidenced a higher amplitude of this seasonality for northern states compared to southern states. This observation suggested that this seasonal trend could be caused by a rapid promotion of tumor growth following environmental UV exposure. This seasonal variation was then retrieved in different countries in both hemispheres (13–21). Some authors suggested that this phenomenon could occur due to an increase diagnosis of melanoma in summer when less clothes are worn and when people are more aware of potential hazard of solar UV exposure. However, no difference in amplitude of seasonality was observed by anatomical localization or by histologies or skin phototype (15,16).

The more probable hypothesis to explain such variation is the biological hypothesis for which this trend results from a recent promotion effect of solar exposure able to launch rapid tumor progression. Indeed, UV is known to have rapid biological effects on melanocytes such as the ability to decrease in vivo the density of dendritic cells in neavi (22), or changing pigmentation distribution within nevi after intense exposure (23).

If this seasonal variation was only due to the change in detection during summer, the seasonal variation should have been different by anatomical body site, with an higher amplitude for unexposed body sites. But the amplitude does not seems to vary by body site (16). Furthermore, this trend exists also in Hawaï where temperature is stable during all year and there is no change in clothing habits. However, there is an important seasonal variation of the amount of solar UV (18,24). This seasonal variation was not in evidence for in situ melanoma, whereas it is not visually possible to distinguish and invasive form from in situ melanoma (17). Moreover, if this seasonal variation resulted from an increase of diagnosis, we would expect to observe a greater amplitude of seasonality for non-invasive forms of melanoma.

Finally an analysis of the incidence of cutaneous melanoma was conducted in Europe using registries participating to Eurocare (25). As suspected on the basis of the earlier U.S. work (12), there was a significant correlation between the amplitude of seasonal variation and the latitude of the registry.

Hence, seasonal variation of the incidence of cutaneous melanoma seems to be in part due to seasonal fluctuation of solar UV radiation. This hypothesis would also suggest that minimizing environmental UV exposure among adults could have a rapid effect on the risk of cutaneous melanoma.

Temporal Trends

In most countries with a majority of the population Caucasian, an important increase of the incidence of cutaneous melanoma was observed during the last decades. In U.S., this was considered as the cancer presenting the more rapid increase in incidence (26). The rate of increase was estimated to be 4.3% annually during the last 50 years (5). This percentage change of incidence was also estimated in France between 1980 and 2000 at 5.9% annually for men, and 4.3% for women (27).

To verify the validity of this observed increase in the incidence of melanoma, a large study reviewed the histological diagnosis of melanoma for various periods of time. No major changes in diagnostic criteria were observed, and the small changes observed were unlikely to explain the importance of melanoma incidence (28).

This increase of incidence of cutaneous melanoma, that is observed in different place of the world was often correlated to decrease in the average thickness of tumors diagnosed. Some authors suggested that this was due to a better, and earlier diagnosis (29). More careful analysis permitted to the demonstration that the increase of incidence of melanoma was mainly due to an increase of thin lesion, whereas incidence of thicker remained stable or slightly increasing with time (30). There is also an increase of diagnosis of in situ forms of melanoma: in Surveillance Epidemiology and End Result registries, between 1995 and 1997, the annual increase of invasive melanoma was 4.5% for men and 3.6% for women, whereas for in situ melanoma the annual increase was 15.8% for men and 15.6% for women (31). This trend was observed for different ages and different birth cohorts. As mean age at diagnosis was older for in situ forms, these non-invasive forms of melanoma were not considered to be precursors of invasive melanoma and would have probably never evolved to invasive melanoma.

Analysis of these trends in recent years permit to evidence a slowdown of the increase of incidence and a stabilization in countries that had the highest rates (Australia, U.S.A., Canada) (32–34). In New South Wales, the incidence even recently decreased for women. This trend was found in Canada for women aged lower than 55 years and for men aged lower than 45 years. In Europe, rates for Nordic countries appear to have stabilized (Finland, Norway, Sweden).

SURVIVAL FROM CUTANEOUS MELANOMA

Melanoma was originally described as the "black cancer" for which no treatment existed to avoid death (35). And the rapid growth of these tumors and the high fatality rate was observed until 20th century. In 1932, melanoma was considered as the cancer having the worst prognosis (36). This bad prognosis was repeated in 10 studies between 1916 and 1947 with a five year survival ranging between less than 1% and 48% (37). With the rapid increase in incidence of melanoma during the last 50 years, and whereas no new treatment appeared, the prognosis of melanoma has considerably changed. In the United States, the five years survival rose from 49% in 1950–1954 to 89.8% in 1992–1999 (5).

The most important prognostic factor for melanoma survival is Breslow's thickness of the tumor (38). This factor is correlated to other prognosis factors such as sex, age, anatomical localization, and histology. Thick melanoma are more often diagnosed among older men, and for nodular histologies. When there are a lymph node metastasis, Breslow's thickness is no longer a key prognosis factor and the survival rate is low. In this case, prognosis is determined by the number of lymph nodes with a metastasis (39).

MORTALITY FROM CUTANEOUS MELANOMA

Geographical Variations

As for melanoma incidence, there is a clear geographical pattern of melanoma death rate. Mortality is higher for developed countries and for Caucasian populations. Age-standardized mortality rate was estimated in 2002 at 1.8 and 1.2 per 100,000 person-years in developed countries for men and women, respectively, and at 0.3 per 100,000 person-years in developing countries for men and

Table 3 Mortality in 2002 in Different Regions of the World
Including an Important Minority or More Caucasian Populations

Regions	Males	Females
Australia and New Zealand	5.2	2.8
South Africa	2.9	2.2
North America	2.5	1.3
Northern Europe	2.2	1.6
Western Europe	1.8	1.3
Eastern Europe	1.6	1.2
Southern Europe	1.6	1.1
South America	0.9	0.6

Note: Mortality rates age-standardized on the world population expressed
as number of annual deaths per 100,000 person-years.
Source: From Ref. 6.

women (6). Among Caucasian populations, the highest mortality rates are found
in Australia and New Zealand (Table 3).

There is a latitude gradient of mortality rates of melanoma. This was
demonstrated in the United States with southern states having the highest mortality rates. However, this geographical pattern has slowly decreased since
1950 to 1954 and was nearly inexistent in 1990 to 1994, whereas there was no
temporal trend in the quantity of UV received by these states (40).

In Europe, these geographical variations have been investigated in an
International Agency for Research on Cancer program in an atlas of mortality
by cancer for the period 1993 to 1997. Figures 1 and 2 present the distribution
of mortality rate for men and women observed in the European community
including the members of the European Economic Area (Switzerland, Iceland,
and Norway). The main map represents the relative distribution of rates using
a scale from lower rates in light gray to highest rates in dark gray using percentiles of the distribution of rates (5, 15, 35, 65, 85, and 95). The second map
represents the distribution of rates using an absolute scale and the upper right
sub-figure contains the distribution of rates and boxplots of rates by country.

Melanoma mortality presents similar geographical distribution as melanoma incidence. There is an inverse latitude gradient for western Europe with
greatest rates for west of northern Europe. In central Europe, the gradient of mortality is more important for southern countries than northern countries.

Temporal Trends

In Europe, mortality has been rising steadily during the last 50 years, but less
quickly than incidence. This increase was more marked for older men (41). In
U.S., where 7000 deaths are yearly attributed to melanoma (42), there was a
191% increase for men and 84% for women between 1950 to 1954 and 1990
to 1994 (40).

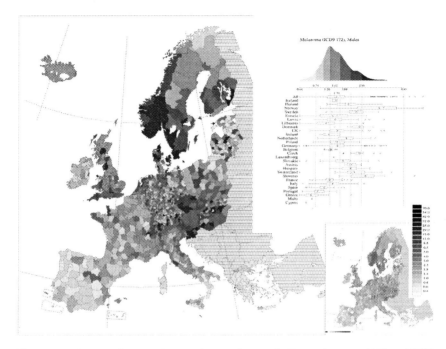

Figure 1   The mortality rates from melanoma for men in Europe between 1993 and 1997.

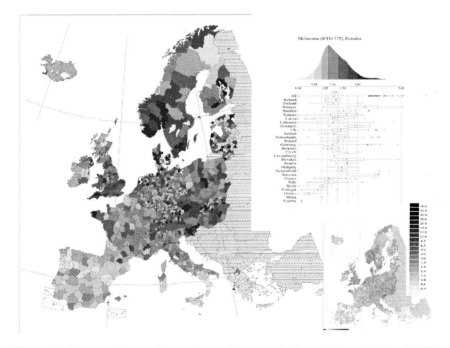

Figure 2   The mortality rates from melanoma for women in Europe between 1993 and 1997.

A survival analysis conducted in Finland showed that the five year survival rate rose from 66.9% between 1975 and 1977 to 81.3% between 1990 and 1992 (43). In the United States, where survival is relatively better, this trend was also observed: the five years survival rose from 82% between 1975 and 1979 to 89.8% in 1995 (5). These observations permit a better understanding of the important differences between temporal trends in incidence and mortality. Indeed, we can observe an improvement in survival with time, whereas no changes in treatment occurred during the last 50 years. This observation is due to an important increase of incidence of the less aggressive forms of melanoma probably coupled with a tendency towards earlier detection. Melanoma incidence increased more rapidly than mortality because the increase of the potentially fatal forms of melanoma was moderate compared to the less aggressive forms.

Melanoma incidence in western Europe is twice that of central Europe. However, melanoma diagnosed in central Europe has a greater thickness at diagnosis, and mortality rates are comparable between central Europe and western Europe. With the recent change to a more market-oriented economy in central Europe, health indicators showed a rapid general improvement. This improvement is correlated with a change in lifestyle with the adoption of a western lifestyle. Thus, we can also foresee that sun exposure habits of Western countries could be adopted by these central European countries, and we can forecast the development of an epidemic of melanoma in these countries. It is therefore of importance to start prevention campaigns in these countries, to prevent worn the population of the hazards associated with intense sun exposure (44).

NONMELANOMA SKIN CANCER

Nonmelanoma skin cancer share similar etiological factors with melanoma, but epidemiological studies show that contrary to melanoma, these tumors are essentially influenced by chronic solar exposure (45). Two main forms of nonmelanoma skin cancer exist: basal cell carcinomas (BCCs) and squamous cell carcinomas (SCCs). Owing to their epidemiological status and anatomical distribution, BCC seems to have etiology close to melanoma, whereas SCC clearly differs from melanoma.

Incidence of Nonmelanoma Skin Cancer

Due to the simple clinical management of nonmelanoma skin cancer, the registration of this cancer is a difficult task, the main issue being the lack of an histological examination in many cases and the high probability of an individual having multiple tumors and a high probability of having tumors diagnosed at different points in their lifetime. This registration is especially more a concern for older people diagnosed with a BCC (10). Hence, for nonmelanoma skin cancer registration, there is a need to involve clinicians responsible of nonmelanoma skin cancer and to conduct extensive surveys to obtain a good registration with histological confirmation of the tumor registered (46,47). In places where these efforts are made, the percentage of histological confirmation for skin cancer can be high, for example, in West Glamorgan it was 74% for BCC and 98.5% for SCC in 1990 (48).

Nonmelanoma skin cancer is essentially a cancer of white populations, it is less frequent for Hispanic and Asian populations, and even less common for blacks (49,50).

BCC represent the cancer with the highest incidence, around 80% of all incidence nonmelanoma skin cancers are BCC (47,51).

Nonmelanoma skin cancer presents a high rate of recurrence (52). In Tazmania, nonmelanoma skin cancer patients had a 12-fold increase among males and 15-fold increase risk of development of a new nonmelanoma skin cancer within five years (53). In a survey in Queensland, about 20% of patients had multiple nonmelanoma skin cancer during the year following diagnosis of nonmelanoma skin cancer (54).

Considering that the incidence of all cancer except nonmelanoma skin cancer is estimated to be 314/100,000 person-years for males and 228/100,000 person-years for females in 2002 in more developed countries (6), the incidence estimated in different countries largely exceeds that of all other forms of cancer (Table 4).

There is a wide range of rates of nonmelanoma skin cancer incidence around the world, and rates exceed 500/100,000 in Australia. When comparing Norwegian and Australian incidence data (46), incidence of nonmelanoma skin cancer in Australia was 11.1 greater for BCC and 22.4 greater for SCC. This suggests that BCC and SCC are more dependant to chronic solar exposure than melanoma (10). Incidence rates of nonmelanoma skin cancer showed a gradient with respect to latitude (10,46).

Nonmelanoma skin cancers develop more frequently among men than women (53,60). In the United States, the sex ratio (male/female) was 3:1 for SCC and 2:1 for BCC (52). This difference is observable mainly for incidence among older adults, whereas before the age of 65, rates of nonmelanoma skin cancer were comparable between males and females (46).

The age-specific incidence of BCC and SCC presents an exponential increase of rates with increasing age when compared to melanoma (60). The age-specific incidence of BCC starts at an earlier age than SCC age-specific incidence. The age-specific incidence of SCC has a more pronounced exponential shape than of BCC (47,53,62,65). Hence, the median age at presentation is roughly between 60 and 70 years for BCC and between 70 and 80 years for SCC (59,66,67).

Rates of SCC and BCC were high for chronically exposed anatomical body sites. Head and neck were the most common localization with 70% to 80% of SCC and BCC occurring on the face, scalp, and neck (48,59,60,62,65).

Table 4 Incidence per 100,000 Person-Years of Basal and Squamous Cell Carcinoma Reported in Different Places in the World

Publication	Geographical area	Years	BCC Male	BCC Female	SCC Male	SCC Female
	North America					
Scotto et al. (52)	Dallas[a]	1971–1972	394	205	124	51
	Iowa[a]	1971–1972	123	69	47	13
	Minneapolis—Saint Paul[a]	1971–1972	165	103	35	12
	San Francisco[a]	1971–1972	198	117	45	15
Harris et al. (55)	Southeastern Arizona[a]	1996	936	497	271	112
Miller and Weinstock (56)	U.S.A.		407	212	65	24
Gallagher et al. (57)	Canada	1973–1987	120	92	31	17
	Australia					
Giles et al. (46)	Australia (survey)	1985	735	593	209	122
Marks et al. (58)	Australia (survey)	1990	849	605	338	164
Green et al. (45)	Nambour, Queensland, Australia (survey)[b]	1985–1987	1772	1610	600	298
Kaldor et al. (53)	Tazmania, Australia	1978–1987	145	83	64	20
Buettner and Raasch (59)	Townsville, Australia	1997	2058	1194	1332	755
	Europe					
Osterlind et al. (60)	Denmark	1978–1982	30	24	6.7	2.5
Roberts (48)	South Wales, U.K.	1988	112	54	32	6.2
Holme et al. (61)	South Wales, U.K.	1998	128	105	25	8.6

Reference	Location	Year				
Ko et al. (67)	North Humberside, U.K.[c]	1991	116	104	29	21
Cited in Ref. (62)	Scotland, U.K.	1990–1995	50	37	18	8
Magnus (10)	Finland	1985	44	32	5.6	3.9
Hannuksela-Svahn et al. (63)	Finland	1991–1995	49	45	7	4.2
Magnus (10)	Iceland	1983–1987			7	4.0
	Norway	1982, 1984–1986	43	39	6.4	3.2
	Sweden	1985			10	4.6
Coebergh et al. (47)	Eindhoven, The Netherlands	1975–1988	46	30	11	3.4
De Vries et al. (11)	Eindhoven, The Netherlands[d]	1998–2000	93	82		
Katalinic et al. (51)	Schleswig-Holstein, Germany	1998–2001	54	44	11	5.3
Levi et al. (64)	Vaud, Switzerland	1991–1992	69	62	29	18
Plesko et al. (65)	Slovakia	1993–1995	38	29	6.7	3.8
Omari et al. (62)	North Jordan[e]	1997–2001	20	23	14	4.2
Revenga et al. (66)	Soria, Spain	1998–2000	65	53	23	13
	Asia					
Koh et al. (50)	Singapore (Chinese)	1993–1997	6.4	5.8	3.2	1.8
	Singapore (Malay)	1993–1997	2.3	3.0	1.3	0.5
	Singapore (Indian)	1993–1997	1.2	1.4	1.8	1.9

[a]Standardized on the U.S. population of 1970.
[b]Standardized on the world population truncated to 20–69 years.
[c]Standardized on the England and Wales population of 1991.
[d]Standardized on the European population.
[e]Standardized on the Jordan population.
Abbreviations: BCC, basal cell carcinoma; SCC, squamous cell carcinoma.

Different surveys and analysis in registries evidenced a continuous increase of rates of nonmelanoma skin cancer in various countries. In Australia, after a survey conducted in 1985, a second survey was conducted in 1990 and evidenced a significant increase of rates of nonmelanoma skin cancer in Australia by 11% for BCC and 51% for SCC over the five year period (58). In the Tasmanian cancer registry, there was a 7.3% annual increase for males and 6.9% for females of incidence of nonmelanoma skin cancer between 1978 and 1987. This increase was more marked for BCC than for SCC (53). This trend was also observed in Eindhoven (The Netherlands), where the incidence of BCC increased over time from 42 to 53/100,000 person-years for males between 1975 and 1988, and from 24 to 38/100,000 person-years for females. The incidence of SCC also increased, but mainly among males (47). This trend was further described in U.K. (67), Switzerland (64), Finland (63), Slovakia (65) and Singapore (50). The analysis of the most recent statistics for BCC in Eindhoven showed that the increase of incidence still continues with no sign of leveling of (68).

To estimate the total burden of nonmelanoma skin cancer in Europe, the International Agency for Research on Cancer conducted a study to estimate the incidence of BCC and SCC for year 2000. Representative Cancer Registry for BCC and SCC registration (registries which published in peer-reviewed journals their incidence statistics, and registries with similar to the previous in term of proportion of BCC and SCC compared to melanoma) were used to estimate the age-specific ratio of BCC/melanoma incidence and SCC/melanoma incidence. These ratios were then multiplied to age-specific melanoma incidence by geographical areas to obtain an estimate of BCC and SCC incidence for existing registries with only good data on melanoma and no relevant data for SCC and BCC. BCC and SCC incidence were then further estimated by country using population age distribution. Tables 5 and 6 present the estimated number of cases and incidence of BCC, SCC, and melanoma in Europe for 2000. In the 25 European member states and the European Free Trade Association (EFTA) member states (Iceland, Norway, and Switzerland), we estimated that there was 195048 BCC and 52556 SCC diagnosed among males, and 210717 BCC and 42295 SCC among females.

Mortality from Nonmelanoma Skin Cancer

Mortality from nonmelanoma skin cancer is rare and less than 1% of nonmelanoma skin cancers are fatal (69). The estimated lethality was between 1.2% to 6.5% for SCC and 0.1% to 0.4% for BCC (70). The SCC form of nonmelanoma skin cancer is more invasive and account for around 75% of all nonmelanoma skin cancer deaths (71). Whereas BCC and SCC seem to have different aetiological characteristics, nonmelanoma skin cancer mortality is coded in registries under one International Classification of Disease (ICD) code and rarely presented by histology.

Table 5 Number and Age Adjusted Rate of Incidence of Basal and Squamous Cell Carcinoma, and Melanoma in Europe Estimated[a] for 2000 for Males

	BCC		SCC		Melanoma	
	N	ASR(w)	N	ASR(w)	N	ASR(w)
Central Europe	38637	21.5	6464	3.5	6303	3.8
Belarus	909	16.5	146	2.7	130	2.5
Bulgaria	1296	18.7	237	3.1	158	2.8
Czech Republic	5399	74.6	958	12.2	657	10.2
Hungary	3504	46	631	7.6	433	6.5
Moldova	430	23.4	61	3.3	76	4.2
Poland	3046	12.5	662	2.6	1274	5.8
Romania	3520	23.3	539	3.3	528	4
Russian	13346	16.9	2029	2.6	2035	2.7
Slovakia	1490	47	287	8.6	186	6.2
Ukraine	5697	20.2	914	3.1	826	3.2
Northern Europe	50811	66.1	13109	14.4	5381	8.6
Denmark	2751	65.6	495	9.8	498	13.9
Estonia	222	25.3	34	3.7	38	4.9
Finland	1899	48	371	8.3	322	9.3
Iceland	70	34.7	14	5.6	14	8.3
Ireland	1709	69.9	453	16.3	163	7.5
Latvia	519	35.2	115	7.5	47	3.5
Lithuania	645	29.4	169	7.2	61	3.1
Norway	2895	78.7	617	13.3	463	15.2
Sweden	4789	57	1041	9.6	753	11.3
U.K.	35312	71.5	9800	16.8	3022	7.7
Southern Europe	53983	45.6	15843	11.4	5868	6.3
Albania	492	35.3	130	9.4	59	4.1
Bosnia	619	28.4	159	7.5	78	3.7
Croatia	2098	64.9	601	17.6	218	7.7
Greece	2203	24.5	637	5.9	245	3.6
Italy	25601	52.1	6863	11.6	3219	8.7
Macedonia	616	51.3	190	15.2	70	6.2
Malta	138	54.1	41	14.9	10	4.5
Portugal	3182	37.5	1045	10.5	264	4
Serbia	1737	23.7	476	6.1	207	3.3
Slovenia	414	30.2	101	7.1	123	10.3
Spain	16883	50.2	5600	14.1	1375	5.2
Western Europe	82377	58.3	22622	13.7	9819	8.6
Austria	2581	41.7	778	10.9	515	10.6
Belgium	1960	26.3	533	6.1	307	4.9
France	32878	73.1	10441	19.8	3066	8.3

(*Continued*)

Table 5 Number and Age Adjusted Rate of Incidence of Basal and Squamous Cell Carcinoma, and Melanoma in Europe Estimated[a] for 2000 for Males (*Continued*)

	BCC		SCC		Melanoma	
	N	ASR(w)	N	ASR(w)	N	ASR(w)
Germany	33661	51.8	7670	10.2	4366	8.5
Luxembourg	177	56.3	48	14.4	22	7.2
Switzerland	3100	57.1	1095	17.1	527	11.5
The Netherlands	8020	71.8	2057	16	1016	10.6

[a]National rates per 100,000 person-years, age-adjusted on the world population, were estimated by extrapolation of statistics from European cancer registries. When data on BCC and SCC were not available for some countries, ratio of age specific incidence of BCC/melanoma and SCC/melanoma from surrounding countries were applied to national statistics.

Abbreviations: BCC, basal cell carcinoma; SCC, squamous cell carcinoma; ASR(w), age-standardized rate on the world population.

In the European atlas of mortality by cancer, it was estimated that the incidence of nonmelanoma skin cancer was 0.57/100,000 person-years for men and 0.27/100,000 person-years for women for the period 1993 to 1997. Figures 3 and 4 present the distribution of mortality rate for men and women observed in the European community including countries of the EFTA (Switzerland, Iceland, and Norway). The main map represents the relative distribution of rates using a scale from lower rates in light gray to highest rates in dark gray using percentiles of the distribution of rates (5,15,35,65,85,95). The second map represents the distribution of rates using an absolute scale and the upper right sub-figure contains the distribution of rates and boxplots of rates by country. Nonmelanoma skin cancer mortality presents a completely different pattern than that of melanoma. There is a latitude gradient of rates with greatest rates for southern Europe. This suggests the importance of chronic solar exposure for this tumor, whereas intermittent exposure seems more important in the aetiology of melanoma.

Contrary to incidence, which showed a continuous increase in different part of the world, mortality did not seem to increase with time (64). On the contrary, in Finland, the rates of BCC and other nonmelanoma skin cancer steadily decreased with time and patients who died were mostly old (63).

CONCLUSION

Incidence of cutaneous melanoma dramatically increased during the last decades whereas no therapeutic improvement emerged to cure this cancer. Nonmelanoma skin cancers present a much lower mortality rate compared to melanoma, but their incidences exceed all other forms of cancer. Recent trends in incidence and mortality from cutaneous melanoma in Australia suggest that interventions could result in decreasing the incidence of both melanoma and

Table 6 Number and Age Adjusted Rate of Incidence of Basal and Squamous Cell Carcinoma, and Melanoma in Europe Estimated[a] for 2000 for Females

	BCC		SCC		Melanoma	
	N	ASR(w)	N	ASR(w)	N	ASR(w)
Central Europe	55454	18.9	7858	2.1	8956	4.2
Belarus	1713	17.7	231	1.9	235	3.2
Bulgaria	1161	14.3	179	1.7	163	2.8
Czech Republic	5033	50.6	704	5.3	678	9.3
Hungary	3740	32.2	609	3.9	480	5.9
Moldova	567	22.4	62	2.1	98	4.5
Poland	4902	12.1	570	1.4	1864	6.8
Romania	3771	18.5	552	2.2	535	3.6
Russian	23890	17	3397	1.9	3385	3.3
Slovakia	1680	37.6	305	5.2	234	6.7
Ukraine	8997	19.4	1249	2.1	1284	3.9
Northern Europe	50119	51	8112	5.8	6796	10.5
Denmark	2743	60.3	274	4	603	18.6
Estonia	325	22.3	39	2.3	80	7.6
Finland	1903	35.7	224	2.9	332	8.7
Iceland	93	50.4	7	2.9	26	17.3
Ireland	2002	66.5	321	8.1	272	11.8
Latvia	792	29.4	118	3.5	93	4.8
Lithuania	908	26	135	3.1	117	4.5
Norway	3014	69.4	375	5.6	529	17.1
Sweden	4585	49	553	3.8	795	12.2
U.K.	33754	53.1	6066	6.7	3949	9.9
Southern Europe	39413	27.4	8379	3.8	6065	5.9
Albania	212	12.8	49	2.5	35	2.3
Bosnia	534	18.9	92	2.9	87	3.4
Croatia	1431	32.5	298	4.8	221	6.9
Greece	1761	16.1	372	2.4	258	3.3
Italy	17811	29.3	3512	3.5	2915	7.4
Macedonia	442	32.1	81	5.1	71	5.8
Malta	91	33.1	20	5.2	13	5.2
Portugal	2720	27.1	621	4.2	383	5
Serbia	1572	17.9	276	2.6	243	3.3
Slovenia	464	23.6	105	3.9	117	8.4
Spain	12375	31.1	2953	4.7	1722	5.8
Western Europe	110021	58.5	24412	8.4	13779	11
Austria	3727	48.4	712	6.2	702	12.2
Belgium	3645	35.2	910	6.2	471	6.2
France	35936	65.5	8457	9.5	4165	10.8

(Continued)

Table 6 Number and Age Adjusted Rate of Incidence of Basal and Squamous Cell Carcinoma, and Melanoma in Europe Estimated[a] for 2000 for Females (*Continued*)

	BCC		SCC		Melanoma	
	N	ASR(w)	N	ASR(w)	N	ASR(w)
Germany	51916	54.2	11352	7.5	6157	10.3
Luxemburg	332	89.2	80	13.6	59	22.4
Switzerland	5103	78.3	1522	16.2	807	16.9
The Netherlands	9362	69.9	1379	7.9	1418	14.7

[a]National rates per 100,000 person-years, age-adjusted on the world population, were estimated by extrapolation of statistics from European cancer registries. When data on BCC and SCC were not available for some countries, ratio of age specific incidence of BCC/melanoma and SCC/melanoma from surrounding countries were applied to national statistics.

Abbreviations: BCC, basal cell carcinoma; SCC, squamous cell carcinoma; ASR(w), age-standardized rate on the world population.

nonmelanoma skin cancer. But these promising results are to put in perspective with the recent changes in incidence of cutaneous melanoma observed in central Europe. Whereas the incidence in central Europe is twice less compared to western Europe, we could expect a real public health problem in a few decades if incidence reaches the level observed in Western countries.

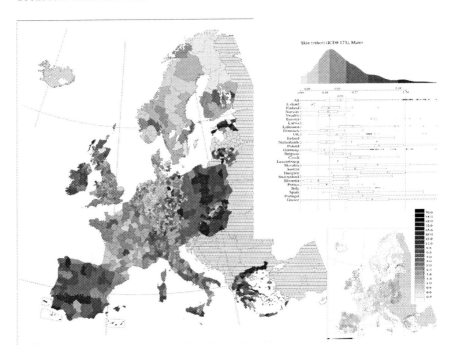

Figure 3 The mortality rates from nonmelanoma skin cancer for men in Europe between 1993 and 1997.

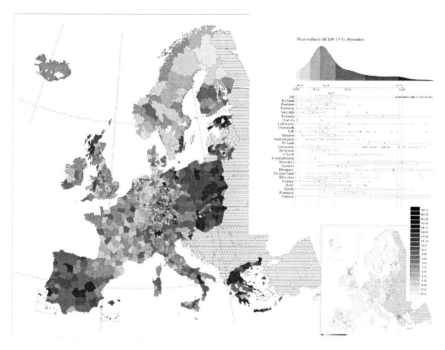

Figure 4 The mortality rates from nonmelanoma skin cancer for women in Europe between 1993 and 1997.

Data concerning nonmelanoma skin cancer are unfortunately sparse. Although it is estimated to be the most common cancer and the most costly to treat (72), it still is not of sufficient importance in cancer recording in registries. Despite the low fatality of this disease, because of aging of populations, this cancer will become a real concern for white populations (73). Emphasis should be given to primary prevention to be able to avoid this cancer and reallocate resources on fatal cancers.

REFERENCES

1. Urteaga OB, Pack GT. On the antiquity of melanoma. Cancer 1966; 19(5):607–610.
2. Laennec RTH. Sur les mélanoses. Bulletin de la Faculté de Médecine de Paris 1806. Premier serie 1804–1808 (Tome premier):2–22.
3. Carswell R. Illustrations of the elementary forms of disease. Londres: Longman, Orme, Brown, Green and Longman, 1838.
4. Norris W. Eight cases of melanosis with pathological and therapeutical remarks on that disease. Londres: Longman, Brown, Green, Longman and Roberts, 1857.
5. Ries LAG, Eisner MP, Kosary CL, et al., eds. SEER Cancer Statistics Review, 1975–2000, National Cancer Institute. Bethesda, MD, http://seer.cancer.gov/csr/1975_2000, 2003.

6. Ferlay J, Bray F, Pisani P, Parkin DM. GLOBOCAN 2002: Cancer Incidence, Mortality and Prevalence Worldwide. IARC CancerBase No. 5, version 2.0, Lyon: IARC Press, 2004.
7. Nguyen HL, Armstrong BK, Coates M. Cutaneous melanoma in NSW in 1983 to 1995. New South Wales: Sydney Cancer Council, 1997.
8. Lee JA, Scotto J. Melanoma: linked temporal and latitude changes in the United States. Cancer Causes Control 1993; 4(5):413–418.
9. Eklund G, Malec E. Sunlight and incidence of cutaneous malignant melanoma. Effect of latitude and domicile in Sweden. Scand J Plast Reconstr Surg 1978; 12(3):231–241.
10. Magnus K. The Nordic profile of skin cancer incidence. A comparative epidemiological study of three main types of skin cancer. Int J Cancer 1991; 47:12–19.
11. De Vries E, Boniol M, Dore JF, Coebergh JWW for the EUROCARE working group. Lower incidences rates but thicker melanomas in Eastern Europe before 1992: a comparison with Western Europe. Eur J Cancer 2004; 40(7):1045–1052.
12. Scotto J, Nam JM. Skin melanoma and seasonal patterns. Am J Epidemiol 1980; 111(3):309–314.
13. Holman CDJ, Armstrong BK. Skin melanoma and seasonal patterns. Am J Epidemiol 1981; 113:202.
14. Poldenak AP. Seasonal patterns in the diagnosis of malignant melanoma of skin and eye in upstate New York. Cancer 1984; 54(11):2587–2594.
15. Swerdlow AJ. Seasonality of presentation of cutaneous melanoma, squamous cell cancer and basal cell cancer in the Oxford region. Br J Cancer 1985; 52(6):893–900.
16. Schwartz SM, Armstrong BK, Weiss NS. Seasonal variation in the incidence of cutaneous malignant melanoma: an analysis by body site and histologic type. Am J Epidemiol 1987; 126(1):104–111.
17. Akslen LA, Hartweit F. Cutaneous melanoma—season and invasion? A preliminary report. Acta Derm Venereol 1988; 68(5):390–394.
18. Braun M, Tucker A, Devesa S, Hoover R. Seasonal variation in frequency of diagnosis of cutaneous malignant melanoma. Melanoma Res 1994; 4:235–241.
19. Akslen LA. Seasonal variation in melanoma progress. J Natl Cancer Inst 1995; 87(13):1025–1026.
20. Blum A, Ellwanger U, Garbe C. Seasonal patterns in the diagnosis of cutaneous malignant melanoma: analysis of the data of the German Central Malignant Melanoma Registry. Br J Dermatol 1997; 136(6):968–969.
21. Lambe M, Blomqvist P, Bellocco R. Seasonal variation on the diagnosis of cancer: a study based on national cancer registration in Sweden. Brit J Cancer 2003; 88: 1358–1360.
22. Azizi E, Schaaf A, Lazarov A, et al. Decreased density of epidermal dendritic cells in melanocytic naevi: the possible role of in vivo sun exposure. Melanoma Res 1999; 9(5):521–527.
23. Stanganelli L, Bauer P, Bucchi L, et al. Critical effects of intense sun exposure on the expression of epiluminescence microscopy features of acquired melanocytic nevi. Arch Dermatol 1997; 133:979–982.
24. Hinds MW, Lee J, Kolonel LN. Seasonal patterns of skin melanoma incidence in Hawaï. Am J Public Health 1981; 71:496–499.
25. Boniol M, De Vries E, Coebergh JW, Dore JF. EUROCARE Working Group. Seasonal variation in the occurrence of cutaneous melanoma in Europe: influence of latitude. An analysis using the EUROCARE group of registries. Eur J Cancer 2005; 41(1):126–132.

26. Facts and figures 1997. Atlanta: American Cancer Society, 1997.
27. Remontet L, Esteve J, Bouvier AM, et al. Cancer incidence and mortality in France over the period 1978–2000. Rev Epidemiol Sante Publique 2003; 51(1 Pt 1): 3–30.
28. Van der Esch EP, Muir CS, Nectoux J, et al. Temporal change in diagnostic criteria as a cause of the increase of malignant melanoma is unlikely. Int J Cancer 1991; 47:483–489.
29. Garbe C, McLeod GR, Buettner PG. Time trends of cutaneous melanoma in Queensland, Australia and Central Europe. Cancer 2000; 89(6):1269–1278.
30. Lipsker DM, Hedelin G, Heid E, et al. Striking increase of thin melanomas contrasts with stable incidence of thick melanomas. Arch Dermatol 1999; 135(12): 1451–1456.
31. Lee JA. The systematic relationship between melanomas diagnosed in situ and when invasive. Melanoma Res 2001; 11:523–529.
32. Bulliard JL, Cox B, Semenciw R. Trends by anatomic site in the incidence of cutaneous malignant melanoma in Canada, 1969–93. Cancer Causes Control 1999; 10(5):407–416.
33. Marrett LD, Nguyen HL, Armstrong BK. Trends in the incidence of cutaneous malignant melanoma in New South Wales, 1983–1996. Int J Cancer 2001; 92(3):457–462.
34. Jemal A, Devesa SS, Hartge P, Tucker MA. Recent trends in cutaneous melanoma incidence among whites in the United States. J Natl Cancer Inst 2001; 93(9):678–683.
35. Cooper S. First lines of theory and practice of surgery. London: Longman, Orme, Brown, Green and Longman, 1840.
36. Farrell HJ. Cutaneous melanomas with special reference to prognosis. Arch Dermatol Syph 1932; 26:110–124.
37. Davis NC, Shaw HM, McCarthy WH. Melanoma: an historical perspective. In: Thompson JF, Morton DL, Kroon BBR, eds. Textbook of Melanoma. London: Martin Dunitz, 2004:1–12.
38. Keefe M, Mackie RM. The relationship between risk of death from clinical stage 1 cutaneous melanoma and thickness of primary tumour: no evidence for steps in risk. Scottish Melanoma Group. Br J Cancer 1991; 64(3):598–602.
39. Buzaid AC, Ross MI, Balch CM, et al. Critical analysis of the current American Joint Committee on Cancer staging system for cutaneous melanoma and proposal of a new staging system. J Clin Oncol 1997; 15(3):1039–1051.
40. Jemal A, Devesa SS, Fears TR, Hartge P. Cancer surveillance series: changing patterns of cutaneous malignant melanoma mortality rates among whites in the United States. J Natl Cancer Inst 2000; 92(10):811–818.
41. De Vries E, Bray FI, Coebergh JW, Parkin DM. Changing epidemiology of malignant cutaneous melanoma in Europe 1953–1997: rising trends in incidence and mortality but recent stabilizations in western Europe and decreases in Scandinavia. Int J Cancer 2003; 107(1):119–126.
42. Landis SH, Murray T, Bolden S, Wingo PA. Cancer statistics, 1999. CA Cancer J Clin 1999; 49:8–31.
43. Brenner H, Hakulinen T. Long-term cancer patient survival achieved by the end of the 20th century: most up-to-date estimates from the nationwide Finnish cancer registry. Br J Cancer 2001; 85(3):367–371.
44. Boyle P, Autier P, Bartelink H, et al. European code against cancer and scientific justification: third version (2003). Ann Oncol 2003; 14(7):973–1005.

45. Green A, Battistutta D, Hart V, Leslie D, Weedon D, The Nambour Study Group. Skin cancer in a subtropical Australian population: incidence and lack of association with occupation. Am J Epidemiol 1996; 144:1034–1040.

46. Giles GG, Marks R, Foley P. Incidence of non-melanocytic skin cancer treated in Australia. Br Med J (Clin Res Ed) 1988; 296(6614):13–17.

47. Coebergh JWW, Neumann HAM, Vrints LW, Van Der Heijden L, Meijer WJ, Verhagen-Teulings MT. Trends in the incidence of nonmelanoma skin cancer in the SE Netherlands 1975–1988: a registry-based study. Br J Dermatol 1991; 125:353–359.

48. Roberts DL. Incidence of nonmelanoma skin cancer in West Glamorgan, South Wales. Br J Dermatol 1990; 122(3):399–403.

49. Scotto J, Fears TR, Fraumeni JF. Incidence of Non-melanoma skin cancer in the United States. NCI NIH Publication, 1983:n.83–n.2433.

50. Koh D, Wang H, Lee J, Chia KS, Lee HP, Goh CL. Basal cell carcinoma, squamous cell carcinoma and melanoma of the skin: analysis of the Singapore cancer registry data 1968–1997. Br J Dermatol 2003; 148:1161–1166.

51. Katalinic A, Kunze U, Schafer T. Epidemiology of cutaneous melanoma and nonmelanoma skin cancer in Schleswig–Holstein, Germany: incidence, clinical sub-types, tumour stages and localization (epidemiology of skin cancer). Br J Dermatol 2003; 149:1200–1206.

52. Scotto J, Kopf AW, Urbach F. Non-melanoma skin cancer among caucasians in four areas of the United States. Cancer 1974; 34:1333–1338.

53. Kaldor J, Shugg D, Young B, Dwyer T, Wang YG. Non-melanoma skin cancer: ten years of cancer-registry-based surveillance. Int J Cancer 1993; 53:886–891.

54. Green A, Battistutta D. Incidence and determinants of skin cancer in a high-risk Australian population. Int J Cancer 1990; 46:356–361.

55. Harris RB, Griffith K, Moon TE. Trends in the incidence of nonmelanoma skin cancers in southeastern Arizona, 1985–1996. J Am Acad Dermatol 2001; 45: 528–536.

56. Miller DL, Weinstock MA. Non melanoma skin cancer in the United States: inci-dence. J Am Acad Dermatol 1994; 30:774–778.

57. Gallagher RP, Ma B, McLean DI, et al. Trends in basal cell carcinoma, squamous cell carcinoma, and melanoma of the skin, 1973–87. J Am Acad Dermatol 1990; 23:413–421.

58. Marks R, Staples M, Giles GG. Trends in non-melanocytic skin cancer treated in Australia: the second national survey. Int J Cancer 1993; 53:585–590.

59. Buettner PG, Raasch BA. Incidence rates of skin cancer in Townsville, Australia. Int J Cancer 1998; 78:587–593.

60. Osterlind A, Hou-Jensen K, Moller Jensen O. Incidence of cutaneous malignant melanoma in Denmark 1978–1982. Anatomic site distribution, histologic types, and comparison with nonmelanoma skin cancer. Br J Cancer 1988; 58:385–391.

61. Holme SA, Malinovszky K, Roberts DL. Changing trends in nonmelanoma skin cancer in South Wales, 1988–98. Br J Dermatol 2000; 143:1224–1229.

62. Omari AK, Khammash MR, Matalka I. Skin cancer trends in northern Jordan. Int J Dermatol 2004:1–5.

63. Hannuksela-Svahn A, Pukkala E, Karvonen J. Basal cell skin carcinoma and other nonmelanoma skin cancers in Finland from 1956 through 1995. Arch Dermatol 1999; 135:781–786.

64. Levi F, Francesci S, Te VC, Randimbison L, La Vecchia C. Trends of skin cancer in the Canton of Vaud, 1976–1992. Br J Cancer 1995; 72:1047–1053.
65. Plesko I, Severi G, Boyle P. Trends in the incidence of nonmelanoma skin cancer in Slovakia, 1978–1995. Neoplasma 2000; 47(3):137–142.
66. Revenga FA, Paricio JFR, Mar Vazquez MS, del Villar VS. Descriptive epidemiology of basal cell carcinoma and cutaneous squamous cell carcinoma in soria (north-eastern Spain) 1998–2000: a hospital-based survey. J Eur Acad Dermatol Venereol 2004; 18:137–141.
67. Ko CB, Walton S, Keczkes K, Bury HPR, Nicholson C. The emerging epidemic of skin cancer. Br J Dermatol 1994; 130:269–272.
68. De Vries E, Louwman M, Bastiaens M, de Gruijl F, Coeabergh JW. Rapid and continuous increases in incidence rates of basal cell carcinoma in the southeast Netherlands since 1973. J Invest Dermatol 2004; 123:634–638.
69. Marks R, Rennie G, Selwood TS. Malignant transformation of solar keratoses to squamous cell carcinoma. Lancet 1988; 8589:795–797.
70. Osterlind A, Hjalgrim H, Kulinsky B, Frentz G. Skin cancer as a cause of death in Denmark. Br J Dermatol 1991; 125:580–582.
71. Dunn JE, Levin EA, Linden G, Hartzfeld L. Skin cancer as a cause of death. Calif Med 1965; 102:361–363.
72. Housman TS, Feldman SR, Williford PM, et al. Skin cancer is among the most costly of all cancers to treat for the Medicare population. J Am Acad Dermatol 2003; 48:425–429.
73. Diffey BL, Langtry JAA. Skin cancer incidence and the ageing population. Br J Dermatol 2005; 153(3):679.

11

Molecular Epidemiology of Skin Cancer

Rajiv Kumar

*Division of Molecular Genetic Epidemiology, German Cancer
Research Center, Heidelberg, Germany and Department of Bioscience,
Karolinska Institute, Huddinge, Sweden*

INTRODUCTION

Human skin provides mechanical protection to the host against various physical, biological, and chemical environmental agents (1). The skin in the process is itself a potential target of environmental toxins and carcinogens. However, being at the primary interface between the environment and the body, it carries several inherent defense mechanisms. The eventual failure of the defense mechanisms, manifested by deficient repair of DNA damage, fixation of mutations in critical genes, immune suppression, and a host of other events, may ultimately lead to carcinogenesis (2). Different cells in skin upon transformation result in cancers of various types. Most common forms of skin cancers are basal cell carcinoma, squamous cell carcinoma, and melanoma. Basal cell carcinoma originates in basal cells and squamous cell carcinoma in keratinocytes within epidermis. Melanoma results from the transformation of the pigment producing melanocytes that are distributed in the dermal layer (3).

The major etiological factor associated with all types of skin cancers is sun exposure (4). The changed lifestyle in the Western countries, which includes an increase in leisurely sun exposure, has resulted in an ever-increasing number of skin cancers. Nonmelanoma skin cancers occur primarily on sun-exposed parts of the body. Both basal and squamous cell carcinoma are associated with chronic sun exposure and account for 80% and 16% of skin cancers respectively (5). On the other hand, childhood and intermittent sun exposure and severe sunburns are the most critical factors for melanoma development (6). Malignant melanoma constitutes only about 4% of all skin cancers; it is associated with poor outcome and is most fatal of all skin malignancies (7).

Individuals with sun-sensitive skin have a high risk of nonmelanoma skin cancer. The nonmelanoma skin cancer is more common in men than women and exhibits a steep rise in incidence with increasing age. The incidence of nonmelanoma skin cancer has increased at the rate of 3–8% since 1960s in Europe, the United States, Canada, and Australia (8–10). The estimated age-adjusted incidence rates of basal cell carcinoma in the United States are 400 to 500 for men and 200 to 250 per 100,000 for women (11). The incidence rates for basal cell carcinoma are estimated at 1000 to 2000 per 100,000 per year in Australia (12,13). Squamous cell carcinoma is less common and its estimated incidence rates vary from 30 to 1000 per 100,000, depending on the geographical region. The estimated annual increase in incidence of malignant melanoma has been around 3% to 7% in Caucasian populations (14). The frequency of occurrence of melanoma is associated with melanocytic nevi, skin freckles, constitutive color of skin and it is also dependent on the geographic zone (15).

SUN EXPOSURE AND DNA DAMAGE

Epidemiological and molecular data strongly suggest that different forms of skin cancers are caused by exposure to sunlight (16). Sunlight comprises a continuous spectrum of electromagnetic radiation that is divided into ultraviolet (UV), visible and infrared radiations, according to the wavelength. High-energy UVC radiation (wavelength below 280 nm) and a part of UVB radiation (wavelength between 280 nm and 290 nm) are blocked by the stratospheric ozone layer from reaching the surface of the earth. However, a part of UVB radiation (wavelength 290–315 nm) and UVA (315–400 nm) is able to reach the earth surface. The radiation reaching the surface of the earth is about 1% to 10% UVB and the rest 90% to 99% is UVA. The exposure of human skin to these components of sunlight may result in sunburn inflammation (erythema), immune suppression, DNA damage, gene mutation, and ultimately cancer (17).

Types of DNA Damage

At the molecular level, UV radiation causes DNA damage. DNA is a chromophore for UVB radiation and exposure to it results in direct lesions (18). UVB radiation primarily induces cyclobutane-type pyrimidine dimers and pyrimidine (6-4) pyrimidone photoproducts (19). Both photoproducts are formed exclusively in tandem pyrimidine residues along a DNA strand. Cyclobutane pyrimidine dimers are the dominant DNA lesions formed by UVB radiation from a [2 + 2] cycloaddition of the C5-C6 double bonds of two adjacent pyrimidine bases.

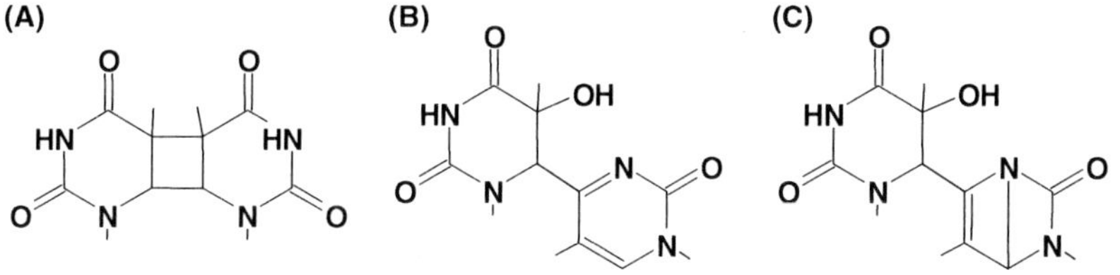

Figure 1 Structure of UV-induced photoproducts. (**A**) Cyclobutane pyrimidine dimer, (**B**) 6,4-photoproduct, and (**C**) Dewar valence isomer.

The torsional flexibility and the bending angle of the DNA helix are important determinants in the formation of cyclobutane dimers in a given dipyrimidine sequence (20). Pyrimidine (6-4) pyrimidone photoproducts (referred to as 6,4-photoproducts) are less common and are formed at a 5- to 10-time lower levels than cyclobutane dimers. These photoproducts are formed from a [2 + 2] cycloaddition involving C5-C6 double bond of the 5'-end pyrimidine and C4 carbonyl group of the 3'-end thymine through an oxetane or azetidine four-membered ring intermediate (20). 6,4-Photoproducts are easily converted into Dewar valence isomers upon UVB radiation (Fig. 1). Dewar photoproducts are more efficiently formed by solar simulated light than by the UVB (21). At a very low quantum yield, purine bases adjacent to pyrimidine bases also form photoproducts in addition to photo-hydrations and photo-oxidations (20). The mechanism of DNA damage by UVA radiation is rather complex and evidently involves photosensitization in oxidation reactions (22). This includes absorption of UVA photons by unidentified endogenous photosensitizers. UVA radiation in cells results in exalted formation of reactive oxygen species, which are implicated in oxidative damage to DNA and skin cancer risk (20). The UVA radiation at a dose used in artificial sunlamps induces cyclobutane pyrimidine dimers in human skin DNA at a level lower than by UVB radiation (23,24).

In Vivo DNA Photoproducts and Consequences

The formation of DNA photoproducts in vivo in human skin upon exposure to sunlight is a common occurrence. In situ irradiation of unexposed skin of human volunteers with solar-simulated radiation at erythema threshold induces DNA damage (2 lesions per 100,000 nucleotides) that far exceeds in levels measured for any other carcinogen (25). The formation of DNA photoproducts is dose-dependent. The measurement of in situ DNA photoproducts based on ^{32}P-postlabelling detected a linear relationship between the lesions in irradiated skin with the UV doses from 40 to 400 J/m (2,25,26). Additional studies based on the same technique detected 15- to 30-fold inter-individual variation in the formation of TC cyclobutane pyrimidine dimers at TTC sequences after irradiation with either uniform UVB or with minimal erythema doses (27). Inter-individual variation in the levels of DNA photoproducts can, in part, explain the observed inter-individual differences in susceptibility to skin carcinogenesis (28).

UV-induced DNA damage in skin is influenced by a number of host factors. The pattern of UV-induced lesions in DNA is also dependent on the nucleosome structure (29). The level of TC and TT cyclobutane pyrimidine dimers (at TTC and TTT sequences), but not 6-4 photoproducts formed, was observed to be higher in individuals with skin type I/II than in those with skin type III/IV (28). One important determinant of DNA damage that has emerged from recent in situ measurements is age (28). The in situ level of TC cyclobutane pyrimidine dimers at TTC sequences upon irradiation of skin has been shown to be significantly higher in individuals above 50 years of age than those below 50 years (30). Age has been estimated to have a systematic effect on the induction on all photoproducts, with a regular increase in levels with the increase in age (28). This is in consonant with a 10% to 20% decrease of active melanocytes in each decade of life, resulting in decreased protection against UV radiation (31). In addition, aging also results in changes in skin morphology, histology, and physiology (32). Sun-protection factors are considered to protect skin from the risk of cancer. In the studies carried out to measure the protection of DNA from the UV-induced photoproducts, it has been found that protection against both erythemal response and DNA damage varied from 5- to 10-fold (26). The sunscreens protect individuals against DNA in accordance with sun-protection factor. However, inter-individual variability can leave some individuals at a high risk of UV-induced damage and consequently skin cancer (33).

The consequences of the formation of UV photoproducts in situ on exposure to solar radiation are manifold. Erythema or sunburn, which is an inflammatory reaction, is the most visible effect of UVB radiation on human skin with varying degrees of severity. Erythema is likely initiated by the release of cytokines like IL-6, IL-10, and TNF-α in the epidermis. The release of these cytokines is linked to UV-mediated DNA damage as demonstrated by the reduction in levels upon stimulation of DNA repair (34–36). The formation of both cyclobutane pyrimidine dimers and 6,4-photoproducts in the promoter region of different genes inhibit DNA-protein interaction, in vitro transcription and trans-activation of reporter genes (37). The most significant consequence of DNA photoproducts, if those are left unrepaired, is fixation of mutations and initiation of skin carcinogenesis.

Repair of DNA Photoproducts

Eukaryotic cells are equipped with evolutionarily conserved repair pathways capable of removing different kinds of DNA damages (38). Two major photoproducts formed as a consequence of UV irradiation in skin cells are repaired by the complex multistep process of *nucleotide excision repair* (39). This repair process comprises two distinct pathways and involves about 30 different proteins (40). The three steps that are specific to nucleotide excision repair are (*i*) recognition of base damage, (*ii*) bimodal incision of DNA, and (*iii*) the excision of oligo-nucleotide fragments. The type of the photoproduct, the sequence context, and the nucleosome structure determine the efficiency of nucleotide excision repair (29,41). DNA lesions in actively transcribed genes are removed rapidly by *transcription-coupled repair*. On the other hand, the *global genome repair* of DNA lesions in noncoding sequences and nontranscribed strand is a slow process (39). The deleterious defects in the genes encoding nucleotide excision repair enzymes result in the severe genetic syndrome xeroderma pigmentosum (XP) (42). In XP individuals, the inability to repair DNA photoproducts results in enhanced mutational burden and neoplastic transformation. The syndrome is characterized by extreme sun-sensitivity and 1000- to 2000-fold higher inci-dences of all types of skin cancers (43).

A number of assays have been described to measure DNA repair capacity, which have been based on DNA strand break, mass spectra, unscheduled DNA synthesis, host-cell reactivation, immunochemical detection, and ^{32}P-postlabelling of DNA photoproducts (27,44–47). Many studies based on host cell reactivation, which involves the use of cultured cells from surrogate tissues, have shown DNA repair capacity to be age-dependent (45,48). Individ-uals with low repair capacity are at an increased risk of skin cancer (48,49). However, no age-specific effect has been detected by studies, which measured kinetics of removal of DNA photoproducts in skin (30). In general, 6,4-photopr-oducts are repaired faster than cyclobutane dimers. Moreover, dependent on the sequence context, TC cyclobutane pyrimidine dimers at TTC sequences may be repaired faster than TT dimers at TTT sequences (50). Dewar photoproducts are repaired slowly and inefficiently; their repair rates in mammalian cells match that of cyclobutane pyrimidine dimers (21). Most photoproducts are repaired within 24 hours of exposure. However, persistence of photoproducts shows a large inter-individual variation. In a study population, the percentage of repaired TC cyclobutane pyrimidine dimers at TTC sequences 24 hours after UV radiation ranged from 0% to 82% (27). Another in situ experiment on human volunteers demonstrated persistence of TT dimers at TTT sequences three weeks after exposure to minimal erythema dose (51). The removal of DNA photoproducts has been shown to be independent of skin type or gender.

Skin cancer patients, in studies mostly based on surrogate tissues, have gen-erally been associated with the reduced DNA repair capacities compared with healthy controls (52,53). In studies on the removal of in situ DNA photoproducts in skin after UV irradiation, no differences in repair kinetics were observed between patients with melanoma or basal cell carcinoma and healthy controls (28,54). From the studies on in situ repair kinetics, it emerged that the two major determinants of individual skin cancer susceptibility are (*i*) inter-individual variation in formation of UV photoproducts and (*ii*) inter-individual variation in repair capacity. An estimated 30-fold variation in the formation of DNA photo-products and a 15-fold variation in DNA repair would translate into 10^3- to 10^4-fold differences in inter-individual susceptibility (28).

UV SIGNATURE MUTATIONS IN CRITICAL GENES

The closest realization of the metaphor "carcinogens leave fingerprints" comes from the study of mutational spectra of critical genes in skin cancers (55). Skin cancers, particularly nonmelanoma, provided the first direct molecular evidence for the role of environmental agents in carcinogenesis. In nonmelanoma skin cancers, *p53* is the most commonly altered gene and mutations occur in about 50% of the tumors (56). The frequency of C>T transitions at dipyrimidinic sites in the *p53* gene is about 61% and that of CC>TT tandem mutations about 17% (17,57). Consistent with the levels of DNA photoproducts, sunlight has been shown to induce mutations to such an extent that sun-exposed skin cells have mutant fractions about a thousand times higher than those observed in peripheral T-cells (58–60).

In human skin, cancers about 35% of all mutations in the *p53* gene are transitions at dipyrimidines within the sequence 5'-TCG and 5'-CCG, which are localized within several mutational hotspots (57). These hot spots include codons 248, 278, and 282. Irradiation of cells with UVB or sunlight results in preferential formation of cyclobutane pyrimidine dimers at dipyrimidinic sites containing 5-methylcytosine (61). Evidence suggests that 5-methylcytosine absorbs about 15-fold higher near UV than unmethylated cytosine, implying that UV light could preferentially affect cytosines at CpG sites (62). Two models for UV mutagenesis have been proposed to explain the predominance of C>T transitions at dipyrimidine sites (Fig. 2). The first one involves bypass of lesions by a DNA polymerase that incorporates adenine opposite to a cytosine or 5-methyl cytosine or both within a cyclobutane pyrimidine dimer. The second pathway involves deamination of cytosine or 5-methylcytosine or both within the CPD lesion, followed by a correct bypass during DNA replication. In the context of 5-methylcytosine, the latter pathway plays an important role in UVB mutagenesis in mammalian cells (57,63).

The *p53* mutations are less common in melanoma and occur with a frequency of less than 10%. However, the frequency of mutations in the gene in melanomas from XP patients is about 60%. XP patients develop melanoma mainly on sun-exposed parts (64). Basal cell carcinoma from both XP and non-XP patients contains a high frequency of UV signature mutations in the *p53* gene (65). Squamous cell carcinomas occur mainly at chronically sun-exposed parts of the body and arise from premalignant lesions (actinic keratosis) with a transformation rate of 1 in 1000. Frequent C>T mutations at dipyrimidines in the *p53* gene occur in both SCC and actinic keratosis (58).

Although UV induces the mutations in the *p53* gene in both basal and squamous cell carcinoma, the mutational spectra and hotspots in the two types of skin cancers are different. Typical mutational hotspots in basal cell carcinoma involve codons 177, 196, and 245. In squamous cell carcinoma, the codon 278 is specifically mutated. Evidence from in vitro experiments suggests a slow repair of UV photoproducts at p53 mutational hotspots. The hotspots for mutations in

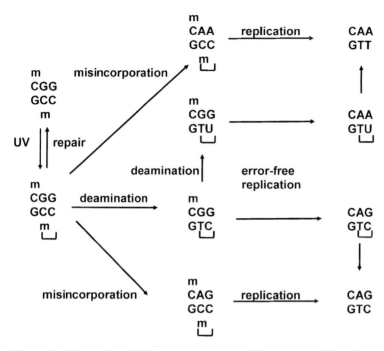

Figure 2 Mechanism of UV mutagenesis at a cyclobutane pyrimidine dimer. The cyclo-butane pyrimidine dimmer (CPD) is indicated by a bracket. The sequence context 5′CmCG is prone to CPD formation by irradiation with sunlight due to the presence of the 5-methylcytosine (mC). *Source*: From Ref. 63; courtesy of Elsevier.

melanoma are different from the other two skin cancer types and include codons 213, 286, 290, and 296 (57). Essentially, different types of skin cancers show a similarity of mutation spectra in both XP and non-XP cases, however, CC>TT tandem mutations are more frequent in skin cancers from XP patients than in non-XP patients (Fig. 3) (57).

In skin cancers, UV-specific mutations also occur in other critical genes. The human homolog of the *PTCH* gene is frequently mutated in sporadic tumors as well as in the rare genetic syndromes such as nevoid basal cell carcinoma (Gorlin's syndrome) and XP (66). Basal cell carcinoma tumors from XP patients reportedly contain significantly higher frequency of UV tandem mutations in the *PTCH* gene than those from the non-XP cases (65). Similarly, UV-specific mutations in basal cell carcinoma from XP patients are also found in the *smoothened* gene (67). At molecular level, the evidence for UV signature mutations in melanoma compared with nonmelanoma skin cancers has been rather feeble. However, the melanoma susceptibility gene *CDKN2A*, which carries disease segregating germline mutations in familial melanoma, is to a certain extent also altered in sporadic melanomas. C > T transitions at dipyrimidine sites in the *CDKN2A* gene are

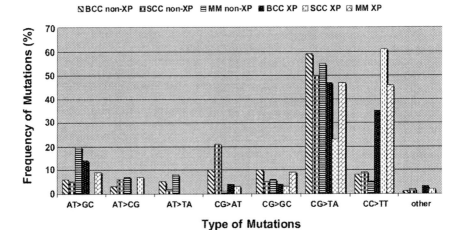

Figure 3   Distribution of different types of base substitutions in *p53* gene in XP and non-XP skin cancers. *Abbreviations*: BCC, basal cell carcinoma; SCC, squamous cell carcinoma; MM, malignant melanoma. *Source*: From Ref. 57; courtesy of Wiley-Liss, Inc., a subsidiary of John Wiley & Sons, Inc.

frequent and CC > TT tandem mutations have also been regularly reported in tumors and melanoma cell lines (68–70). UV-specific mutations in the *CDKN2A* gene have also been detected in squamous cell carcinomas, particularly, in cases from psoralen-plus-UVA-treated psoriasis patients (71,72).

More recently, 60% to 70% of sporadic melanomas and melanocytic nevi have been shown to carry oncogenic mutations in the *BRAF* gene (73–76). Mutations in the *BRAF* gene occur on a mutual exclusive basis with *N-RAS* mutations (74). The predominant *BRAF* mutation, T1799A transversion at codon 600, accounts for over 90% of all alterations detected in the gene (73). The major oncogenic mutation in the *BRAF* gene has been speculated to be a consequence of oxidative damage (75). Incidentally, mutations in the *N-RAS* gene occur mainly in melanomas localized on sun-exposed parts and involve a dipyrimidinic site at codon 61 (77,78).

GENETIC DETERMINANTS OF RISK MODULATION

Inter-individual differences in susceptibility to various skin cancers implicate the involvement of genetic factors in risk modulation. Many repair genes that encode enzymes involved in DNA repair carry nonsynonymous single nucleotide polymorphisms that can potentially modulate function (79). A population-based study on screening of 37 DNA repair genes identified 127 single nucleotide polymorphisms, with frequencies of variant alleles between 0.01 and 0.50 (80). The majority of single nucleotide variants identified cause exchanges of amino acid residues with dissimilar chemical and physical properties. It is postulated that the single nucleotide polymorphisms in different repair genes could, in part, be associated with altered susceptibility to cancers including that of skin (81,82). Many of the single nucleotide polymorphisms in DNA repair genes have been tested for modulation of risk of skin cancer in population-based case-control studies (83). A number of studies have shown association between variant alleles and risk of various skin malignancies (Table 1). Polymorphisms in the *XPC*, *XPD*, *XRCC1*, *XRCC3*, and *NBS1* genes have been associated with modulation of risk of different skin cancers (84–88). Several studies also provided the evidence for a gene–environment interaction. In some studies on skin cancers, the polymorphisms in the *XRCC1* and *XRCC3* gene were shown to be associated with a life-time risk of sunburns (85,89).

The functional relevance of some polymorphisms in DNA repair genes is supported by a number of studies. In a study on DNA repair kinetics in human skins, individuals older than 50 years with the K751Q *XPD* polymorphism showed decreased repair rate of UV photoproducts (90). Similarly, in host cell reactivation assays, polymorphisms in *XPC* and *XPD* were associated with a reduced repair capacity (91). Two separate studies found that the common allele for the K751Q polymorphism in the *XPD* gene was associated with

Table 1 Single Nucleotide Polymorphisms in Some of the DNA Repair Genes and Associated Effect on the Risk of Different Skin Cancers

Gene	Exon	Base change	Amino acid change	Variant allele frequency	Effect of variant allele	References
XPC	15	A > C	K939Q	0.38	Risk of melanoma and multiple primary melanomas	(86)
	8	C > T	A499V	0.24		
XPD	10	G > A	D312N	0.40	Protective haplotype combination in BCC; risk of subsequent skin cancer	(84,87)
	23	A > C	K751Q	0.32		
XRCC1	6	C > T	R194W	0.13	Protective in NMSC; association with risk of sunburns	(89)
	10	G > A	R399Q	0.24		
NBS1	5	G > C	Q185E	0.34	Risk of BCC in men	(Kumar et al., Unpublished data)
XRCC3	7	C > T	T241M	0.43	Protective in BCC	(85)

Abbreviations: BCC, basal cell carcinoma; NMSC, nonmelanoma skin cancer.

increased micronuclei in radiation workers and chromosomal aberrations in lymphocytes from general population (92,93). Lymphoblastoid cell lines with variant allele for the D312N polymorphism in the *XPD* gene showed increased apoptotic response upon UV or ionized radiation exposure (94).

In addition to the DNA repair genes, polymorphisms in specific susceptibility genes have also been associated with modulation of skin cancer risk. In some studies, the polymorphisms in the *PTCH* gene were associated with the rate of developing BCC and with skin pigmentation (95,96). An increased risk of melanoma on the other hand has been associated with polymorphisms in the *CDKN2A* gene (97,98). Similarly, carriers of the common allele in the promoter region of the *vitamin D receptor* gene have been associated with increased risk of melanoma and with the risk of metastasis (99). Polymorphisms in the *melanocortin-1 receptor* (*MC1R*) gene are associated with the variation in human pigmentation phenotypes and skin types. More than 65 human *MC1R* variant alleles with varying physiological activity have been identified (100). Three variant alleles reportedly increase the risk of all forms of skin cancers and in melanoma families modulate penetrance and the age of onset in *CDKN2A* mutation carriers (101).

ARSENIC AS A SKIN CARCINOGEN

Skin cancers of all types are overwhelmingly associated with UV exposure, but other environmental factors may also play a role in the risk modulation. In specific situations, such factors can become major determinants of the risk (102). One such factor associated with an increased risk of skin cancer is arsenic exposure. Inorganic arsenic is one of the earliest identified human carcinogens, with both basal and squamous cell carcinoma being associated with arsenic ingestion (102). Exposure to arsenic through drinking water results in skin lesions, which are preceded by nonmalignant lesions as hyperkeratosis. The evidence for its role in human carcinogenesis has come from epidemiological studies on exposed populations in Bangladesh, Taiwan, Argentina, and Mexico (102–104). Arsenic is metabolized in vivo by the reduction of pentavalent form to trivalent form and the addition of methyl groups (105). The mechanism of skin carcinogenesis by arsenic is still not completely understood, the evidence from in vitro experiments suggests interference with repair systems (106). Moreover, arsenic enhances mutagenecity or clastogenicity of UV and other carcinogens in mammalian cells (107). At low doses, arsenic has been shown to inhibit the incision step of nucleotide excision repair and also blocks base excision repair, causing increased strand breaks in human cells (108). On the basis of evidence from animal models, it is hypothesized that inorganic arsenic acts as a co-carcinogen by enhancement of UV-induced skin cancers through several mechanisms (102,107).

CONCLUSIONS

The etiology of human skin cancer is mainly linked to sun exposure and, in certain situations, with arsenic exposure. The development of skin cancer involves interplay between the DNA damage caused by the UV component of the sunlight, repair of the damage, fixation of the mutations in critical genes, and a host of other critical factors. Many of the factors critical for skin carcinogenesis display vast inter-individual variations that lead to differences in susceptibilities. It is postulated that the inter-individual variations are genetically determined, with a possible role for the polymorphisms in the DNA repair and other critical genes. Many of the polymorphisms in different genes have been shown to modulate risk of different skin cancers at population level. However, many more determinants of the risk modulation remain unknown. Ultimately, the cancer susceptibility depends on interaction between environmental and individual genetic factors.

ACKNOWLEDGMENTS

I express my gratitude to Professor Kari Hemminki, Drs Asta Försti, Dan Segerbäck, Justo Lorenzo Bermejo, and Lei Haixin for critical reading of the manuscript and for their comments and suggestions.

REFERENCES

1. Mancini AJ. Skin. Pediatrics 2004; 113:1114–1119.
2. Moodycliffe AM, Nghiem D, Clydesdale G, et al. Immune suppression and skin cancer development: regulation by NKT cells. Nat Immunol 2000; 1:521–525.
3. Einspahr JG, Stratton SP, Bowden GT, et al. Chemoprevention of human skin cancer. Crit Rev Oncol Hematol 2002; 41:269–285.
4. Armstrong BK, Kricker A. The epidemiology of UV induced skin cancer. J Photochem Photobiol B 2001; 63:8–18.
5. Bowden GT. Prevention of non-melanoma skin cancer by targeting ultraviolet-B-light signalling. Nat Rev Cancer 2004; 4:23–35.
6. Gandini S, Sera F, Cattaruzza MS, et al. Meta-analysis of risk factors for cutaneous melanoma: II. Sun exposure. Eur J Cancer 2005; 41:45–60.
7. Gilchrest BA, Eller MS, Geller AC, et al. The pathogenesis of melanoma induced by ultraviolet radiation. N Engl J Med 1999; 340:1341–1348.
8. Diepgen TL, Mahler V. The epidemiology of skin cancer. Br J Dermatol 2002; 146(suppl 61):1–6.
9. Green A. Changing patterns in incidence of non-melanoma skin cancer. Epithelial Cell Biol 1992; 1:47–51.
10. Glass AG, Hoover RN. The emerging epidemic of melanoma and squamous cell skin cancer. JAMA 1989; 262:2097–2100.
11. Miller DL, Weinstock MA. Nonmelanoma skin cancer in the United States: incidence. J Am Acad Dermatol 1994; 30:774–778.

12. Buettner PG, Raasch BA. Incidence rates of skin cancer in Townsville, Australia. Int J Cancer 1998; 78:587–593.
13. Green A, Battistutta D, Hart V, et al. Skin cancer in a subtropical Australian population: incidence and lack of association with occupation. The Nambour Study Group. Am J Epidemiol 1996; 144:1034–1040.
14. Jemal A, Devesa SS, Hartge P, et al. Recent trends in cutaneous melanoma incidence among whites in the United States. J Natl Cancer Inst 2001; 93:678–683.
15. Tucker MA, Goldstein AM. Melanoma etiology: where are we? Oncogene 2003; 22:3042–3052.
16. Matsumura Y, Ananthaswamy HN. Toxic effects of ultraviolet radiation on the skin. Toxicol Appl Pharmacol 2004; 195:298–308.
17. Melnikova VO, Ananthaswamy HN. Cellular and molecular events leading to the development of skin cancer. Mutat Res 2005; 571:91–106.
18. Cleaver JE, Crowley E. UV damage, DNA repair and skin carcinogenesis. Front Biosci 2002; 7:d1024–d1043.
19. Cadet J, Sage E, Douki T. Ultraviolet radiation-mediated damage to cellular DNA. Mutat Res 2005; 571:3–17.
20. Ravanat JL, Douki T, Cadet J. Direct and indirect effects of UV radiation on DNA and its components. J Photochem Photobiol B 2001; 63:88–102.
21. Perdiz D, Grof P, Mezzina M, et al. Distribution and repair of bipyrimidine photoproducts in solar UV-irradiated mammalian cells: possible role of Dewar photoproducts in solar mutagenesis. J Biol Chem 2000; 275:26732–26742.
22. Cadet J, Berger M, Douki T, et al. Oxidative damage to DNA: formation, measurement, and biological significance. Rev Physiol Biochem Pharmacol 1997; 131:1–87.
23. Young AR, Potten CS, Nikaido O, et al. Human melanocytes and keratinocytes exposed to UVB or UVA in vivo show comparable levels of thymine dimers. J Invest Dermatol 1998; 111:936–940.
24. Xu G, Marcusson JA, Hemminki K. DNA photodamage induced by UV phototherapy lamps and sunlamps in human skin in situ and its potential importance for skin cancer. J Invest Dermatol 2001; 116:194–195.
25. Bykov VJ, Jansen CT, Hemminki K. High levels of dipyrimidine dimers are induced in human skin by solar-simulating UV radiation. Cancer Epidemiol Biomarkers Prev 1998; 7:199–202.
26. Bykov VJ, Marcusson JA, Hemminki K. Ultraviolet B-induced DNA damage in human skin and its modulation by a sunscreen. Cancer Res 1998; 58:2961–2964.
27. Bykov VJ, Sheehan JM, Hemminki K, et al. In situ repair of cyclobutane pyrimidine dimers and 6-4 photoproducts in human skin exposed to solar simulating radiation. J Invest Dermatol 1999; 112:326–331.
28. Hemminki K, Xu G, Le Curieux F. Ultraviolet radiation-induced photoproducts in human skin DNA as biomarkers of damage and its repair. IARC Sci Publ 2001; 154:69–79.
29. Thoma F. Repair of UV lesions in nucleosomes—intrinsic properties and remodeling. DNA Repair (Amst) 2005; 4:855–869.
30. Xu G, Snellman E, Bykov VJ, et al. Effect of age on the formation and repair of UV photoproducts in human skin in situ. Mutat Res 2000; 459:195–202.
31. Gilchrest BA, Blog FB, Szabo G. Effects of aging and chronic sun exposure on melanocytes in human skin. J Invest Dermatol 1979; 73:141–143.

32. Yaar M, Gilchrest BA. Ageing and photoageing of keratinocytes and melanocytes. Clin Exp Dermatol 2001; 26:583–591.
33. Bykov VJ, Marcusson JA, Hemminki K. Protective effects of tanning on cutaneous DNA damage in situ. Dermatology 2001; 202:22–26.
34. Vink AA, Roza L. Biological consequences of cyclobutane pyrimidine dimers. J Photochem Photobiol B 2001; 65:101–104.
35. Wolf P, Maier H, Mullegger RR, et al. Topical treatment with liposomes containing T4 endonuclease V protects human skin in vivo from ultraviolet-induced upregulation of interleukin-10 and tumor necrosis factor-alpha. J Invest Dermatol 2000; 114:149–156.
36. Petit-Frere C, Clingen PH, Grewe M, et al. Induction of interleukin-6 production by ultraviolet radiation in normal human epidermal keratinocytes and in a human keratinocyte cell line is mediated by DNA damage. J Invest Dermatol 1998; 111:354–349.
37. Ghosh R, Tummala R, Mitchell DL. Ultraviolet radiation-induced DNA damage in promoter elements inhibits gene expression. FEBS Lett 2003; 554:427–432.
38. Friedberg EC. DNA damage and repair. Nature 2003; 421:436–440.
39. Friedberg EC. How nucleotide excision repair protects against cancer. Nature Reviews Cancer 2001; 1:22–33.
40. Wood RD, Mitchell M, Lindahl T. Human DNA repair genes. Mutat Res 2005. www.cgal.icnet.uk/dna_repair_genes.html.
41. Tornaletti S, Pfeifer GP. Slow repair of pyrimidine dimers at *p53* mutation hotspots in skin cancer. Science 1994; 263:1436–1438.
42. Friedberg EC, Walker GC, Siede W. DNA Repair and Mutagenesis. Washington: ASM Press, 1995.
43. Daya-Grosjean L, Sarasin A. The role of UV-induced lesions in skin carcinogenesis: an overview of oncogene and tumor suppressor gene modifications in xeroderma pigmentosum skin tumors. Mutat Res 2005; 571:43–56.
44. Gao S, Drouin R, Holmquist GP. DNA repair rates mapped along the human PGK1 gene at nucleotide resolution. Science 1994; 263:1438–1440.
45. Wei Q, Matanoski GM, Farmer ER, et al. DNA repair and aging in basal cell carcinoma: a molecular epidemiology study. Proc Natl Acad Sci USA 1993; 90:1614–1618.
46. Mu D, Sancar A. DNA excision repair assays. Prog Nucleic Acid Res Mol Biol 1997; 56:63–81.
47. Kelly CM, Latimer JJ. Unscheduled DNA synthesis: a functional assay for global genomic nucleotide excision repair. Methods Mol Biol 2005; 291:303–320.
48. Wei Q. Effect of aging on DNA repair and skin carcinogenesis: a minireview of population-based studies. J Invest Dermatol. Symposium Proc 1998; 3:19–22.
49. Goukassian D, Gad F, Yaar M, et al. Mechanisms and implications of the age-associated decrease in DNA repair capacity. Faseb J 2000; 14:1325–1334.
50. Xu G, Snellman E, Bykov VJ, et al. Cutaneous melanoma patients have normal repair kinetics of ultraviolet-induced DNA repair in skin in situ. J Invest Dermatol 2000; 114:628–631.
51. Hemminki K, Xu G, Kause L, et al. Demonstration of UV-dimers in human skin DNA in situ 3 weeks after exposure. Carcinogenesis 2002; 23:605–609.
52. Wei Q, Lee JE, Gershenwald JE, et al. Repair of UV light-induced DNA damage and risk of cutaneous malignant melanoma. J Natl Cancer Inst 2003; 95:308–315.

53. Berwick M, Vineis P. Markers of DNA repair and susceptibility to cancer in humans: an epidemiologic review. J Natl Cancer Inst 2000; 92:874–897.
54. Hemminki K, Thilly WG. Implications of results of molecular epidemiology on DNA adducts, their repair and mutations for mechanisms of human cancer. IARC Sci Publ 2004; 217–235.
55. Vogelstein B, Kinzler KW. Carcinogens leave fingerprints. Nature 1992; 355:209–210.
56. Boukamp P. Non-melanoma skin cancer: what drives tumor development and progression? Carcinogenesis 2005; 26:1657–1667.
57. Giglia-Mari G, Sarasin A. *TP53* mutations in human skin cancers. Hum Mutat 2003; 21:217–228.
58. Ziegler A, Jonason AS, Leffell DJ, et al. Sunburn and *p53* in the onset of skin cancer. Nature 1994; 372:773–776.
59. Zhang W, Remenyik E, Zelterman D, et al. Escaping the stem cell compartment: sustained UVB exposure allows *p53*-mutant keratinocytes to colonize adjacent epidermal proliferating units without incurring additional mutations. Proc Natl Acad Sci USA 2001; 98:13948–13953.
60. Thilly WG. Have environmental mutagens caused oncomutations in people? Nat Genet 2003; 34:255–259.
61. Tornaletti S, Pfeifer GP. Complete and tissue-independent methylation of CpG sites in the *p53* gene: implications for mutations in human cancers. Oncogene 1995; 10:1493–1499.
62. Lee DH, Pfeifer GP. Deamination of 5-methylcytosines within cyclobutane pyrimidine dimers is an important component of UVB mutagenesis. J Biol Chem 2003; 278:10314–10321.
63. Pfeifer GP, You YH, Besaratinia A. Mutations induced by ultraviolet light. Mutat Res 2005; 571:19–31.
64. Spatz A, Giglia-Mari G, Benhamou S, et al. Association between DNA repair-deficiency and high level of *p53* mutations in melanoma of Xeroderma pigmentosum. Cancer Res 2001; 61:2480–2486.
65. Ling G, Ahmadian A, Persson A, et al. PATCHED and *p53* gene alterations in sporadic and hereditary basal cell cancer. Oncogene 2001; 20:7770–7778.
66. D'Errico M, Calcagnile A, Canzona F, et al. UV mutation signature in tumor suppressor genes involved in skin carcinogenesis in xeroderma pigmentosum patients. Oncogene 2000; 19:463–467.
67. Couve-Privat S, Bouadjar B, Avril MF, et al. Significantly high levels of ultraviolet-specific mutations in the smoothened gene in basal cell carcinomas from DNA repair-deficient xeroderma pigmentosum patients. Cancer Res 2002; 62:7186–7189.
68. Kumar R, Lundh Rozell B, Louhelainen J, et al. Mutations in the CDKN2A (p16INK4a) gene in microdissected sporadic primary melanomas. Int J Cancer 1998; 75:193–198.
69. Pollock PM, Yu F, Qiu L, et al. Evidence for UV induction of CDKN2 mutations in melanoma cell lines. Oncogene 1995; 11:663–668.
70. Ruas M, Peters G. The p16INK4a/CDKN2A tumor suppressor and its relatives. Biochim Biophys Acta 1998; 1378:F115–F177.
71. Soufir N, Moles JP, Vilmer C, et al. P16 UV mutations in human skin epithelial tumors. Oncogene 1999; 18:5477–5481.
72. Kreimer-Erlacher H, Seidl H, Back B, et al. High frequency of ultraviolet mutations at the INK4a-ARF locus in squamous cell carcinomas from psoralen-plus-ultraviolet-A-treated psoriasis patients. J Invest Dermatol 2003; 120:676–682.

73. Davies H, Bignell GR, Cox C, et al. Mutations of the BRAF gene in human cancer. Nature 2002; 417:949–954.

74. Kumar R, Angelini S, Hemminki K. Activating BRAF and N-Ras mutations in sporadic primary melanomas: an inverse association with allelic loss on chromosome 9. Oncogene 2003; 22:9217–9224.

75. Kumar R, Angelini S, Snellman E, et al. BRAF mutations are common somatic events in melanocytic nevi. J Invest Dermatol 2004; 122:342–348.

76. Pollock PM, Harper UL, Hansen KS, et al. High frequency of BRAF mutations in nevi. Nat Genet 2003; 33:19–20.

77. Jiveskog S, Ragnarsson-Olding B, Platz A, et al. N-ras mutations are common in melanomas from sun-exposed skin of humans but rare in mucosal membranes or unexposed skin. J Invest Dermatol 1998; 111:757–761.

78. Omholt K, Karsberg S, Platz A, et al. Screening of N-ras Codon 61 mutations in paired primary and metastatic cutaneous melanomas: mutations occur early and persist throughout tumor progression. Clin Cancer Res 2002; 8:3468–3474.

79. Shen MR, Jones IM, Mohrenweiser H. Nonconservative amino acid substitution variants exist at polymorphic frequency in DNA repair genes in healthy humans. Cancer Res 1998; 58:604–608.

80. Mohrenweiser HW, Xi T, Vazquez-Matias J, et al. Identification of 127 amino acid substitution variants in screening 37 DNA repair genes in humans. Cancer Epidemiol Biomarkers Prev 2002; 11:1054–1064.

81. Mohrenweiser HW, Wilson DM, 3rd, Jones IM. Challenges and complexities in estimating both the functional impact and the disease risk associated with the extensive genetic variation in human DNA repair genes. Mutat Res 2003; 526:93–125.

82. Xi T, Jones IM, Mohrenweiser HW. Many amino acid substitution variants identified in DNA repair genes during human population screenings are predicted to impact protein function. Genomics 2004; 83:970–979.

83. Goode EL, Ulrich CM, Potter JD. Polymorphisms in DNA repair genes and associations with cancer risk. Cancer Epidemiol Biomarkers Prev 2002; 11:1513–1530.

84. Lovatt T, Alldersea J, Lear JT, et al. Polymorphism in the nuclear excision repair gene ERCC2/XPD: association between an exon 6-exon 10 haplotype and susceptibility to cutaneous basal cell carcinoma. Hum Mutat 2005; 25:353–359.

85. Han J, Colditz GA, Samson LD, et al. Polymorphisms in DNA double-strand break repair genes and skin cancer risk. Cancer Res 2004; 64:3009–3013.

86. Blankenburg S, Konig IR, Moessner R, et al. Assessment of 3 xeroderma pigmentosum group C gene polymorphisms and risk of cutaneous melanoma: a case-control study. Carcinogenesis 2005; 26:1085–1090.

87. Brewster AM, Alberg AJ, Strickland PT, et al. XPD polymorphism and risk of subsequent cancer in individuals with nonmelanoma skin cancer. Cancer Epidemiol Biomarkers Prev 2004; 13:1271–1275.

88. Han J, Colditz GA, Liu JS, et al. Genetic variation in XPD, sun exposure, and risk of skin cancer. Cancer Epidemiol Biomarkers Prev 2005; 14:1539–1544.

89. Nelson HH, Kelsey KT, Mott LA, et al. The XRCC1 Arg399Gln polymorphism, sunburn, and non-melanoma skin cancer: evidence of gene-environment interaction. Cancer Res 2002; 62:152–155.

90. Hemminki K, Xu G, Angelini S, et al. XPD exon 10 and 23 polymorphisms and DNA repair in human skin in situ. Carcinogenesis 2001; 22:1185–1188.

91. Qiao Y, Spitz MR, Guo Z, et al. Rapid assessment of repair of ultraviolet DNA damage with a modified host-cell reactivation assay using a luciferase reporter

gene and correlation with polymorphisms of DNA repair genes in normal human lymphocytes. Mutat Res 2002; 509:165–174.

92. Vodicka P, Kumar R, Stetina R, et al. Genetic polymorphisms in DNA repair genes and possible links with DNA repair rates, chromosomal aberrations and single-strand breaks in DNA. Carcinogenesis 2004; 25:757–763.

93. Angelini S, Kumar R, Carbone F, et al. Micronuclei in humans induced by exposure to low level of ionizing radiation: influence of polymorphisms in DNA repair genes. Mutat Res 2005; 570:105–117.

94. Seker H, Butkiewicz D, Bowman ED, et al. Functional significance of xpd polymorphic variants: attenuated apoptosis in human lymphoblastoid cells with the xpd 312 asp/asp genotype. Cancer Res 2001; 61:7430–7434.

95. Strange RC, El-Genidy N, Ramachandran S, et al. PTCH polymorphism is associated with the rate of increase in basal cell carcinoma numbers during follow-up: preliminary data on the influence of an exon 12-exon 23 haplotype. Environ Mol Mutagen 2004; 44:469–476.

96. Asplund A, Gustafsson AC, Wikonkal NM, et al. PTCH codon 1315 polymorphism and risk for nonmelanoma skin cancer. Br J Dermatol 2005; 152:868–873.

97. Kumar R, Smeds J, Berggren P, et al. A single nucleotide polymorphism in the 3′untranslated region of the CDKN2A gene is common in sporadic primary melanomas but mutations in the *CDKN2B, CDKN2C, CDK4* and *p53* genes are rare. Int J Cancer 2001; 95:388–393.

98. Debniak T, Scott RJ, Huzarski T, et al. *CDKN2A* common variants and their association with melanoma risk: a population-based study. Cancer Res 2005; 65:835–839.

99. Halsall JA, Osborne JE, Potter L, et al. A novel polymorphism in the 1A promoter region of the vitamin D receptor is associated with altered susceptibilty and prognosis in malignant melanoma. Br J Cancer 2004; 91:765–770.

100. Rees JL. The genetics of sun sensitivity in humans. Am J Hum Genet 2004; 75:739–751.

101. Sturm RA. Skin colour and skin cancer—MC1R, the genetic link. Melanoma Res 2002; 12:405–416.

102. Rossman TG, Uddin AN, Burns FJ. Evidence that arsenite acts as a cocarcinogen in skin cancer. Toxicol Appl Pharmacol 2004; 198:394–404.

103. Chen YC, Guo YL, Su HJ, et al. Arsenic methylation and skin cancer risk in southwestern Taiwan. J Occup Environ Med 2003; 45:241–248.

104. Tondel M, Rahman M, Magnuson A, et al. The relationship of arsenic levels in drinking water and the prevalence rate of skin lesions in Bangladesh. Environ Health Perspect 1999; 107:727–729.

105. Yu RC, Hsu KH, Chen CJ, et al. Arsenic methylation capacity and skin cancer. Cancer Epidemiol Biomarkers Prev 2000; 9:1259–1262.

106. Hartwig A, Pelzer A, Asmuss M, et al. Very low concentrations of arsenite suppress poly(ADP-ribosyl)ation in mammalian cells. Int J Cancer 2003; 104:1–6.

107. Burns FJ, Uddin AN, Wu F, et al. Arsenic-induced enhancement of ultraviolet radiation carcinogenesis in mouse skin: a dose-response study. Environ Health Perspect 2004; 112:599–603.

108. Hartwig A, Groblinghoff UD, Beyersmann D, et al. Interaction of arsenic(III) with nucleotide excision repair in UV-irradiated human fibroblasts. Carcinogenesis 1997; 18:399–405.

12

The Usefulness of Sunscreens

Jean-François Doré

*International Agency for Research on Cancer and INSERM Unit 590,
Centre Léon Bérard, Lyon, France*

Mathieu Boniol

International Agency for Research on Cancer, Lyon, France

Marie-Christine Chignol

INSERM Unit 590, Centre Léon Bérard, Lyon, France

Philippe Autier

International Agency for Research on Cancer, Lyon, France

INTRODUCTION

Skin cancers, both nonmelanoma and melanoma, are being influenced by genetically determined host factors and by exposure to an environmental carcinogen,
solar ultraviolet (UV) radiation. However, while squamous cell carcinomas
(SCCs) of the skin and solar keratoses (an actinic precursor skin lesion) are
clearly induced by chronic and cumulative exposure of body surfaces to sunlight,
substantial proportions of basal cell carcinomas (BCCs) and melanomas are
associated with intermittent exposure of usually covered body parts, such as
recreative sun exposure during holidays, more especially during childhood,
rather than with chronic sun exposure (1). Furthermore, while wavelengths
responsible for the induction of SCC lie within the UVB range of the UV spectrum, wavelengths responsible for the induction of BCC and melanoma are not
yet fully identified and may involve UVB as well as UVA (2).

Hence, prevention of skin tumors should rely on avoidance of sun exposure, more especially for individuals with a high susceptibility to solar UV radiation. In many countries, sun-protection programs were developed to prevent skin cancers. Adequate protection may be achieved by limiting exposure during hot hours of the day, by seeking shade, wearing protective clothes, and by using sunscreens. High sun protection factor (SPF) sunscreens have therefore been and are still widely advocated as part of sun protection in the prevention of human skin cancers.

As pointed out by Hill (3), the justification for the recommendation of sunscreen use in the prevention of skin cancers rested not so much on hard "evidence of efficacy" as on a line of "evidence-based reasoning" leading to a highly plausible basis for action. This recommendation was based on laboratory evidence showing that UV rays are carcinogenic, and that sunscreens provide a barrier to UV rays. Sunscreens are remarkably free of adverse reactions, efficiently prevent sunburn in humans, and have the capacity to prevent skin cancer in animals. As epidemiological studies have shown an association between sunburn and skin cancer, advising people to buy and use sunscreens is of very little expense to the health system, and effective solar-protection campaigns may lead to potentially large savings in direct health-care costs.

But attitudes toward sun exposure have changed during the twentieth century (4–6). While during the ninetieth century, many individuals, particularly women of the upper social classes, were vigilant in avoiding excessive sunlight, in the 1930s the suntanning fashion exploded among light-skinned populations, and suntan, which had previously been considered as characteristic of lower social classes, was viewed as de rigueur in the United States and Europe. Nowadays, in spite of increased public awareness of the carcinogenicity of sunlight exposure, favorable societal views of suntanning serve as an obstacle to skin cancer prevention.

Sunscreens that appeared on the market in the late 1920s were originally developed to prevent sunburn. During World War II, dark red veterinary petrolatum was found to be an effective physical sunscreen agent by the U.S. military, becoming standard equipment on life rafts and in vehicles in tropical areas (7). But during the second half of the twentieth century, with the explosion of holidays in sunny resorts, sunscreens gradually became to be used as a tanning aid, to acquire a "safe tan" without suffering from a sunburn.

Numerous surveys in Europe and North America have shown that across all age groups, sunscreen is the most frequently used sun-protection method, more especially among children (8,9), adolescents, and young adults. Younger adults are declared to be more likely to sunbathe deliberately than other people (10). Sun seekers tend to use sunscreen as a tanning aid (8,11,12), and sunscreen use when on the beach appears to be associated with more time spent in the sun, and, paradoxically, with more sunburns (13–15).

The efficacy of sunscreens in the prevention of skin cancers has been recently reviewed by the International Agency for Research on Cancer

(IARC), the U.S. Preventive Services Task Force, and the U.S. National Cancer Institute (16–18).

NONMELANOMA SKIN CANCERS

Surprisingly, few studies have addressed the issue of efficacy of sunscreen use in the primary prevention of nonmelanoma skin cancers.

Case-Control and Cohort Studies

Two case-control studies (19,20) and one cohort study (21) failed to demonstrate any protective effect of sunscreen use on the risk of SCC. However, it is worth mentioning that these studies suffer from several weaknesses, for example, the sun exposure and sunscreen use of persons in an old-age center is not representative of the Spanish population, and only a two-year sunscreen use was assessed in the nurses' cohort (Table 1).

One case-control study (22) and one cohort study (23) have studied the effect of using sunscreens when outdoors in summer on BCC risk. Both studies showed little evidence that the use of sunscreens protects against BCC. A slightly elevated risk persisting after adjustment for host factors was even noticed for persons who had used sunscreens in the years preceding diagnosis of BCC (Table 2).

Randomized Trial

Only one randomized trial evaluated the use of sunscreens in the prevention of nonmelanoma skin cancer (24). This trial was performed in Queensland, Australia, in a population living in an area with high ambient sunshine all the year round, and where skin cancer incidence is the highest in the world. In 1992, 1850 residents aged 20 to 69 of the town of Nambour, who had participated in 1986 in a skin cancer survey, were invited to participate in a randomized trial of daily application of SPF 16 sunscreen and use of 30 mg β-carotene. Among them, 1647 eligible subjects attended the baseline survey and 1621 agreed to be randomized in one of the four groups comparing sunscreen versus no sunscreen and β-carotene versus placebo. Participants were followed every three months for 4.5 years, and in 1994 and 1996 the subjects were again examined, and all skin cancers diagnosed and removed were histologically confirmed. In 1996, 1383 subjects remained in the study and 789 new skin cancers had been diagnosed in 250 subjects. The end points were the incidence of BCCs and SCCs both in terms of people treated for newly diagnosed disease and in terms of the numbers of tumors that occurred. This trial showed a reduction in newly diagnosed SCC tumors but not in the number of subjects treated for a newly diagnosed disease. Sunscreen use had no effect on BCC incidence (Table 3).

Table 1 Sunscreen Use and Cutaneous Squamous Cell Carcinoma

Study design	Place and date of study	Subjects	Exposure assessment	RR (95% CI)	Comments	Reference
Case-control (from population cohort)	Geraldton, Western Australia, 1987–1994	132 prevalent and incident cases 1031 controls	Use of SPF >10 versus no use Age 8–14 Age 15–19 Age 20–24	0.61 (0.08–4.7) 1.9 (0.82–4.4) 0.99 (0.44–2.2)	Included prevalent cases in 1987 and new cases diagnosed up to 1994	(67)
Case-control	Valencia, Spain, 1990–1992	260 cases 552 hospital controls	Use of solar protective "creams"	Men 0.6 (0.3–1.1) Women 0.7 (0.4–1.4)	Controls recruited in a hospital and an old-age center. Few subjects used sunscreens. Data were not analyzed by histological type; separate risk estimates for SCC and BCC not available	(20)
Cohort study	U.S. nationwide nurses' health cohort	191 SCC from a cohort of 107,900 female nurses	Use of sunscreen over a 2-yr period by women spending ≥8 hrs/wk in the sun	1.1 (0.83–1.7)		(21)

Abbreviations: BCC, basal cell carcinoma; CI, confidence interval; SCC, squamous cell carcinoma; SPF, sun protection factor; RR, relative risk.

Table 2 Sunscreen Use and Cutaneous Basal Cell Carcinoma

Study design	Place and date of study	Subjects	Exposure assessment	RR (95% CI)	Comments	Reference
Case-control (from a population cohort of 4103 subjects aged 40–64 yrs)	Geraldton, Western Australia, 1987–1994	226 cases 1021 controls	Use of SPF >10 sunscreen half the time or more while in the sun in the 10 yrs before diagnosis versus no use or less than half of the time		Included prevalent cases diagnosed at inclusion in the cohort in 1987 or in the preceeding year	(22)
			1–9 yrs	1.8 (1.1–2.9)		
			10 yrs	1.1 (0.69–1.7)		
			Use of SPF >10 sunscreen half the time or more while in the sun in the 11–30 yrs before diagnosis versus no use or less than half of the time			
			1–9 yrs	1.2 (0.69–2.1)		
			≥10 yrs	0.72 (0.40–1.3)		
Cohort study	U.S. nationwide nurses' health cohort	771 BCC from a cohort of 73,366 female nurses aged 34–59 in 1980	Usual use of sunscreen when outdoors during summer	1.4 (1.2–1.7)	Sunscreen use analyzed only among women spending ≥8 hrs/wk in the sun RR declined but remained elevated after adjustment for hair color, sun sensitivity, and history of sunburn	(23)

Abbreviations: BCC, basal cell carcinoma; CI, confidence interval; SPF, sun protection factor; RR, relative risk.

Table 3 Randomized Trial of Daily Sunscreen Use in the Prevention of Squamous Cell and Basal Cell Carcinoma of the Skin

Place and date of study	Subjects	Intervention	Tumor	Cases	Rate ratio (95% CI)	Comments	Reference
Nambour, Queensland, Australia, 1992–1996	1850 participants to a skin cancer survey, aged 20–69 in 1986, invited	Daily sunscreen application to head, neck, arms, and hands	SCC	Sunscreen arm: 28 tumors in 22 subjects No sunscreen arm: 46 tumors in 25 subjects	SCC lesions 0.61 (0.46–0.81) SCC subjects 0.88 (0.50–1.6)	789 new skin cancers in 250 subjects Analysis restricted to 758 new lesions	(24)
	1621 subjects randomized 1383 subjects followed 4.5 yrs		BCC	Sunscreen arm: 153 tumors in 65 subjects No sunscreen arm: 146 tumors in 63 subjects	BCC lesions 1.0 (0.82–1.3) BCC subjects 1.03 (0.73–1.5)	diagnosed after 1993 and histologically confirmed Analysis concentrated only on skin cancers occuring on body sites where sunscreen had been applied	

Abbreviations: BCC, basal cell carcinoma; CI, confidence interval; SCC, squamous cell carcinoma.

Precursor Lesions: Actinic (Solar) Keratoses

Actinic (solar) keratoses are risk factors for BCC and melanoma and precursor lesions for SCC, although the rate of transformation is low. They are known to be related to sun exposure and frequently regress spontaneously in the absence of exposure. They have been used as intermediary end points in studies of prevention of SCC by sunscreens.

Two cross-sectional studies (25,26) and two randomized trials (27,28) in relatively aged volunteers with a history of sun-induced skin damage, and non-habitual sunscreen users (27), showed the ability of sunscreen use to reduce the development of new solar keratoses (Table 4) [a 36% reduction in average annual rate of incidence of actinic keratoses ($P = 0.001$) was observed in the study by Naylor et al., while a reduction of 38% was observed by Thompson et al.], and even to decrease the number of pre-existing keratoses (28).

MELANOMA

Case-Control Studies

Twenty-one case-control studies have addressed the impact of sunscreen use on the risk of cutaneous melanoma (Table 5). Three of these (29–31, Berwick, unpublished) were not fully published in peer-review journals, and will not be further considered in this chapter. An in-depth analysis of studies published before 2000 was conducted by the IARC (16).

The results of these studies show great variations. Among the seven studies published before 1995, some, such as the well-controlled population-based studies by Holman et al. (29,30) in Australia and by Osterlind et al. (32) in Denmark, showed no effect; others eventually showed an increased risk or a non-significant trend, but suffered from methodological limitations which prevented reaching any firm conclusion (33–36), and none suggested a reduction in melanoma risk associated with the use of sunscreen.

The publication in 1995 by Westerdahl et al. (37) and Autier et al. (38) of two European studies, showing an increased melanoma risk associated with the use of sunscreen and suggesting that the use of sunscreen could actually lead to increase sun exposure, fired a controversy (39–40).

Among the nine studies published after 1995, some showed no effect of sunscreen use on melanoma risk (41), including a study in adolescent melanoma patients (42), or an effect restricted to subsets of cases (43). A study conducted with dermatology patients as controls showed an elevated risk (44), and a second study in the same area of Southern Sweden again showed an elevated risk, more especially among patients who used sunscreens to prolong sunbathing (45). Three studies reported a reduced melanoma risk associated with the use of sunscreens (46–48).

Most studies reporting attenuated melanoma risk among sunscreen users are unusual. The study by Holly et al. [published in 1995 (49), but conducted

(*Text continued on page 255.*)

Table 4 Sunscreen Use and Actinic Keratoses

Study design	Place and date of study	Subjects	Exposure	End point	Risk ratio (95% CI)	Comments	Reference
Randomized trial	Lubbock, Texas, U.S.A., 1987–1990	50 persons with clinically diagnosed keratoses	SPF 29 sunscreen daily versus placebo (base cream)	Average annual rate of actinic keratoses incidence	Sunscreen: 21 keratoses Placebo: 28 keratoses $P = 0.001$	Participants were told to avoid sun exposure and encouraged to use physical protections (hats, clothing)	(83)
Cross-sectional	County of South Glamorgan, Wales, U.K., 1988–1992	560 subjects of both genders, aged ≥ 60	Normal use of sunscreen	Prevalent actinic keratoses or SCC	Sunscreen use versus no use: 0.56 (0.34–0.82) (unadjusted for age)	137 actinic keratoses confirmed on pictures by a panel of three dermatologists Univariate analysis showed that subjects who had used sunscreens had a reduced risk for prevalent actinic	(25,26)

Randomized trial	Maryborough, Southern Australia	431 persons aged ≥40 with 1–30 actinic keratoses	SPF 17 sunscreen daily versus placebo (base cream)	Prevalent actinic keratoses on head, neck, hands, and forearms	Placebo versus sunscreen: 1.5 (0.81–2.2)	keratoses; but this effect is largely confounded by age in multivariate analysis
				No. of new actinic keratoses	Sunscreen versus placebo: 0.62 (0.54–0.71)	Participants were told to avoid mid-day sun and to wear hats [28]
				No. of remissions	Sunscreen versus placebo: 1.5 (1.3–1.8)	

Abbreviations: CI, confidence interval; SCC, squamous cell carcinoma; SPF, sun protection factor.

Table 5 Sunscreen Use and Cutaneous Melanoma: Case-Control Studies

Place and date of study	Subjects	Exposure assessment	OR[a] (95% CI)	Comments	Reference
Oslo, Norway, 1974–1975	78 hospital cases 131 controls (other cancer patients) Age ≥20	Categories: sometimes, often, or almost always use of sun oil/lotion	Males: 2.8[b] (1.2–6.7) Females: 1.0[b] (0.42–2.5) Total: 2.3[b] (1.3–4.1)	Sunscreens poorly characterized, not differentiated from sun lotions Risk elevated only for males	(33)
Buffalo, New York, U.S.A., 1974–1980	404 hospital cases 521 controls (other cancer patients from the same hospital)	Use versus no use: sunscreen Sun-tanning lotion	Males: 2.2[b] (1.2–4.1) Males: 1.7 (1.1–2.7)	Risk elevated only for males "No added risk for females"	(34)
Queensland, Australia, 1979–1980	183 population cases 183 population controls Age 14–86	Use of "sun lotions"	Not reported	"Possible protective effect when any kind of preparation is applied to the skin prior to sun exposure"	(92)
Western Australia, 1980–1981	507 population cases 507 population controls Age ≤80	Use of sunscreens for ≤ 10 yrs	1.1 (0.71–1.6)		(29,30)

Denmark, 1982–1985	474 population cases 926 population controls Age 20–79	Ever versus never use of sunscreens: <10 yrs ≥10 yrs Always versus ever or hardly ever	1.3 (0.9–1.7) 1.2 (0.9–1.5) 1.1 (0.8–1.5)	High participation rates (cases: 92%, controls: 82%) Control for sun sensitivity Information on duration and frequency of sunscreen use	(32)
Stockholm, Sweden, 1978–1983	523 hospital cases 505 population controls	Often or very often versus never use of "sun-protection agents"	1.8 (1.2–2.7)	Postal questionnaire. High response rates (cases: 99.6%, controls: 92.2%) Poor definition of "sun-protection agents"	(35)
Upstate, New York, U.S.A., 1977–1979	324 male cases with melanoma of the trunk 415 population controls Age ≥18	"Always" use of "suntan lotion" versus less frequent or never	2.6[b] (1.4–4.7) Not significant in logistic regression analysis (risk ratios not given)	Telephone interview; response rates cases: 82%, but 38% respondents were patient's relatives, controls: 62% No differentiation in questionnaire between sunscreens and tanning oils	(36)

(Continued)

Table 5 Sunscreen Use and Cutaneous Melanoma: Case-Control Studies (*Continued*)

Place and date of study	Subjects	Exposure assessment	OR[a] (95% CI)	Comments	Reference
San Francisco, CA, U.S.A., 1981–1986	452 female population cases 930 female population controls Age 25–59	"Almost always" sunscreen use versus never	All melanomas: 0.62[b] (0.49–0.83) Superficial spreading melanoma: 0.43 (CI not available)	Surprisingly, sun exposure does not appear as a risk factor Risk for SSM adjusted for host factors and sun exposure	(49)
Southern Sweden, 1988–1990	400 population cases 640 population controls Age 15–75	"Almost always" sunscreen use versus never	1.8 (1.1–2.0) Trunk melanomas: 1.4 (0.6–3.2) Other sites: 2.0 (1.1–3.7)	Similar elevation of risk by use before the age of 15, or 15–19, or >19	(37)
Belgium, Germany, France, 1991–1992	418 hospital cases 438 neighborhood controls Age ≥20	Ever use of psoralen sunscreen Ever use of regular sunscreens	2.3 (1.3–4.0) 1.5 (1.1–2.1) Males: 1.8 (1.1–2.7) Females: 1.3 (0.87–2.0)	Highest risk among sun-sensitive subjects using sunscreens to tan: OR 3.7 (1.0–7.6)	(38)
Andalusia, Spain, 1989–1993	105 hospital cases 138 hospital controls (visitors) Age 20–79	Always use of sunscreens	0.2 (0.04–0.79)	Low prevalence of sunscreen use	(46)
U.S.A.	70 cases 109 controls		0.3 (0.1–0.8)	Abstract No full publication available	(31)

Queensland, Australia, 1987–1994	50 population cases (adolescents) 156 controls from the same school Age ≤15	Always use of sunscreens	On holidays: 2.2 (0.4–12) At school: 0.7 (0.1–6.0)	Small study, only 11 patients reported sunscreen use on holidays and two at school	(42)
Styria, Austria, 1993–1994	193 hospital cases 319 dermatology controls Age 15–89	Often use of sunscreens versus never	3.5 (1.8–6.6)	Controls were patients with other dermatological conditions	(44)
Western Canada Melanoma Study, 1979–1981	369 population cases 369 population controls	"Almost always" or "sometimes" use of sunscreens Only in the first hours	1.1 (0.75–1.6) 1.6 (1.0–2.5)	Analysis of a subset of cases with melanoma of the trunk or lower limbs. Information on sunscreen use relevant only to sites intermittently sun exposed Elevated risk restricted to patients who use sunscreens only in the first hours of sun exposure	(43)
Multicentric study (27 centers) in Italy, 1992–1995	542 hospital cases 538 hospital cases	Often use of sunscreens versus never Sometimes use of sunscreens	0.80 (0.54–1.17) 0.97 (0.69–1.35)	Non-specific trend of increasing association with high SPF sunscreens	(41)

(Continued)

Table 5 Sunscreen Use and Cutaneous Melanoma: Case-Control Studies (*Continued*)

Place and date of study	Subjects	Exposure assessment	OR[a] (95% CI)	Comments	Reference
Southern Sweden, 1995–1997	571 population cases 913 population controls	Always used sunscreens	1.8 (1.1–2.9)		(45)
		Used sunscreens to prolong sunbathing	8.7 (1.0–75.8)		
Porto Alegre, Brazil, 1995–1998	103 hospital cases 206 hospital controls Age 20–80	Ever versus never sunscreen use	0.5[b] (0.3–0.9)	Progressive protection with increasing SPF. Only SPF15 or greater (SPF15+) showed significant protection	(48)
Queensland, Australia, 1987–1994	201 population cases (adolescents) 205 population controls Age 15–19	Sunscreen use at home ≤5 yrs: Never/rarely versus always Sometimes versus always	2.2 (0.7–7.1) 1.6 (1.05–5.3)	No association with reported sun exposure in this high genetic susceptibility group	(93)
Connecticut, U.S.A. 1987–1989	Not stated	Always/sometimes versus never Sometimes Almost always	1.2 (0.9–1.6) 1.1 (0.8–1.5) 1.3 (0.9–1.6)	Unpublished, used in meta-analysis by Dennis et al. (52)	Berwick (unpublished)

[a]Adjusted for other risk factors.
[b]Only crude OR available.
Abbreviations: CI, confidence interval; SPF, sun protection factor; OR, odd's ratio; SSM, superficial spreading melanoma.

10 years before], among 25 to 59 years old female melanoma patients of the Bay area in San Francisco, is unusual in showing the highest levels of risk for melanoma among women with the least sun exposure. It is not unlikely that this study could have been among the first to experience a bias analyzed in a recent European case-control study where awareness of risk factors led patients, and also controls, to under-report their sun exposure and overestimate their protection (50). The two Spanish studies are relatively small hospital-based studies with either low prevalence of sunscreen use (46) or a surprisingly high risk factor for skin sensitivity to sun exposure (47).

To examine the sunscreen controversy, meta-analyses were conducted. However, one can think that the analyzed studies may actually have been as different as chalk and cheese. A meta-analysis based on 11 studies found a summary relative risk of 1.11 but with considerable heterogeneity (51). Data from 4800 patients enrolled in population-based case-control studies showed no such heterogeneity, indicating that they could reliably be included in a meta-analysis, and the resulting summary relative risk was 1.01 [95% confidence interval (CI), 0.46–2.28].

More recently, another meta-analysis analyzed 18 case-control studies (52). The pooled odds ratio for the 18 studies was 1.0 (95% CI, 0.8–1.2) with significant heterogeneity; when only the 9 studies adjusting for sun sensitivity were considered, the pooled odds ratio decreased to 0.8 (0.6–1.0). However, this study used a quality score, which may be viewed as the most insidious source of bias that can be imported in a meta-analysis: "Quality scoring adds the analyst's subjective bias to the results, wastes information and can prevent the recognition of key sources of heterogeneity" (53).

Overall, case-control studies of sunscreen use and melanoma have failed to convincingly demonstrate a reduction in risk, and some well-controlled studies have even suggested an increased risk, particularly among sun seekers using sunscreens to prolong sunbathing.

Nevus Development (in Children)

Nevi are focal collections of melanocytes, usually found at the junction of the epidermis and dermis or at various depths in the dermis. Although it is not currently known whether nevi represent pre-malignant lesions or risk factors, many melanomas arise in acquired nevi, and the number of nevi constitutes the best predictor of individual risk of melanoma. Common acquired nevi arise after birth, both spontaneously and in response to sun exposure (54), and can be considered both as an exposure and as an intermediate effect biomarker (55). In a case-control study conducted in Europe in 418 melanoma cases and 438 controls (38), the use of sunscreen was associated with a higher density of pigmented lesions of the skin in controls. The nevus count in both arms in control subjects significantly increased from no sunscreen use to ever use of sunscreen [rate ratio, 1.31 (95% CI, 1.19–1.43) adjusted for age, sex, hair color, and sun exposure].

Children seem particularly vulnerable to sun-induced biological events involved in the genesis of melanoma, and the greatest increase in nevus numbers per unit of skin surface takes place before adolescence. Therefore, the development of nevi in children is relevant to understanding melanoma occurrence in adults. To further explore the relation between sunscreen use and melanoma, nine cross-sectional studies and two randomized trials have investigated the development of nevi in children as a function of sun exposure, sun protection, and sunscreen use (Table 6).

Cross-Sectional and Cohort Studies

While two studies failed to demonstrate a significant protective effect of applying sunscreen on number of nevi (54,56), seven studies found a positive association between nevus numbers and the use of sunscreens (57–63).

The most complete cross-sectional study to date on the relationship between sunscreen use and the prevalence of nevi was conducted among elementary school children in Belgium, Germany, France, and Italy (59). A retrospective cohort examined the number of nevi in 631 children aged six to seven years in Brussels, Bochum, Lyons, and Rome, according to their sun-exposure history, physical protection, sunscreen use, and sunburn history from birth to the moment of skin examination. In all study places, the median numbers of nevi tended to increase with total or average sunscreen use during holidays, whereas the reverse was true for average wearing of clothes in the sun. Median nevus counts increased with both increasing sun exposure and average sunscreen use. After adjustment for sun exposure and host characteristics, the relative risk for high nevus count on the trunk was 1.68 (95% CI, 1.09–2.59) for the highest level of sunscreen use and 0.59 (95% CI, 0.36–0.97) for the highest level of wearing clothes while in the sun. The average SPF of the sunscreen used had no demonstrable effect on nevus counts. Interestingly, the highest risk of nevi on the trunk associated with sunscreen use was seen in children who never suffered from sunburn (relative risk, 2.21; 95% CI, 1.33–3.67).

The most recent of these studies (63), similar to that of Autier et al. (59), found the highest nevus number in children using only sunscreen as a protection against sun and showed that clothing is an excellent protective agent.

Prospective Intervention Trials

The prospective intervention study by Gallagher et al. (64) is the only study to have shown a moderate 15% reduction in new nevus development. Sunscreen use attenuated nevus development on intermittently sun-exposed body sites (trunk) (65). However, all the effects are concentrated in children with numerous freckles and no effect was observed in children without freckles. The reason for the interaction with freckles is still obscure and could be attributed to a specific susceptibility to UV radiation in children with freckles. Most recently, a prospective randomized intervention study in 1232 German children followed up for three years did not show any reduction in nevus number associated with

(*Text continued on page 263.*)

Table 6 Studies of Nevus Development in Children as a Function of Sun Exposure, Sun Protection, and Sunscreen Use

Study type	Place and date of study	Subjects	Exposure	End point/main outcome	Comments	Reference
Cross-sectional	West Midlands, U.K.	2140 children (1010 boys, 1130 girls) Age 4–11	Always or often use of sunscreens	Nevi ≥2 mm. Significantly higher nevus count in children using sunscreen ($P < 0.001$)		(57)
Cross-sectional	Townsville, North Queensland, Australia	506 children Age 1–6	Use of sunscreen during summer	Nevi ≥2 mm. Use of sunscreen "not associated with nevus number or density"		(54)
5-yr cohort	Bochum, Germany, 1988–1993	357 children (170 boys, 187 girls) 1–6 yrs at inclusion	Regular, seldom, or never use sunscreen	Whole body nevus counts at inclusion and 5 yrs later (age: 7–11 yrs; median: 9 yrs) RR of increase in nevi ≥1 mm: 1, 0.81 (0.65–1.01), and 0.41 (0.23–0.75) for regular, seldom, or never use of sunscreen	Univariate analysis. Regular use as reference category. Similar figures but less significant for nevi ≥2 mm	(58)

(Continued)

Table 6 Studies of Nevus Development in Children as a Function of Sun Exposure, Sun Protection, and Sunscreen Use (*Continued*)

Study type	Place and date of study	Subjects	Exposure	End point/main outcome	Comments	Reference
Cross-sectional (retrospective cohort)	Brussels (B), Bochum (D), Lyons (F), Rome (I), 1995–1997	631 children (321 boys, 310 girls) Age 6–7	Total and average sunscreen use, wearing of clothes, sun exposure	Whole body nevus count Median number of nevi increased with total and average sunscreen use, and decreased with average wearing clothes Adjusted RR of high nevus count on the trunk 1.68 (95% CI, 1.09–2.59) for the highest level of sunscreen use and 0.59 (95% CI, 0.36–0.97) for the highest level of wearing clothes	SPF of sunscreen has no effect on nevus count Highest risk of nevi on the trunk in children using sunscreen and who never suffered from sunburns (RR, 2.21, 95% CI, 1.33–3.67)	(59)

Cross-sectional	Israel, Ramat Gan, 1992–1993, Jerusalem, 1994–1995	974 pupils Age 7: 489 Age 12: 485	Regular, seldom, or never use sunscreen	Whole body nevus count (≥ 2 mm). In Ramat Gan, regular sunscreen use contributes to increased nevus risk at age 7: RR = 1.7 (1.3–2.2), and at age 12: RR = 1.5 (1.2–2.0). Similar figures in Jerusalem	Differences in sun-exposure behavior more frequent in Ramat Gan (sea level) than in Jerusalem (elevation: 700 m). Nevus counts decreased with less-frequent recreational sun exposure	(60)
Randomized trial 3-yr follow-up	Vancouver, BC, Canada, 1993–1996	Intervention group: 145 children Control group: 164 children Age 6–10 at inclusion	Sunscreen SPF 30 when sun exposed for >30 min, and instructions on sunscreen use	Significantly fewer new nevi in children in the intervention group (0.85). Sunscreen use attenuated nevus development on intermittently sun-exposed body sites	Effect concentrated in children with numerous freckles, no effect observed in children without freckles	(64,65)

(Continued)

Table 6 Studies of Nevus Development in Children as a Function of Sun Exposure, Sun Protection, and Sunscreen Use (*Continued*)

Study type	Place and date of study	Subjects	Exposure	End point/main outcome	Comments	Reference
5-yr cohort	Brisbane, Queensland, Australia, 1990–1994	111 school children (63 boys, 48 girls) Age 12–13 at baseline	Use sunscreen on shoulders: always, most times, sometimes/rarely	Full body nevus counts. Adjusted means ratios (counts 1994/1990): always: 1 (Reference) most times: 1.82 (1.27–2.61) sometimes/rarely 1.08 (0.83–1.46)	Summer holiday sun exposure was not significantly associated with development of nevi in this adolescent cohort. School lunchtime in the sun was associated with nevus development	(61)
Cross-sectional	Hamburg, Germany, 1993–1994	11,478 children Age 5–6	Sunscreen usage: never, occasionally, on summer holidays, or regular, also at home	In children who used sunscreens more frequently the nevus counts were higher than in children who used sunscreens never or only occasionally	No significant association of nevus count with daily sun exposure at home. Major impact of holiday activities in southern climates on the number of nevi	(62)

Cross-sectional	Yorkshire and Surrey, U.K.	103 monozygous, 118 dizygous twin pairs Age 10–18	Sun exposure, use of sunscreen or clothing	"Not able to demonstrate a protective effect for either sun protection cream or shirt wearing"	In this twin study, 66% of total variance of nevus count is attributable to genetic effects, only 25% is attributable to environmental influences and ≈8% is estimated to result from sun holidays exposure	(56)
Cross-sectional	Stuttgart and Bochum, Germany March–October, 1998	1812 children Age 2–7	Scores for extent and frequency of sunscreen use, and for clothing worn at the beach or outdoor swimming pool	Whole body nevus counts using standard protocol Multivariate analyses: no significant protective effect of applying sunscreen on number of nevi Highest nevus number in children using only sunscreen as a protection against sun	95% of children had used sunscreen previously Children who used sunscreens and wore more clothing spent significantly longer periods on holidays in sunny climates Inverse dose–response relationship between number of clothes worn and number of nevi ($P < 0.001$)	(63)

(Continued)

Table 6 Studies of Nevus Development in Children as a Function of Sun Exposure, Sun Protection, and Sunscreen Use (*Continued*)

Study type	Place and date of study	Subjects	Exposure	End point/main outcome	Comments	Reference
Randomized trial 3-yr follow-up	Stuttgart and Bochum, Germany, 1998–2001	Control group: 398 children Educational group: 369 children Education and sunscreen group: 455 children	Education letter three times yearly 800 ml free broad-spectrum sunscreen SPF 25	Whole body naevus counts using standard protocol Main outcome: number of incident (new) nevi No significant differences between the three study arms	Sunscreen use in the entire cohort: no impact on number of incident nevi	(66)

Abbreviations: RR, relative risk; CI, confidence interval; SPF, sun protection factor.

sunscreen use (66). It is worthy of note that a school-based non-randomized sun-protection intervention, Kidskin, conducted in the area of Perth, Western Australia, over four years (1995–1999) and combining a specially designed sun-protection curriculum (moderate intervention) and Kidskin program materials and sun-protective swimwear (high intervention), resulted only after 6-year follow-up in a relative increase in number of new nevi on the back of 0.94 (95% CI, 0.86–1.04) for the moderate intervention group and of 0.89 (95% CI, 0.81–0.99) for the high intervention group (67).

SUNSCREEN USE AND DURATION OF SUN EXPOSURE

Compensation Hypothesis

In contrast to laboratory data, retrospective and prospective epidemiological studies have shown that sunscreen use is associated with a moderately higher risk for cutaneous melanoma, BCC, and with higher numbers of nevi. To explain this discrepancy between the ability of sunscreens to prevent sunburn, actinic keratoses, and SCCs and their inability to reduce melanoma risk or nevus development in children, a "compensation hypothesis" was put forward (68). This hypothesis assumes that because sunscreens protect primarily against UVB radiations, which induce tanning and cause sunburn, sunscreen users would increase the time they spend in the sun to achieve an equivalent suntan. Hence, sunscreen users would be exposed to more UVA radiations than that if they had not used a sunscreen. It also assumes that the melanoma action spectrum differs from the erythema action spectrum and is shifted toward the longer wavelengths, and that UVA may be involved in the induction of cutaneous melanoma, this view being supported by the spectrum of melanoma induction in an experimental model in *Xiphophorus maculatus* × *Xiphophorus helleri* hybrids (platyfish × swordtail hybrids). Interspecies hybrids of these freshwater fishes spontaneously develop melanomas, known as the Gordon-Kosswig melanoma model. In this model, melanoma can be induced by UVB, UVA, and also visible light irradiation (69).

Compensation Hypothesis: Sunscreen Use and Exposure to UVA Radiation

However, the hypothesis that sunscreen use would expose to a higher level of irradiation by UVA, a wavelength responsible for melanoma induction, is highly unlikely. Whereas earlier studies may have, in fact, examined the effect of low SPF sunscreens, this is no longer true, and sunscreens used in the more recent studies of nevus development in children, for instance, were of higher SPF. It is not possible to obtain an SPF higher than 10 with only pure UVB filters because of the erythemogenic activity of the shorter UVA wavelengths, and modern high SPF sunscreens usually contain both UVB and UVA filters or inorganic zinc or titanium oxides that block UVA.

Although it has recently been shown that UVA may be mutagenic (70), and that UVA and UVB cause similar number of *p53* gene mutations in actinic keratoses and SCCs (71), there is currently little evidence to support a major role of UVA in the induction of cutaneous melanoma. The melanoma action spectrum in humans is not known. However, there is indirect evidence that melanoma may be caused by UVB. Firstly, patients with Xeroderma pigmentosum, who have a genetic defect in DNA repair and are extremely susceptible to UVB, develop all kinds of skin tumors, BCCs, and SCCs and melanomas, with an exceptionally high incidence (72). Recent epidemiological evidence tends to indicate that melanoma risk may be positively influenced by short periods of high UVB exposure (73), more especially during childhood (74). In addition, melanoma patients have recently been shown to display an impaired reactivity to UVB (75–77).

Sunscreen Paradox: Sunscreen Use Increases Duration of Sun Exposure

Occasionally, epidemiological studies had observed that sunscreen users tend to spend more time in the sun and, paradoxically, to get more sunburns than non-users (11,63). To investigate what has been termed the "sunscreen paradox," several studies have tried to evaluate the impact of sunscreen use on duration of sun exposure, or on exposure to UV radiation using specifically designed UV-dosimeters.

Observational Studies

Observational studies (Table 7) have indicated that sunscreen use may (*i*) actually increase sunburn risk (8,15,78,79), (*ii*) increase time spent in the sun (8,12,14,15), and (*iii*) increase exposure to UV radiation (12,13). A more detailed study of UV exposure in relation to sunscreen use was conducted in Denmark over three consecutive summer seasons by Thieden et al. (12), using a convenience sample of 340 volunteers (children, adolescents, indoor workers, sun worshippers, golfers, and gardeners) who recorded their sunscreen use and sun-exposure behavior in diaries and carried personal electronic UV-dosimeters continuously recording UV doses with a spectral response similar to the erythema action spectrum, during a median of 119 days, corresponding to 346 subjects participating for a summer season. Table 7 summarizes the UV exposure data in Southern Europe (Mediterranean area) for 93 subjects engaging in risk behavior (sunbathing or exposing the upper body), and shows that the UV dose per risk behavior day with sunscreen was greater than that of days without sunscreen, except for gardeners, and more especially for children and sun worshippers.

Randomized Trials

While observational studies may at best only be indicative, their design is inadequate to reach firm conclusions. Probably, the more suitable design to

Table 7 Observational Studies of Sunscreen Use and Duration of Sun Exposure and/or Exposure to Ultraviolet Radiation

Study design	Place and date of study	Subjects	Data collection	End point	Sunscreen use	Time spent in the sun or UV dose	% difference	% subjects with sunburn	Reference
Cross-sectional	Connecticut, U.S.A., 1988	153 adults participants to a skin cancer screening campaign	Retrospective questionnair on summer of previous years	Average sun exposure duration per weekend day	Never Always	2.57 hrs 2.9 hrs	13% $P = 0.06$	NR	(14)
Cross-sectional	Denmark, July 1994	805 sunbathers (mean age 28) on four beaches and in one park	Questionnaire	(1) Difference in minutes between time of arrival on the beach and time of expected departure	No Yes	197 min 206 min	5% $P = 0.19$	34 42	(13,78,79)
			UV-dosimeter on the location	(2) UV dose recorded between arrival and departure times	No Yes	4.5 SED 4.8 SED	7% $P = 0.04$	NR	
Cross-sectional	Galveston beaches, Texas, U.S.A., July 1997	55 beachgoers (age 16–59)	Questionnaire on sunbathing activities of the day	Duration of sunbathing (hrs)	No SPF ≤ 15 SPF > 15	2.8 hrs 3.2 hrs 3.5 hrs	15% 25%	54 50 73	(15)

(Continued)

Table 7 Observational Studies of Sunscreen Use and Duration of Sun Exposure and/or Exposure to Ultraviolet Radiation (*Continued*)

Study design	Place and date of study	Subjects	Data collection	End point	Sunscreen use	Time spent in the sun or UV dose	% difference	% subjects with sunburn	Reference
Cross-sectional	Nationwide, U.S.A., July–August 1997	503 children <13 years	Telephone survey questionnaire on five successive weekend	Mean number of hours spent outside between 10 am and 4 pm during the past weekend	No Yes	4.6 hrs 5.7 hrs	23 % *P* < 0.05	7 20 *P* < 0.05	(8)
Prospective study	Denmark, three summer seasons, 1999–2001	340 volunteers Age 4–68	(1) Daily diaries	Hours of sun exposure per "risk behavior" day	No Yes	4.1 hrs 5.7 hrs	39 %	4.8 % 9.5 %	(12)
		93 subjects	(2) Personal UV-dosimeters (during risk behavior days in southern Europe)	Median SED per risk behavior day					

Group				
Total (93)	No	3.5 SED	Reference	NR
	Yes	7.8 SED	223%	NR
	Test for difference between groups		NR	
Children (19)	No	1.5 SED	Reference	NR
	Yes	7.4 SED	393%	NR
	Test for difference between groups		$P < 0.05$	
Sun worshippers (22)	No	1.8 SED	Reference	NR
	Yes	9 SED	400%	NR
	Test for difference between groups		NR	
Gardeners (8)	No	8.1 SED	Reference	NR
	Yes	10.2 SED	26%	NR
	Test for difference between groups		NR	

Abbreviations: NR, not reported; SED, standard erythemal dose (1 SED = 100 J/m^2).

address the issue of sun-exposure duration as a function of sunscreen use would be a randomized prospective trial (Table 8). Two such double-blind prospective randomized trials were conducted in Europe by the European Organization for Research and Treatment of Cancer (EORTC) Melanoma Group (80,81). To either a low SPF or a high SPF sunscreen group, 87 French and Swiss volunteers, aged 18 to 24 years, were randomly assigned. They were given free commercially available sunscreen of either SPF 10 or SPF 30, reconditioned in tubes with no SPF indication, and were asked to complete daily records of their sunscreen use and sun-exposure behavior during their usual holidays in sunny resorts. Neither medical personnel nor study participants were aware of their sunscreen assignment. To avoid influencing the recreational sun-exposure habits of the study participants, no recommendation was made about sun exposure or sun protection. Furthermore, participants were told that the trial end point was the number of pigmented skin lesions before and after the holidays. Duration of outdoor activities, distinguishing the diverse recreative activities from actual sunbathing, was calculated from the diaries. The overall results of this study shows that SPF 10 ($n = 44$) and SPF 30 ($n = 42$) groups had equivalent mean holiday durations (19.4 days versus 20.2 days) and mean quantities of sunscreen used (72.3 g versus 71.6 g). The mean cumulative sun exposures for the two groups were 58.2 and 72.6 hours, respectively ($P = 0.011$). The mean daily durations of sunbathing were 2.6 and 3.1 hours, respectively ($P = 0.0013$), and, for outdoor activities, they were 3.6 and 3.8 hours, respectively ($P = 0.62$). There was no difference in sunburn experience between the two groups (80).

The same group conducted a second trial with the same protocol on a smaller sample. Volunteers in this trial carried electronic personal UV-dosimeters continuously recording UVA and UVB doses (81). The median daily sunbathing duration was 2.4 hours in the SPF 10 group and 3 hours in the SPF 30 group ($P = 0.054$). The increase in daily sunbathing duration was paralleled by an increase in daily UVB exposure, but not by changes in UVA or UVB accumulated over all sunbathing sessions, or in daily UVA exposure. Of all participants, those who used the SPF 30 sunscreen and had no sunburn spent the highest number of hours in sunbathing activities. Differences between the two SPF groups in total number of sunbathing hours, daily sunbathing duration, and daily UVB exposure were largest among participants without sunburn during holidays. Among those with sunburn, the differences between the two groups tended to reduce.

Hence, use of higher SPF sunscreen seems to increase the duration of recreational sun exposure of young white Europeans and tends to increase the duration of exposures to doses of UV radiation below the sunburn threshold.

Recently, a randomized trial, funded by a major sunscreen manufacturer, appeared to contradict EORTC results, finding no difference in the duration of time spent in the sun according to sunscreen SPF (82). It was even considered that the sunscreen controversy has come to an end (83). However, this study is

Table 8 Randomized Trials on Sunscreen Use and Sun-Exposure Duration

Study design	Place, season, and year of study	Subjects	Data collection	End point	Sunscreen use	Time spent in the sun or UV dose	% difference	% with sunburn	Quantity of sunscreen used (g)	Reference
Double-blind randomized trial	Sunny resorts where students spent holidays, July–August 1997	87 French and Swiss students 18–24 yrs	Self-administered daily diaries	Mean hours of sun bathing per day with sunbathing (average of 11 days)	SPF 10	2.6 hrs	Ref.	47%	72.3 (mean)	(80)
					SPF 30	3.1 hrs	19% P = 0.0013	43% P = 0.90	71.6 (mean) P = 0.95	
					Test for difference between groups					
Double-blind randomized trial	Sunny resorts where students spent their holiday in July–August, 1998	48 French and Belgian students 18–24 yrs old taking holidays in sunny resorts in July–August	(1) Self-administered daily diaries	Mean hours of sun bathing per day with sunbathing (average of nine days)	SPF 10	2.4 hrs	Ref.	38%	67 (mean)	(81)
					SPF 30	3.0 hrs	25% P = 0.054	41% P = 0.46	77 (mean) P = 0.22	
					Test for difference between groups					
			(2) Individual UVB- and UVA-dosimeters		SPF 10	UVB: 841 J/m², UVA: 136 KJ/m²	Ref.	—	—	

(Continued)

Table 8 Randomized Trials on Sunscreen Use and Sun-Exposure Duration (*Continued*)

Study design	Place, season, and year of study	Subjects	Data collection	End point	Sunscreen use	Time spent in the sun or UV dose	% difference	% with sunburn	Quantity of sunscreen used (g)	Reference
					SPF 30	UVB: 984 J/m²; UVA: 812 KJ/m²	UVB: +17%; UVA: +11%	—	—	
					Test for difference between groups		UVB: $P = 0.15$; UVA: $P = 0.70$			
Randomized trial with sunscreen tubes labeled as "basic" or "high protection"	Summer villages located on the sea in France in July–August 2001	367 adults 18–78 yrs old (mean =39) during one week of holidays in July–August	Daily diaries and question-naires (completed with help of on-site investigator)	Duration (hours) of sun exposure over one week while wearing a swimming suit or equivalent	SPF 12, "basic protection"	14.6 hrs	Ref.	24%	109 (median)	(82)
					SPF 40 "basic protection"	12.9 hrs	−12%	14%	30 (median)	
					SPF 40 "high protection"	14.2 hrs	−3%	16%	26 (median)	
					Test for difference between groups[a]		$P = 0.06$	$P = 0.049$	$P < 0.001$	

[a]Test for difference between SPF 12 "basic protection" and SPF 40 "basic protection."

in no way comparable to the EORTC studies, and the trial design and conduct were likely to produce a negative result, that is, no difference in sun-exposure duration according to SPF of sunscreen used. First, the target population was different. Trial participants were mainly females of older age than in the EORTC trials (18–78 years versus 18–24 years), with low interest in sunbathing or getting a tan: only 25% of participants reported being interested in sun exposure, while most participants in EORTC studies were eager to engage in intentional sun exposure during their holidays. Methodological weaknesses prevent this study from reaching firm conclusions. More especially, "sunbathing" was defined as a period of exposure with light clothing and could thus include actual sunbathing as well as other outdoor activities, and thus duration of "sunbathing" activities were probably more influenced by scheduled holiday activities than by willingness to lay down on the beach. Reporting of "sunbathing" activities was collected by fixed 30-minute periods, so that short duration exposures were a priori, considered as of 30-minute duration. (This way of recording introduced measurement errors likely to make sun-exposure duration equal between randomization groups.) Sunscreens were labeled according to a suggested protection category but had different textures, which may explain the huge (3.6-fold) difference in amount of sunscreen used between the randomization groups. Hence, the French sunscreen trial was improper to investigate whether the use of sunscreen among young "sun seekers" could increase the duration of sun exposure.

CONCLUSION

From this rapid review, the usefulness of sunscreens in the prevention of skin cancer appears rather limited. Currently, the only convincing evidence is that daily sunscreen use on exposed body surfaces may prevent the development of new solar keratoses, favor the remission of pre-existing keratoses, and prevent the development of new SCC in patients. Moreover, this prevention effect is a modest one (a nearly 40% reduction in risk), and the U.S. Preventive Services Task Force has even calculated that, based on the Australian randomized trial, 140 people would need to use sunscreen daily for 4.5 years to prevent one case of squamous cell cancer (17). Sunscreen had no effect on basal cell cancer.

There is no direct data about the effect of sunscreen on melanoma incidence. Several epidemiologic studies have found higher melanoma risk among sunscreen users than among non-users, and a recent meta-analysis of population-based case-control studies failed to demonstrate any effect of sunscreen use on melanoma risk (51). When nevus development in children was used as surrogate end point to evaluate the possibility that sunscreens may prevent melanoma, several studies found a positive association between nevus numbers and the use of sunscreens. These conflicting results may actually reflect the fact that sunscreen use is more common among fair-skinned people, who are at higher risk for melanoma, or, they may reflect the fact that sunscreen use could be harmful if it encourages longer stays in the sun without protecting completely against cancer-causing radiation. And indeed, two prospective randomized studies demonstrated that high SPF sunscreen prolongs sun exposure, enhances risk behavior such as sunbathing during hot hours of the day, and exposure to UVB.

All three U.S. National and IARC expert groups who reviewed available evidence reached similar conclusions, and presented their overall evaluation in terms stressing the importance of learning more about potential harms of counseling for sunscreen use: "Sunscreens probably prevent SCC of the skin when used mainly during unintentional sun exposure. No conclusion can be drawn about the cancer preventive activity of topical use of sunscreens against BCC and cutaneous melanoma. Use of sunscreens can extend the duration of intentional sun exposure, such as sunbathing. Such an extension may increase the risk for cutaneous melanoma" (16).

The conviction that sunscreens may have the potential of reducing the incidence of both nonmelanoma and melanoma is reflected by recommendations from clinical organizations: the American Cancer Society (84), the American Academy of Dermatology (85), the American Academy of Pediatrics (86), the American College of Obstetricians and Gynecologists (87), and a National Institutes of Health consensus panel (88). All recommend patient education concerning sun avoidance and sunscreen use. The American Academy of Family Physicians (89) recommends sun protection for all with increased sun exposure, whereas the American College of Preventive Medicine (ACPM) concluded that sun-protective measures (e.g., clothing, hats, opaque sunscreens) are probably effective in reducing skin cancer but that the evidence does not support discussion of sunscreen and sun protection with every patient. ACPM concluded that evidence is insufficient to advise patients that chemical sunscreens protect against malignant melanoma and that their use may actually lead to increased risk (90). The Task Force on Community Preventive Services found insufficient evidence to determine the effectiveness of a range of population-based interventions to reduce unprotected UV light exposure and recommended additional research on educational policy approaches, media campaigns, and both health-care setting and community-based interventions (91).

Overall, it seems clear that, although sunscreens have the capacity to prevent actinic keratoses and SCC, their capacity to reduce incidence of melanoma remains to be determined, ideally through intervention studies in groups of patients at very high risk of developing melanoma.

It also appears that among young adults, sunscreens are being used not as a protection against detrimental effects of sun exposure but as a means of acquiring a "safe tan." Indeed, a recent survey of UV exposure across different populations in Denmark clearly indicates that, among young people, sunscreens are used to increase sun exposure without sunburn. Unfortunately, this behavior is being backed-up by commercial advertising promoting "safe sun." Prevention messages should be specifically tailored to address this population, melanoma being a disease that strikes young adults.

REFERENCES

1. International Agency for Research on Cancer. Solar and ultraviolet radiation. IARC Monogr Eval Carcinog Risks Humans. Vol. 55. Lyon, France: IARC Press, 1992.
2. Doré JF, Boniol M. Environmental influences on cutaneous melanoma. In: Thompson JF, Morton DL, Kroon BBR, eds. Textbook of Melanoma. Andover, UK: Martin Dunitz, 2003:43–55.
3. Hill D. Efficacy of sunscreens in protection against skin cancer. Lancet 1999; 354:699–700.
4. Albert MR, Ostheimer KG. The evolution of current medical and popular attitudes toward ultraviolet light exposure: part 1. J Am Acad Dermatol 2002; 47:930–937.
5. Albert MR, Ostheimer KG. The evolution of current medical and popular attitudes toward ultraviolet light exposure: part 2. J Am Acad Dermatol 2003; 48:909–918.
6. Albert MR, Ostheimer KG. The evolution of current medical and popular attitudes toward ultraviolet light exposure: part 3. J Am Acad Dermatol 2003; 49:1096–1106.
7. MacEachern WN, Jillson OF. A practical sunscreen—"red vet pet." Arch Dermatol 1964; 89:147–150.
8. Robinson JK, Rigel DS, Amonette RA. Summertime sun protection used by adults for their children. J Am Acad Dermatol 2000; 42:746–753.
9. Severi G, Cattaruzza MS, Baglietto L, et al. European Organization for Research Treatment of Cancer (EORTC) Melanoma Cooperative Group. Sun exposure and sun protection in young European children: an EORTC multicentric study. Eur J Cancer 2002; 38:820–826.
10. Stanton WR, Janda M, Baade PD, Anderson P. Primary prevention of skin cancer: a review of sun protection in Australia and internationally. Health Promot Int 2004; 19:369–378.
11. Garbe C, Buettner PG. Predictors of the use of sunscreen in dermatological patients in Central Europe. Prev Med 2000; 31:134–139.
12. Thieden E, Philipsen PA, Sandby-Møller J, Wulf HC. Sunscreen use related to UV exposure, age, sex, and occupation based on personal dosimeter readings and sun-exposure behavior diaries. Arch Dermatol 2005; 141:967–973.
13. Wulf HC, Stender IM, Lock-Andersen J. Sunscreens used at the beach do not protect against erythema: a new definition of SPF is proposed. Photodermatol Photoimmunol Photomed 1997; 13:129–132.
14. Berwick M, Fine JA, Bolognia JL. Sun exposure and sunscreen use following a community skin cancer screening. Prev Med 1992; 21:302–310.
15. McCarthy EM, Ethridge KP, Wagner RF Jr. Beach holiday sunburn: the sunscreen paradox and gender differences. Cutis 1999; 64:37–42.
16. International Agency for Research on Cancer (IARC). Handbooks of Cancer Prevention: Sunscreens. Vol. 5. Lyon, France: IARC Press, 2001.

17. U.S. Preventive Services Task Force. Counseling to Prevent Skin Cancer. Recommendations and Rationale of the U.S. Preventive Services Task Force. MMWR 2003; 52:13–17.
18. National Cancer Institute. Skin Cancer (PDQ) Prevention. www.cancer.gov.
19. English DR, Armstrong BA, Kricker A, Winter MG, Heenan PJ, Randell PL. Case-control study of sun exposure and squamous cell carcinoma of the skin. Int J Cancer 1998; 77:347–353.
20. Suarez-Varela MM, Gonzalez AL, Caraco EF. Non-melanoma skin cancer: A case-control study on risk factors and protective measures. J Environ Pathol Toxicol Oncol 1996; 15:255–261.
21. Grodstein F, Speizer DE, Hunter DJ. A prospective study of incident squamous cell carcinoma of the skin in the nurses' health study. J Natl Cancer Inst 1995; 87:1061–1066.
22. Kricker A, Armstrong BK, English DR, Heenan PJ. Does intermittent sun exposure cause basal cell carcinoma? A case-control study in Western Australia. Int J Cancer 1995; 60:489–494.
23. Hunter DJ, Colditz GA, Stampfer MJ, Rosner B, Willett WC, Speizer FE. Risk factors for basal cell carcinoma in a prospective cohort of women. Ann Epidemiol 1990; 1:13–23.
24. Green A, Williams G, Neal R, et al. Daily sunscreen application and betacarotene supplementation in prevention of basal-cell and squamous-cell carcinomas of the skin: A randomised controlled trial. Lancet 1999; 354:723–729.
25. Harvey I, Frankel S, Marks R, Shalom D, Nolan-Farrell M. Non-melanoma skin cancer and solar keratoses. I. Methods and descriptive results of the South Wales skin cancer study. Br J Cancer 1996; 74:1302–1307.
26. Harvey I, Frankel S, Marks R, Shalom D, Nolan-Farrell M. Non-melanoma skin cancer and solar keratoses. II. Analytical results of the South Wales skin cancer study. Br J Cancer 1996; 74:1308–1312.
27. Naylor MF, Boyd A, Smith DW, Cameron GS, Hubbard D, Neldner KH. High sun protection factor sunscreens in the suppression of actinic neoplasia. Arch Dermatol 1995; 131:170–175.
28. Thompson SC, Jolley D, Marks R. Reduction of solar keratoses by regular sunscreen use. New Engl J Med 1993; 329:1147–1151.
29. Holman CD, Armstrong BK, Heenan PJ. Relationship of cutaneous malignant melanoma to individual sunlight-exposure habits. J Natl Cancer Inst 1986; 76:403–414.
30. Holman CD, Armstrong BK, Heenan PJ, et al. The causes of malignant melanoma: results from the West Australian Lions Melanoma Research Project. Recent Results Cancer Res 1986; 102:18–37.
31. Fisher J, Schwartzbaum J, Siegle R. A matched case-control study of the effects of chemical sunscreen use on cutaneous malignant melanoma [Abstract]. Am J Epidemiol 1996; 143:S9.
32. Osterlind A, Tucker MA, Stone BJ, Jensen OM. The Danish case-control study of cutaneous malignant melanoma. II. Importance of ultraviolet-light exposure. Int J Cancer 1988; 42:319–324.
33. Klepp O, Magnus K. Some environmental and bodily characteristics of melanoma patients. A case-control study. Int J Cancer 1979; 23:482–486.
34. Graham S, Marshall J, Haughey B, et al. An inquiry into the epidemiology of melanoma. Am J Epidemiol 1985; 122:606–619.

35. Beitner H, Norell SE, Ringborg U, Wennersten G, Mattson B. Malignant melanoma: aetiological importance of individual pigmentation and sun exposure. Br J Dermatol 1990; 122:43–51.

36. Herzfeld PM, Fitzgerald EF, Hwang SA, Stark A. A case-control study of malignant melanoma of the trunk among white males in upstate New York. Cancer Detect Prev 1993; 17:601–608.

37. Westerdahl J, Olsson H, Masback A, Ingvar C, Jonsson N. Is the use of sunscreens a risk factor for malignant melanoma? Melanoma Res 1995; 5:59–65.

38. Autier P, Doré JF, Schifflers E, et al. For the EORTC Melanoma Cooperative Group. Melanoma and use of sunscreens: an EORTC case-control study in Germany, Belgium and France. The EORTC Melanoma Cooperative Group. Int J Cancer 1995; 61: 749–755.

39. Roberts LK, Stanfield JW. Suggestion that sunscreen use is a melanoma risk factor is based on inconclusive evidence. Melanoma Res 1995; 5:377–378.

40. Naylor MF, Farmer KC. The case for sunscreens. A review of their use in preventing actinic damage and neoplasia. Arch Dermatol 1997; 133:1146–1154.

41. Naldi L, Gallus S, Imberti GL, Cainelli T, Negri E, La Vecchia C. Sunscreens and cutaneous malignant melanoma: an Italian case-control study. Int J Cancer 2000; 86:879–882.

42. Whiteman DC, Valery P, McWhirter W, Green AC. Risk factors for childhood melanoma in Queensland, Australia. Int J Cancer 1997; 70:26–31.

43. Elwood M, Gallagher RP. More about: Sunscreen use, wearing clothes and number of nevi in 6- to 7-year old European children. J Natl Cancer Inst 1999; 91:1164–1166.

44. Wolf P, Quehenberger F, Mullegger R, Stranz B, Kerl H. Phenotypic markers, sunlight-related factors and sunscreen use in patients with cutaneous melanoma: an Austrian case-control study. Melanoma Res 1998; 8:370–378.

45. Westerdahl J, Ingvar C, Masback A, Olsson H. Sunscreen use and malignant melanoma. Int J Cancer 2000; 87:145–150.

46. Rodenas JM, Delgado-Rodriguez M, Herranz MT, Tercedor J, Serrano S. Sun exposure, pigmentary traits, and risk of cutaneous malignant melanoma: a case-control study in a Mediterranean population. Cancer Causes Control 1996; 7:275–283.

47. Espinosa Arranz J, Sanchez Hernandez JJ, Bravo Fernandez P, et al. Cutaneous malignant melanoma and sun exposure in Spain. Melanoma Res 1999; 9:199–205.

48. Bakos L, Wagner M, Bakos RM, et al. Sunburn, sunscreens, and phenotypes: some risk factors for cutaneous melanoma in southern Brazil. Int J Dermatol 2002; 41:557–562.

49. Holly EA, Aston DA, Cress RD, Ahn DK, Kristiansen JJ. Cutaneous melanoma in women. I. Exposure to sunlight, ability to tan, and other risk factors related to ultraviolet light. Am J Epidemiol 1995; 141:923–933.

50. deVries E, Boniol M, Severi G, et al. Public awareness about risk factors could pose problems for case-control studies: The example of sunbed use and cutaneous melanoma. Eur J Cancer 2005; 41:2150–2154.

51. Huncharek M, Kupelnick B. Use of topical sunscreens and the risk of malignant melanoma/A meta-analysis of 9067 patients from 11 case-control studies. Am J Pub Health 2002; 92:1173–1177.

52. Dennis LK, Beane Freeman LE, VanBeek MJ. Sunscreen use and the risk for melanoma: A quantitative review. Ann Intern Med 2003; 139:966–978.

53. Greenland S. Invited commentary: A critical look at some popular meta-analytic methods. Am J Epidemiol 1994; 140:290–296.
54. Harrison SL, MacLennan R, Speare R, Wronski I. Sun exposure and melanocytic naevi in young Australian children. Lancet 1994; 344:1529–1532.
55. Doré JF, Pedeux R, Boniol M, Chignol MC, Autier P. Intermediate-effect biomarkers in prevention of skin cancer. In: Miller AB, Bartsch H, Bofetta P, Dragsted L, Vainio H, eds. Biomarkers in Cancer Chemoprevention. IARC Scientific Publication no. 154. Lyon, France: International Agency for Research on Cancer, 2001:81–91.
56. Wachsmuth RC, Turner F, Barrett JH, et al. The effect of sun exposure in determining nevus density in UK adolescent twins. J Invest Dermatol 2005; 124:56–62.
57. Pope DJ, Sorahan T, Marsden JR, Ball PM, Grimley RP, Peck IM. Benign pigmented nevi in children. Prevalence and associated factors: the West Midlands, United Kingdom Mole Study. Arch Dermatol 1992; 128:1201–1206.
58. Luther H, Altmeyer P, Garbe C, et al. Increase of melanocytic nevus counts in children during 5 years of follow-up and analysis of associated factors. Arch Dermatol 1996; 132:1473–1478.
59. Autier P, Doré JF, Cattaruzza MS, et al. European Organization for Research and Treatment of Cancer Melanoma Cooperative Group. Sunscreen use, wearing clothes, and number of nevi in 6- to 7-year-old European children. J Natl Cancer Inst 1998; 90:1873–1880.
60. Azizi E, Iscovich J, Pavlostsky F, et al. Use of sunscreen is linked with elevated naevi counts in Israeli school children and adolescents. Melanoma Res 2000; 10:491–498.
61. Darlington S, Siskind V, Green L, Green A. Longitudinal study of melanocytic nevi in adolescents. J Am Acad Dermatol 2002; 46:715–722.
62. Dulon M, Weichenthal M, Blettner M, et al. Sun exposure and number of nevi in 5-to-6-year-old European children. J Clin Epidemiol 2002; 55:1075–1081.
63. Bauer J, Buttner P, Wiecker TS, Luther H, Garbe C. Effect of sunscreen and clothing on the number of melanocytic nevi in 1,812 German children attending day care. Am J Epidemiol 2005; 161:620–627.
64. Gallagher RP, Rivers JK, Lee TK, Bajdik CD, Mc Lean DI, Coldman AJ. Broad-spectrum sunscreen use and the development of new nevi in white children: a randomized controlled trial. J Am Med Assoc 2000; 283:2955–2960.
65. Lee TK, Rivers JK, Gallagher RP. Site-specific protective effect of broad spectrum sunscreen on nevus development among white schoolchildren in a randomized trial. J Am Acad Dermatol 2005; 52:786–792.
66. Bauer J, Buttner P, Wiecker TS, Luther H, Garbe C. Interventional study in 1,232 young German children to prevent the development of melanocytic nevi failed to change sun exposure and sun protective behavior. Int J Cancer 2005; 116:755–761.
67. English DR, Milne E, Jacoby P, Giles-Corti B, Cross D, Johnston R. The effect of a school-based sun protection intervention on the development of melanocytic nevi in children: 6-year follow-up. Cancer Epidemiol Biomarkers Prev 2005; 14:977–980.
68. Weinstock MA. Sunscreen use can reduce melanoma risk. Photodermatol Photoimmunol Photomed 2001; 17:234–241.
69. Setlow RB, Grist E, Thompson K, Woodhead AD. Wavelengths effective in induction of malignant melanoma. Proc Natl Acad Sci U S A 1993; 90:6666–6670.
70. Robert C, Muel B, Benoit A, Dubertret L, Sarasin A, Stary A. Cell survival and shuttle vector mutagenesis induced by ultraviolet A and ultraviolet B radiation in a human cell line. J Invest Dermatol 1996; 106:721–728.

71. Haliday GM, Agar NS, Barnetson RS, Ananthaswamy HN, Jones AM. UV-A finger-print mutations in human skin cancer. Photochem Photobiol 2005; 81:3–8.
72. Kraemer KH, Lee MM, Andrews AD, Lambert WC. The role of sunlight and DNA repair in melanoma and non-melanoma skin cancer: the xeroderma pigmentosum paradigm. Arch Dermatol 1994; 130:1018–1021.
73. Fears TR, Bird CC, Guerry D, et al. Average midrange ultraviolet radiation flux and time outdoors predict melanoma risk. Cancer Res 2002; 62:3992–3996.
74. Autier P, Doré JF. Influence of sun exposures during childhood and during adulthood on melanoma risk. EPIMEL and EORTC Melanoma Cooperative Group. European Organisation for Research and Treatment of Cancer. Int J Cancer 1998; 77:533–537.
75. Landi MT, Baccarelli A, Tarone RE, et al. DNA repair, dysplastic nevi, and sunlight sensitivity in the development of cutaneous malignant melanoma. J Natl Cancer Inst 2002; 94:94–101.
76. Pedeux R, Boniol M, Autier P, Doré JF. Re: DNA repair, dysplastic nevi, and sunlight sensitivity in the development of cutaneous malignant melanoma. J Natl Cancer Inst 2002; 94:772–773.
77. Pedeux R, Sales F, Pourchet J, et al. Ultraviolet B sensitivity of peripheral lympho-cytes as an independent risk factor for cutaneous melanoma. Eur J Cancer 2006; 42:212–215.
78. Stender IM, Andersen JL, Wulf HC. Sun exposure and sunscreen use among sunbathers in Denmark. Acta Derm Venereol 1996; 76:31–33.
79. Stender IM, Lock-Andersen J, Wulf HC. Sun-protection behaviour and self-assessed burning tendency among sunbathers. Photodermatol Photoimmunol Photomed 1996; 12:162–165.
80. Autier P, Doré JF, Négrier S, et al. European Organization for Research and Treatment of Cancer Melanoma Cooperative Group. Sunscreen use and duration of sun exposure: a double-blind, randomized trial. J Natl Cancer Inst 1999; 91:1304–1309.
81. Autier P, Doré JF, Condé Reis A, et al. EORTC Melanoma Cooperative Group. Sunscreen use and intentional sun exposure to ultraviolet A and B radiation: a double-blind randomized trial using personal dosimeters. Br J Cancer 2000; 83:1243–1248.
82. Dupuy A, Dunant A, Grob JJ. For Réseau d'Epidémiologie en Dermatologie. Randomized controlled trial testing the impact of high-protection sunscreens on sun-exposure behavior. Arch Dermatol 2005; 141:950–956.
83. Naylor MK, Robinson JK. Sunscreen, sun protection, and our many failures. Arch Dermatol 2005; 141:1025–1027.
84. American Cancer Society. Cancer prevention & early detection facts & figures 2003. Atlanta, GA, USA: American Cancer Society. Available at http://www.cancer.org/docroot/STT/content/STT_1x_Cancer_Prevention_Early_Detection_Facts_Figures_2003.asp or at http://www.cancer.org/downloads/STT/CPED2003PWSecured.pdf.
85. Lim HW, Cooper K. The health impact of solar radiation and prevention strategies: report of the Environmental Council, American Academy of Dermatology. J Am Acad Dermotol 1999; 41:81–99.
86. American Academy of Pediatrics, Committee on Environmental Health. Ultraviolet light: a hazard to children. Pediatrics 1999; 104:328–333.
87. American College of Obstetricians and Gynecologists. Primary and Preventive Care: Periodic Assessments. ACOG Committee Opinion 246. Washington, DC: ACOG, 2000.

88. NIH Consensus Development Program. Diagnosis and Treatment of Early Melanoma. NIH Consensus Development Conference, January 27–29, 1992. Vol. 10, No. 1. Bethesda, MD: US Department of Health and Human Services, National Institutes of Health. Available at http://consensus.nih.gov/cons/088/088_intro.htm.

89. American Academy of Family Physicians. "Safe-Sun" Guidelines. Leawood, KS, USA: American Academy of Family Physicians, 2000. Available at http://www.aafp. org/afp/20000715/375ph.html.

90. Ferrini RL, Perlman M, Hill L. Skin protection from ultraviolet light exposure: American College of Preventive Medicine Practice Policy Statement. Am J Prev Med January 1998; 14:83–86. Available at http://www.acpm.org/skinprot.htm.

91. Centers for Disease Control and Prevention. Preventing skin cancer: findings of the task force on community preventive services on reducing exposure to ultraviolet light. MMWR 2003; 52:1–12.

92. Green A, Bain C, McLennan R, Siskind V. Risk factors for cutaneous melanoma in Queensland. Recent Results Cancer Res 1986; 102:76–97.

93. Youl P, Aitken J, Hayward N, et al. Melanoma in adolescents: a case-control study of risk factors in Queensland, Australia. Int J Cancer 2002; 98:92–98.

13

Solaria

Jean-Pierre Césarini

Agence Française de Sécurité Sanitaire de l'Environnement et du Travail—Unité Agents Physiques, Maisons-Alfort, France

More than 2000 years ago, Romans and Greeks were enjoying sunbathing in the nude and even the Egyptians of the oldest dynasty associated life with solar radiation. However, at the beginning of the 20th century, sunbathing was not popular in Europe. Developing a tan was, for a long time, considered to be associated with outdoor and agricultural work and a connotation of low class. Members of high-class society tried to avoid solar exposure as much as possible by wearing gloves and veils and using parasols. It was the social improvement with paid holidays and the associated freedom, which, much later, made the exposure of large parts of the body popular.

By the end of the 19th century, especially in Nordic countries and Germany, the use of ultraviolet radiation (UVR) to improve health status or cure some diseases became popular. The antibacterial, antiviral, or metabolic effects of UV light were also recognized. However, long-term adverse effects were practically denied. It is interesting to note the comment of Saidman (1): "If immediate adverse effects produced by UV are in fact very benign, long-term consequences should not be neglected since some may be unpleasant for the patient. We can observe, on the irradiated teguments some hyperkeratosis, which may evoke the possibility of a late neoplasia. The statement by Guillaume on that subject requests verification since no proof has been provided. If the UV were able to produce, actually, secondary neoplasia, the 30 years of experiences of Institute Finsen's physicians, would have told us."

By the end of the Wold War II, antibiotics and sulfamides had been discovered and their use spread in developing countries. As a counterpart, the use of

UVR to treat human diseases declined greatly but remained essential for the cure of skin diseases such as psoriasis, vitiligo, and special forms of leukemia. In parallel, the lamp industry, responding to the desire of the population to have a tan all around the year, even when solar exposure was not possible, developed several technologies, which in turn had to be controlled by international regulations, as the industry was not able to regulate itself.

HISTORY

In the years before and just after the World War II, devices used for tanning were derived from an old technology that had developed small units for use by medical practitioners or for original over-the-counter sale by pharmacists. These units emitted UVA, UVB, and UVC radiation. These types of lamps were able to produce sunburn of the skin in a few minutes. With the emergence of low-pressure fluorescent lamp tubes and the possibility to control the UV spectral emission by the appropriate selection of different phosphors, it appeared that the risk of burning could be reduced and tanning efficiency could be improved. The indoor tanning industry began to develop in the 1960s, and created a demand and a market with publicity that was essentially based on the safe practice of artificial tanning along with some fallacious promises of improvement in public health. Nowadays, millions of individuals expose themselves to artificial UVR with a clear gradient from north to south, (decreasing at lower latitudes) generating billions of Euros in benefits for the industry making the solaria equipment and for the operators who provide the services.

Most of the users of tanning devices are also "sun-seekers" and, because biological effects of UV are the essentially the same regardless of the origin of the UVR, the total of UVR exposure of this population has increased regularly throughout the years since at least 1950. Along with the steady increase in population exposure to UVR, there has been in parallel (but with some delay), an actual increase in the incidence of all forms of skin cancers. Since 1980, scientists linked to medical societies and health authorities have attempted with little success to draw attention to the uncontrolled growth of the fashion for tanning. After the worldwide recognition of the possible increase of skin cancers and cataracts that would be linked to stratospheric ozone depletion, along with the actual increased incidence of skin cancers (with a doubling of the deadly form, melanoma, every decade, and a doubling of other forms every 15–20 years), the World Health Organization (WHO) launched its INTERSUN program (2,3). As part of the INTERSUN program, there was a general recommendation for the reduction of unnecessary UVR exposure, that is, a reduction of the fashion for tanning. The WHO's latest publication on this subject, "Artificial Tanning Sunbeds: Risk and Guidance," is intended for governmental health authorities to assist them in the development of public health policy in relation to sunbeds (4). WHO does not recommend the use of tanning devices for cosmetic purposes.

TECHNOLOGIES: HOW IS ARTIFICIAL UV PRODUCED?

When a tungsten filament, or any material, is heated to a sufficient temperature, it emits some UVR. This general principle of incandescence has been applied in different technologies to produce a substantial amount of UVR. Compared to other lamp technologies, however, the incandescent lamp is quite inefficient for producing UVR. High-pressure discharge lamps are far more efficient, and include families of lamps such as high-pressure mercury-vapor lamps and metal-halide lamps. High-pressure mercury-vapor lamps were commonly used with little or no UVC filtration for medical purposes and were also sold as well for cosmetic tanning purposes until about 1960. Typically these lamps were 80- to 300-watt lamps and were used individually or in groups. In the 1970s, 500- to 5000-watt lamps have been manufactured with adequate protective filtration (suppression of UVB and UVC) for tanning purposes. High-pressure mercury lamps may also contain additives (metal halides) to increase the UVA output for cosmetic tanning equipment. These high-pressure lamps have been applied as several units for partial-body irradiation (facial units) or in combination with a second type of lamp: low-pressure discharge lamps.

The low-pressure discharge lamps, with appropriate fluorescent phosphors, also called UV-fluorescent lamps, operate by means of an electrical discharge between two electrodes through a mixture of mercury vapor and a rare gas, usually argon. These are actually quite similar to fluorescent tubes used for general lighting, but with different phosphors having peak emissions in the UV region of the spectrum. Light is produced by conversion of the very rich 254.0, 313.0, and 353.7 nm mercury emission radiation produced inside the electric discharge into longer wavelengths radiations by means of excitation of the phosphor coating inside of the lamp wall. The lamp's output spectrum is varied by changing the composition of the phosphor and the quality of the lamp envelope. A wide range of spectral emissions covering visible, UVA and UVB regions can be obtained. The output can be further improved by the introduction of a reflective coating inside one part of the tube. Table 1 shows UVR emission data from UVA fluorescent lamps (5).

Lamps may have different sizes and shapes and are arranged in several types of fixtures, like a canopy, a bed (with acrylic layer to protect the tubes), as vertical panels and as cabins. The electric energy required to operate the devices may vary from about 100 watts to several thousands of watts. Fluorescent tubular lamps and filtered mercury-lamp sources may be used together, especially to irradiate the facial zone.

For cosmetic devices, exposures are controlled by a timer that can be adjusted to deliver a given dose according to a schedule, which has been provided by the manufacturer who assembled the lamp sources and associated parts of the device. It should be noted that after about 600 hours of operation, the lamp sources may lose as much as 50% of their output radiant power. So, the delivered UV exposure dose cannot be calculated with good precision. The same sources

Table 1 UVR Emission (Unweighted) Data for UVA Fluorescent Lamps Used for Tanning Purposes

Lamp type	UVB (mW m^{-2})		UVA (mW m^{-2})	
	280–315 nm	315–400 nm	315–340 nm	340–400 nm
Philips TL09	7.2 (0.7)	1040 (99.3)	210 (20.0)	830 (79.3)
GEC UVA	7.02 (0.7)	970 (99.3)	200 (20.6)	770 (78.7)
Wolff Rapidsonne	35.6 (3.0)	1110 (97.0)	330 (30.0)	770 (67.0)
Wolff Fitsonne	6.9 (1.0)	690 (99.0)	150 (22.0)	540 (77.0)
Wolff Photomed	63.5 (6.0)	1000 (94.0)	390 (36.0)	610 (58.0)
Philips Cleo Natural	(4.5)	(95.5)	(35.5)	(60.0)
Philips Cleo Performa	(0.8)	(99.2)	(20.3)	(78.9)
Wolff Bellarium	(2.7)	(97.3)	(27.1)	(70.2)
Mercury Metal Halide (with special filter)	(0.0)	(100.0)	(0.0)	(100.0)
Tropical sun	(4.8)	(95.2)		

Note: Measurements are made at 50 cm (% emission in parentheses).

are used in medical devices and employed mostly in the form of cabins. The cabins are equipped with electronic dosimeters with at least two probes and the delivered dose is calculated automatically with excellent precision. As a consequence, the price of medical devices is of an order of magnitude higher than the devices used for commercial tanning purposes.

REGULATION

The international sunbed standard IEC 60335-2-27 was first drafted in the mid-1980s by a working group (WG) under the International Electrotechnical Commission (IEC) Technical Committee 61 (TC-61). The need for this international standard was that several countries had introduced differing technical requirements into national regulations concerning sunbed equipment. The IEC WG consisted of experts in dermatology, photobiology, radiation protection, and standardization as well as representatives from the tanning industry. The IEC standard is also reviewed and endorsed by the Committee for the European Community Normalization body (CEN/CENELEC). In this process, the IEC standard is usually endorsed within two years and then later endorsed by national normalization bodies thereafter.

Since the mid-1980s, the norm has been regularly revised to improve the safety for consumers and to avoid deviation from the norm. The standard makes use of the Commission Internationale de l'Eclairage (CIE), erythema reference action spectrum (6). Lamp spectral emissions are subdivided by this standard into "short" and "long" wavelength regions—above and below

320 nm—to categorize UV appliances into four "UV-types," according to their spectral characteristics and UV-power output. There were no upper irradiance limits for UV-types 1, 2, or 4, but a timer-dose requirement for the first exposure (more than one minute and $100 \, \text{J m}^{-2} \, \text{E}_{\text{eff}}$).

The UV classification system along with UV-type marking of the devices is one of the cornerstones of IEC 60335-2-27 (7). This classification system enables national authorities to bar certain IEC product types from the market in their countries should they desire. One reason for not permitting certain types of appliances may be, the objection of medical authorities against certain wavelength ranges used for tanning. The following summarizes the appliance categories.

1. UV type 1 appliance: appliance having a UV emitter such that the biological effect is caused by radiation having wavelengths longer than 320 nm and characterized by a relatively high irradiance in the range 320 to 400 nm.
2. UV type 2 appliance: appliance having a UV emitter such that the biological effect is caused by radiation having wavelengths both shorter and longer than 320 nm and characterized by a relatively high irradiance in the range 320 to 400 nm.
3. UV type 3 appliance: appliance having a UV emitter such that the biological effect is caused by radiation having wavelengths both shorter and longer than 320 nm and characterized by a limited irradiance over the whole UVR band. It should be noted that the maximum effective irradiance has been limited to $0.3 \, \text{W}/\text{m}_{\text{eff}}^{-2}$ equivalent to a tropical sun in blue-sky conditions at midday, that is, UV-index 12 (8).
4. UV type 4 appliance: appliance having a UV emitter such that the biological effect is mainly caused by radiation having wavelengths shorter than 320 nm.
5. Effective irradiance: irradiance of electromagnetic radiation weighted according to a specified action spectrum, that is, the CIE erythema action spectrum.

Appliances having UV emitters shall not emit radiation in hazardous amounts and their effective irradiance shall comply with the values specified in Table 2 of the standard.

Working Group WG8 has been renamed recently as Maintenance Team (MT16) to handle UV-matters concerning the standard. It has convened each year since 1998 and worked on several revisions of the standard some of which are listed here.

1. The CIE nonmelanoma skin cancer (NMSC) action spectrum was introduced to calculate the maximum yearly exposure (a recommendation).

Table 2   Limits of Effective Irradiance

UV type	Effective irradiance W/m^2	
	$250 < \lambda < 320$ nm	320 nm $< \lambda < 400$ nm
1	<0.0005	≥ 0.15
2	0.0005 to 0.15	≥ 0.15
3	<0.15	<0.15
4	≥ 0.15	<0.15
5 (§)	≥ 0.15	≥ 0.15

Note: λ is the wavelength of the radiation; total UV irradiance $= 0.6$ W/m^{-2}.

2. A UV type 5 (9) was introduced to fill a gap that had developed in the 1980s, for products that had not been anticipated to be used for tanning. In violation of the 1990s standard, the industry introduced sources with higher UVB power than type 3. The MT16 was forced to create this type 5 (§):
   UV type 5 appliance: appliance having a UV emitter such that the biological effect is caused by radiation having wavelengths both shorter and longer than 320 nm and characterized by a relatively high irradiance over the whole UVR band.
3. A "cap" was recommended to limit the UV-irradiance levels of the most powerful UV-types 1, 2, 4, and 5 to about twice the natural tropical sun (0.6 W/m$_{eff}^{-2}$).

Attaining a consensus position and compromise between the members who represented public health interests and those representing the tanning industry have always been quite difficult, and there have been a few occasions where procedural rules were used to thwart the recommendations of one group. For example, as a result of a decision of the Secretariat for TC61 (household appliances), a document, which had not been previously approved by the MT16, was issued and adopted by international vote (including countries with no tanning industry or national customers). The medical and radiation protection experts drew the attention of international health authorities to this abnormal practice, which resulted in enquiries from the European Commission (10) within the framework of Council Directive 73/23/EEC, relating to electrical equipment for use within certain voltage limits, safety of tanning devices for cosmetic purposes. The commission requested CEN/CENELEC to re-examine the standard on the basis of the 1997 standard, and to re-evaluate the risks linked to the use of tanning devices.

The International Commission on Non-Ionizing Radiation Protection (11) issued a statement concerning the safety of cosmetic tanning. The recommendations were followed by the World Health Organization (4), which, in the framework of its INTERSUN program, produced a practical document on artificial tanning sunbeds, Risks and Guidance, which was also based on the IEC 60335-2-27, version 2000.

The conclusions of the European Community Scientific Committee, other arguments forwarded to the EC, and the results of the IEC voting on that Amendment 2, were awaited to clarify the confusing status of the international norm created by the procedural actions that had been initiated from certain national delegations, by the reactions (fact-sheets and statements) issued by national, European, and international health authorities.

CONSUMER USE OF TANNING DEVICES

The primary goal for consumers who visit commercial tanning facilities or who use personal tanning devices at home is to develop a tan. The physiological mechanisms to acquire a tan are now well known. The natural production of melanin, which is responsible for the skin color, may be increased by exposure to UVA and UVB (12). Tanning is produced by a chain of events that begins with the production of DNA damage by either direct absorption of UVB or indirectly through UVA absorption by cellular chromophores that produce reactive oxygen species that in turn damage the DNA. This DNA damage is repaired and excised dimers in turn trigger the cascade of events through c-AMP that leads to neo-melanogenesis. Specifically, UVB induces the proliferation of the keratinocytes, which, as a consequence, almost doubles the thickness of the epidermis after repeated exposures. Keratinocytes send messages to melanocytes in order to stimulate melanogenesis. In addition, UVA, when absorbed by chromophores, specifically produce lipoperoxides and membrane damage with activation of tyrosinase as the final step for neo-melanogenesis. A tan is always the consequence of cellular injuries and so, there is no safe way to acquire a tan: "tan is a scar resulting from ultraviolet radiations, artificial or natural, injuries."

For very clear-skin, melano-compromised individuals (13), the doses of UVA or UVB to acquire a tan are equivalent: no tan can be produced without damage at the molecular and cellular level and a "burn." For melano-competent individuals (white skin), the doses of UVB to burn or acquire a tan are equivalent but the doses of UVA to tan are significantly below the "burning" dose.

Surveys in the United Kingdom, Sweden, Holland, and northern European countries indicate that consumers have the desire to have a tan for several reasons (14): to look better (58%), to feel healthier (34%), to obtain a pre-holiday tan (28%), and still other reasons (14%). The tanning industry is "surfing" on those desires and make claims in publicity that a tan is safe, a tan is healthy, and that UVR produces vitamin D that will help to keep a general good health and even prevent cancers, cardiovascular diseases, and many other pathological conditions (15,16,17).

From surveys in these countries, it has been found that young people, especially females, intentionally tan outdoors and/or use sunbeds. Half of those surveyed experienced sunburns in both situations: 37% of the female population, 19% of the males used frequently sunbeds, and almost 70% of the users were under 30 years of age. About one-fifth practiced indoor tanning with a sunbed for more than 10 years. Another 20% of sunbed users reported burning after sunbed use, and 71% of these users experienced sunburns when tanning outdoors in their country or in sunny, mostly Mediterranean countries (18).

RISKS LINKED TO THE USE OF SOLARIA

The risks have to be defined by their nature, their dimension, and finally the proof of a health risk.

It should be stressed that the ultraviolet effects on tissues result from the absorption of the electromagnetic radiation by different cellular components. There is no reason to estimate that natural ultraviolet radiation (solar) may have different effects than those produced by artificial ultraviolet radiation. Of course, depending on the wavelengths, effects may be different. Throughout the day and throughout the year, the composition of solar UVR received on earth shows variations in the ratio of UVA/UVB: morning and afternoon versus midday, winter versus summer. In the same manner, due to technical possibilities, the UVA/UVB ratio of solaria may be changed purposefully.

The progress in the detection and quantification of DNA lesions induced by the absorption of UVR has substantially changed the estimation of the risks linked to UVA and UVB. It should be stressed that, before the Second World War, the carcinogenicity of UVR was not taken into consideration when treating severe rickets or bacterial infections. The recognition of the carcinogenicity of UVB became evident in the 1960s with, as a consequence, the general opinion that UVA was relatively safe. During the past ten years, it became evident that UVA exposures were not so innocent and the progresses in research and technology made UVA-induced lesions detectable, and their consequences were evaluated. Studies of fingerprint mutations in the basal layer of human squamous tumors pointed out that UVA and UVB were responsible for photocarcinogenesis in the skin at the same level as UVB at least for the midday UVA/UVB ratio (19,20,21). Nowadays, it cannot be claimed that UVA exposures are safer than UVB with regard to consideration of the long-term risk. However, for short-term risks, like erythema, UVA exposure in the same midday ratio counts for 20% of the effect. Furthermore, the 0.8% ultraviolet B content of ultraviolet type 3 sunlamp (a so-called UVA lamp) induces 75% of cyclobutane pyrimidine dimers in human keratinocytes in vitro (22).

Nature of the Risk

Sunburning is the principle immediate risk experienced by individuals when exposed to tanning devices. The risk has been minimized by the strict application of the IEC norm; nevertheless, phototoxic and photoallergic reactions to medications or skin-applied chemicals (cosmetics) may always occur. Photo-induced or photo-aggravated diseases have been observed following sun exposures as well as solaria exposures.

As burns have been significantly associated with an increased risk of skin cancer, considering the high probability of burns when exposed to artificial tanning devices, the aggravated risk of skin cancers is not negligible. Furthermore, the increased incidence of skin cancers is related to an increase of natural UV exposure and there is no reason to believe that the further increase of exposures to artificial UV will contribute to the increased incidence.

There is good experimental and epidemiological evidence that UVR exposure (mainly from sunlight) is related to all forms of human skin cancers, including cutaneous malignant melanoma (CMM) (23,24).

Nonmelanoma Skin Cancers

Experimental and epidemiological data on NMSCs have been used to establish a mathematical model able to provide a risk analysis of the NMSCs. The application of multivariate analysis to population-based epidemiology of NMSCs has shown that, for a group of subjects with a given genetic susceptibility, age and environmental UVR exposure are the two most important factors in determining the relative risk (25). The model was improved by introducing a series of experiments with mice and the establishment of the skin cancer action spectrum (26,27,28). Its shape, after normalization to 1, is very similar to the erythema action spectrum. The National Radiological Protection Board (29) evaluated the risk for NMSCs resulting from artificial UV exposure. The observed and calculated age standardized rates for basal cell carcinoma (BCC) and squamous cell carcinoma (SCC) were in good concordance when the mathematical model was applied to different latitudes and country of birth. The same model applied to the relative risk of BCC and SCC at 70 years as a result of whole body exposure to tanning equipment showed that a course of 10 sessions to acquire a tan before going on holiday is associated with a small (<10%) increased risk of inducing NMSCs compared with non-users. Of greater concern are the users of sunbeds at home who may expose themselves to artificial UV two or more times a week throughout the year during several years. For them, the risk jumps to more than 200%. In 2002, a study performed in the United States has shown that the risk for developing SCC was multiplied by 250% and the risk to develop BCC multiplied by 150%, among users of solaria (30).

Cutaneous Malignant Melanoma

A number of studies have been conducted to evaluate the risk of CMM after exposure to sunlamps and/or sunbeds. Gallagher et al. (31) conducted a systematic review and analysis of the relevant melanoma studies through a MEDLINE database search for the years 1984 to 2004. All case-control studies of CMM that reported on use of sunlamps, sunbeds, or both were initially considered for the analysis and inclusion/exclusion criteria were applied. Nine case controls and one cohort study provided the data for the analysis. A positive association was found between exposure and risk. The authors concluded: "results indicate a significantly increased risk of cutaneous melanoma subsequent to sunbed/sunlamp exposure."

The most convincing evidence that the use of artificial UV exposure for cosmetic purposes is responsible, at least in part, for a significant number of CMM, came from a large prospective cohort study (106,379 women) performed in the European Northern Countries (Norway, Sweden) (32). This work confirms previous findings that hair color, number of nevi on the legs, and history of sunburn are risk factors for melanoma and suggest that use of a solarium is associated with melanoma risk. Adolescent, an early adulthood, is among the most sensitive age period for the effects of sunburn and solarium use on CMM risk.

CONCLUSIONS AND RECOMMENDATIONS

Nowadays, there is ample evidence to consider that sunlight exposure is responsible for all forms of skin cancers. There is no biological reason to believe that UVR emitted by artificial sources have different biological consequences from sun-emitted UVR. As a consequence, unnecessary exposure to UVR, that is, exposure to artificial UVR for cosmetic purposes, is responsible in part for the epidemic of skin cancers, including their most deadly form, cutaneous melanoma. It is, indeed, time for the tanning industry to realize that the sales of equipment have to be deeply regulated as well as, for the operators of tanning devices, to provide complete and honest information (claims like vitamin D production as a potential anti-cancer agent have never been significantly substantiated) to the consumers, who should be educated by the health authorities about the general risk associated with excessive sun exposures and tanning fashion. In order to help these actors in their approach to a more common-sense behavior, the recommendations of independent international bodies, like ICNIRP (11) and World Health Organization (4,33), should be recognized and applied.

In particular, people should not use artificial tanning if they

1. have melano-compromised skin (skin phototypes I and II), that is, their skin always sunburns with no ability to tan or has high susceptibility to sunburn with only an ability to develop a light tan (Table 3),
2. are less than 18 years of age,
3. have large numbers of nevi (moles),
4. tend to freckle,
5. have a history of frequent childhood sunburn,
6. have pre-malignant or malignant skin lesions,
7. have sun-damaged skin,
8. are wearing cosmetics, as this may enhance their sensitivity to UV exposure, and

Table 3 Classification of Skin Types Based on Their Susceptibility to Sunburn in Sunlight

Skin phototype	Sunburn susceptibility	Tanning ability	Classes of individuals
I	Always sunburn	No tan	Melano-compromised
II	High	Light tan	
III	Moderate	Medium tan	Melano-competent
IV	Low	Dark tan	
V	Very low	Natural brown skin	Melano-protected
VI	Extremely low	Natural black skin	

    9. are taking medication. In this case, they should seek advice from their physician to determine if the medication will make them UVR-sensitive.

If, however, artificial tanning devices are nevertheless used, then the following points are recommended as a guide for the development of health policy in this area.

    1. *Tanning devices.* Sunbed tanning devices should comply with the requirements of the IEC's standard (1995) or national standards where they exist. Manufacturers should supply exposure schedules based on the tanning device lamp characteristics. Replacement of lamps, filters, or reflectors should not change the IEC classification of the device. Tanning devices should have an appropriate timer.

    2. *Eyewear.* UVR protective eyewear must be worn during tanning exposures.

    3. *Maximum exposure times and irradiance.* Maximum exposure times should ensure that no person suffers erythema (skin reddening) as a result of UVR exposure in a sunbed. Particular caution must be exercised with first-time users to gauge the user's skin response. If adverse reactions occur, further use should be discouraged. No UVC less than 280 nm should be emitted from a sunbed.

    4. *Maximum repeat exposure.* Further artificial sunbed exposure should not be administered before 48 hours after the previous exposure. An occasional break from the regularity of exposure is advisable.

    5. *Promotion.* Claims of health benefits should not be made in the promotion of sunbed use.

    6. *Supervision.* Whether it is a single-purpose retail sunbed facility or a sunbed is part of a hotel, recreation center, beauty parlor and the like; a trained supervisor should be available at all times the sunbed is in operation. Any person who is supervising the operation of a commercial sunbed should be properly trained in the following.

Proper determination of skin types and exposure times
Proper screening for potentially exposure-limiting conditions
Emergency procedures in case of overexposure to UVR
Types and wavelength ranges of UVR
Proper procedures for sanitizing protective eyewear and tanning
   equipment

Unsupervised, self-serviced sunbeds should be banned. Therapeutic use of sunbeds should only be conducted in a medical unit under medical supervision. Products designed to enhance or accelerate tanning should not be used.

   7.   *Client information and client concern form.* In a commercial estab-
        lishment, one or more notices (minimum A4 paper size) should
        present the following information, presented in the immediate view
        of every client entering the establishment, in each sunbed cubicle
        and repeated on the client concern form.

        Exposure to ultraviolet radiation such as from a sunbed contributes to
           the skin aging process and may cause skin cancer.
        People with skin that does not tan in natural light should not use a
           sunbed.
        Intentional exposure to sunlight or other sunbed exposures should be
           avoided for 48 hours after any sunbed exposure.
        UVR protective goggles must be worn at all times while undergoing
           sunbed exposure.
        Additional risk conditions should be taken in to consideration: treat-
           ment for solar keratosis and/or skin cancers, abnormal reactions/
           allergy to UV light, taking medications/applying certain cosmetics
           on the skin.
        No person under the age of 18 should use a sunbed.
        Before beginning a tanning course of one or more exposure sessions,
           the sunbed operator should ensure that a consent form in duplicates,
           containing the above six items, is handed to the client who signs
           and dates the forms, one being kept by the establishment for a
           period not less than two years, the other being retained by the client.

It is the medical view that any use of sun-tanning appliances is likely to raise the risk of skin cancer and international health authorities recommend against the use of UV-emitting appliances for tanning or other non-medical purposes.

REFERENCES

1. Saidman J. Les rayons ultraviolets et associés en thérapeutique. 2d ed, Paris: Doin G et Cie, 1928:465–466.
2. World Health Organization. Ultraviolet Radiation, Environmental Health Criteria 160, Geneva: WHO, 1994.

3. World Health Organization. INTERSUN, The Global UV Project, a Guide and Compendium. Geneva: WHO, 2003.
4. World Health Organization. Artificial Tanning Sunbeds—Risks and Guidance, Geneva: WHO, 2003.
5. National Radiological Protection Board. Board Statement on Effects of Ultraviolet Radiation on Human Health and Health Effects from Ultraviolet Radiation—Report of an Advisory Group on Non-ionising Radiation. Documents of the NRPB, Didcot: National Radiological Protection Board, 1995;6.
6. Commission Internationale de l'Eclairage. Erythemal reference action spectrum and standard erythemal dose: CIE Standard S007-1998, ISO 17166, Vienna, 1999.
7. International Electrotechnical Commission. International standard IEC 60335-2-27. Household and similar electrical appliances—Safety, Part 2-27: particular requirements for appliances for skin exposure to ultraviolet and infrared radiation. Geneva: CEI/IEC, 1995.
8. World Health Organization. Global Solar UV-Index. A practical guide. A joint recommendation of World Health Organization, World Meteorological Organization, United Nations Environmental Program, International Commission on Non-Ionizing Radiation Protection, Geneva: WHO, 2002.
9. International Electrotechnical Commission. International Standard IEC 60335-2-27, Amendment 1. Household and similar electrical appliances—Safety, Part 2-27: particular requirements for appliances for skin exposure to ultraviolet and infrared radiation. Geneva: CEI/IEC, 2004.
10. Official Journal of the European Union, Commission opinion of 27 October 2004 within the framework of Council Directive 73/23/EEC relating to electrical equipment designed for use within certain voltage limits. Safety of tanning devices for cosmetic purposes, 2004/C 275/03, 2004.
11. International Commission on Non-Ionizing Radiation Protection. ICNIRP statement: health issues of ultraviolet tanning appliances used for cosmetic purposes. Health Phys 2003; 84:119–127.
12. Césarini JP. Photo-induced events in the human melanocytic system: photoaggression and photoprotection. Pigment Cell Res 1988; 1:223–233.
13. Fitzpatrick TB, Césarini JP, Young A, Kollias N, Pathak MA, cited by Fitzpatrick TB, Bolognia JL. Human melanin pigmentation: role in pathogenesis of cutaneous melanoma. In: Zeise L, Chedekel MR, Fitzpatrick TB, eds. Melanin: Its Role in Human Photoprotection. KS: Valdenmar Publishing Co, 1995:177–182.
14. Health Education Authority. Sunbeds: what are they, who use them and what are the health effects? Diffey B for Health Education Authority, 1997.
15. Holick MF. Evolution and function of vitamin D. Recent Results Cancer Res 2003; 164:3–28.
16. Holick MF, Jenkins M. The UV Advantage. New York: Ibooks, 2003.
17. Gillie O. Sunlight Robbery. London: Health Research Forum, 2003.
18. Boldeman C, Bränström R, Dal H, et al. Tanning habits and sunburn in Swedish population age 13–50 years. Eur J Cancer 2001; 37:2441–2448.
19. Robert C, Muel B, Benoit A, et al. Cell survival and schuttle vector mutagenesis induced by ultraviolet A and ultraviolet B radiation in a human cell line. J Invest Dermatol 1996; 106:722–728.
20. Agar NS, Halliday GM, Barnetson R, et al. The basal layer in human squamous tumors harbors more UVA than UVB fingerprint mutations: a role for UVA in human skin carcinogenesis. Proc Nat Acad Sci USA 2004; 101:4954–4959.

21. Halliday GM, Agar NS, Barnetson R, et al. UVA fingerprint mutations in human skin cancer. Photochem Photobiol 2005; 81:3–8.
22. Woollons A, Kipp C, Young AR, et al. The 0.8% ultraviolet B content of an ultraviolet sunlamp induces 75% of cyclobutane pyrimidine dimers in human keratinocytes in vitro. Br J Derm 1999; 140:1023–1030.
23. International Agency for Research on Cancer. IARC Monographes on the Evaluation of Carcinogenic Risk to Humans. Vol. 55. Solar and Ultraviolet Radiation. Lyon: IARC Press, 1992.
24. US Department of Health and Human Services. National Toxicology Program. The report on carcinogens tenth edition: ultraviolet radiation related exposures: Broad-spectrum ultraviolet (UV) radiation, UVA, UVB, UVC, solar radiation, and exposure to sunlamps and sunbeds. Section 301 and 262, 2002.
25. Fears TR, Scotto J, Schneiderman MA. Mathematical model for age and ultraviolet effects on the incidence of skin cancer among whites in the United States. Am J Epidemiol 1977; 105:420–427.
26. De Gruijl FR, Sterenborg HJ, Forbes PD, et al. Wavelength dependence of skin cancer induction by ultraviolet irradiation of albino hairless mice. Cancer Res 1993; 53: 53–60.
27. Commission Internationale de l'Eclairage. Action spectrum for photocarcinogenesis (non-melanoma skin cancers). CIE 138/2 report 2000, CIE Vienna.
28. Commission Internationale de l'Eclairage. Photocarcinogenesis action spectrum (non-melanoma skin cancers) CIE DS 019.2/E: 2005, CIE Vienna.
29. National Radiological Protection Board. Board statement on effects of ultraviolet radiation on human health and health effects from ultraviolet radiation—report of an advisory group on non-ionising radiation. Documents of the NRPB, Appendix B: Risk analysis of human skin cancer. Didcot: National Radiological Protection Board, 2002; 13:253–268.
30. Karagas M, Stannard A, Mott LA, et al. Use of tanning devices and risk of basal cell and squamous cell skin cancers. J Natl Cancer Inst 2002; 94:224–266.
31. Gallagher RP, Spinelli JJ, Lee TK. Tanning beds, sunlamps, and risk of cutaneous malignant melanoma. Cancer Epidemiol Biomarkers Prev 2005; 14:562–566.
32. Veierød MB, Weiderpass E, Thörn M, et al. A prospective study of pigmentation, sun exposure, and risk of cutaneous malignant melanoma in women. J Natl Cancer Inst 2003; 95:1530–1538.
33. World Health Organization, Regional Office for Europe. UV Radiation and Health. Geneva: WHO, 2003.

14

Risk Groups for Skin Cancer and Aspects on Preventive Management

Johan Hansson and Ulrik Ringborg

Department of Oncology-Pathology, Karolinska Institute and Karolinska University Hospital Solna, Stockholm, Sweden

INTRODUCTION

The design of efficient preventive programs for skin cancer requires the identification of high-risk groups of individuals appropriate for participation in preventive interventions. The prevention of cutaneous malignant melanoma (CMM) is a task of utmost importance, as this is a potentially lethal tumor which shows a rapid increase in Caucasian populations (1). This chapter will therefore focus mainly on risk groups for CMM. However, from the perspective of both individual suffering and health economics at the societal level, prevention of the more common, although rarely lethal, nonmelanoma skin cancers, basal cell carcinoma (BCC) and squamous cell carcinoma (SCC) is also important. High-risk groups for nonmelanoma skin cancers will therefore also be briefly discussed.

HIGH-RISK GROUPS FOR CUTANEOUS MELANOMA

Risk groups for melanoma have previously been identified mainly by phenotypic characteristics and/or the presence of a personal or family history of CMM. More recently, progress has been made in the understanding of gene alterations that predispose for melanoma. In this chapter, the main focus will be on rare gene alterations that are associated with a markedly increased risk of melanoma, as these can be used to identify individuals and families with an inheritable high risk for CMM. However, at the population level, such rare alterations in high-risk genes probably play a minor role for CMM incidence. Therefore, in order to make a significant impact on CMM in the population, other groups of individuals with a more moderate risk elevation should also be identified. Recent studies have shown that more common gene variants that moderately increase the risk for CMM can be defined. Further studies of these and other presently undefined genetic variants should enhance future possibilities to define further risk groups for CMM in the population.

PHENOTYPIC CHARACTERISTICS

Skin, Hair and Eye Color, Freckling: Skin Type

Numerous studies have confirmed that risk of CMM is moderately increased in individuals with light skin and blond or red hair color. In general, these risk factors give a relative CMM risk of approximately two to four (2–7). Eye color has not, however, been firmly established as a risk factor for melanoma. Freckling is associated with a two- to three-fold increased risk of CMM (3).

Likewise, skin type, characterized by the tendency to burn and the ability to tan following sun exposure, is also correlated to risk of CMM: individuals with skin type I who never tan but always burn have the highest risk and those with type IV who never burn but always tan have the lowest CMM risk (3). More recently, these phenotypic pigment-related traits have been partly associated with variants in the risk-modifying *MC1R* gene (described subsequently).

Nevi

Nevus Numbers

Melanocytic nevi are benign skin lesions, which occur normally in healthy individuals. The number of common nevi is inversely proportional to the extent of cutaneous pigmentation and the average number of nevi varies between approximately 15 and 35 in young Caucasian adults in different studies (8,9). The development of nevi is enhanced by sun exposure in early life and nevi among young individuals are most frequent on body sites with intermittent sun exposure (10). Twin studies have indicated a higher correlation of nevus counts in monozygotic twins than in dizygotic twins, supporting that the number of nevi is under genetic control [(11), Bataille, 2000 (50), Zhu, 1999 (51)]. Numerous case-control investigations have shown that total nevus counts are significantly correlated to melanoma risk. Thus, individuals with more than 50 nevi have five- to 17-fold increased risk of CMM (12–14).

Dysplastic Nevi—Atypical Moles

Dysplastic nevi (DN) or atypical moles are melanocytic skin lesions that are both markers for melanoma risk and potential precursors for melanoma. These lesions were initially described in the members of families with familial melanoma

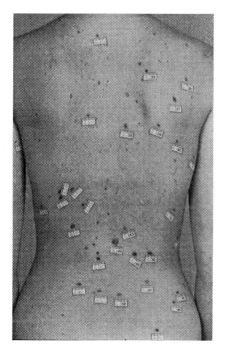

Figure 1   The dysplastic nevus syndrome phenotype. The back of a young woman belonging to a kindred with familial melanoma, which exhibits numerous dysplastic nevi. *Source*: Photo courtesy of Dr. Boel Ragnarsson-Olding.

(described subsequently), but have been shown to be relatively frequent in the general population. Thus the proportion of individuals with DN has been reported in frequencies varying between 1% and 18% in different populations (14,15). These differences may be partially due to varying diagnostic criteria but may also reflect differences in patterns of sun exposure and the genetic background in different populations. The clinical characteristics of DN resemble those of superficial spreading melanomas and can be summarized in the ABCD criteria: asymmetry, border irregularity, color variegation, and diameter over 6 mm (16) (Figs. 1 and 2). Histologically, DN exhibits architectural disorder and melanocyte atypia. Several studies show an increased melanoma risk in individuals with DN, but estimates of relative risk vary considerably between approximately two- and three-fold up to 30-fold in different studies (17,18).

Likewise, it is also controversial whether the presence of DN or a large number of common nevi show the strongest association with CMM (13,17,18,19,20,21,22). There is considerable evidence that DN may be precursor lesions for melanoma (Fig. 2). For instance, one study reported that 23% of melanomas had an associated nevus and of these 38% were histologically classified as DN (23).

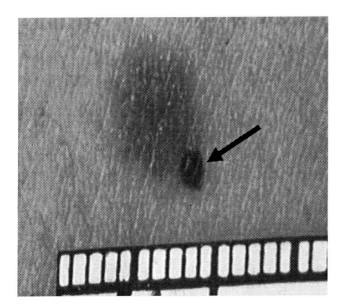

Figure 2 Development of an early melanoma in a dysplastic nevus. During follow-up of this member of a kindred with familial melanoma, a dark pigmentation arose in the lower part of this dysplastic nevus (*arrow*). Histopathological examination of the excised nevus showed that the darkly pigmented area corresponds to an early cutaneous malignant melanoma: a superficial spreading melanoma with a tumor thickness of 0.5 mm, T1a according to the American Joint Committee on Cancer classification. *Source*: Photo courtesy of Dr. Boel Ragnarsson-Olding.

PREVIOUS MELANOMA

A personal history of a previous CMM significantly increases the risk of a second primary melanoma. Thus, a large population-based study in Sweden of over 20,000 CMM patients showed a 10-fold-increased risk of a second primary CMM (24). Interestingly, the same group showed that the risk of CMM was at least as elevated in patients diagnosed with a melanoma in situ, which showed a 22-fold relative risk of developing an invasive melanoma (25).

HEREDITARY FACTORS

A proportion of melanoma cases occur in kindreds with a hereditary predisposition for CMM. In addition, the risk of CMM is increased in a number of other hereditary syndromes. These conditions will be reviewed in this section.

Familial Melanoma

It is estimated that 5% to 10% of all cases of CMM occur in kindreds with hereditary predisposition for CMM (26) and in population-based studies 1% to 13% of melanoma cases report melanoma in at least one first-degree relative (27,28).

Whereas individuals with a single first-degree relative with CMM have only a 2.2-fold increase of developing the disease themselves (27), members of families with multiple CMM cases have a much higher risk. The occurrence of families with increased melanoma risk has been recognized for nearly two centuries. Thus, in the first description of CMM in the English language, Norris reported a family where two members had CMM and several relatives had large moles (29). In 1978, Clark reported six melanoma-prone families where both patients with CMM and relatives had large "funny-looking" nevi, which were designated as potential precursors of CMM (30) (Figs. 1 and 2). The syndrome was subsequently entitled the "dysplastic nevus syndrome" (DNS) (28). In parallel, Lynch reported the same syndrome, which he entitled the "familial atypical multiple mole melanoma" syndrome (31). The syndrome is also called the "atypical mole syndrome" (32).

In 1985, a study of 14 DNS families was reported (33). Approximately, 95% of the melanoma patients and 50% of the family members had DN and during follow-up new cases of CMM were diagnosed only in individuals with DN. In an another early report, DNS families were defined as so called D-2 kindreds, with at least two family members with CMM and also two or more with DN (34). The lifetime risk of CMM in family members with DN was estimated to be 150-fold increased over the general population. A later study of 23 D-2 kindreds indicated that family members with DN had an 89-fold increased melanoma risk and those with a previous CMM a 229-fold increased risk for a second CMM (35). However, as more recent data indicate that a proportion of melanoma kindreds do not show the classical DNS phenotype, the focus today in familial melanoma is less on clinical phenotype and more on melanoma inheritance. In the last decade, important advances in the understanding of the molecular genetics of familial melanoma have been achieved.

Molecular Genetics of Familial Cutaneous Melanoma

In recent years, considerable efforts have been made to unravel the genetic alterations responsible for familial CMM. For instance, the Melanoma Genetics Consortium, GenoMEL has been active as a nonprofit consortium since 1997 in this area. GenoMEL is comprised of the majority of research groups worldwide, working on the genetics of familial CMM. The mission of GenoMEL is to develop and support collaborations between member groups to identify melanoma susceptibility genes, to evaluate gene-environment interactions, and to assess the risk of CMM and other cancers related to variations in these genes. More detailed information on GenoMEL and its activities can be obtained at its website (36).

CDKN2A: In 1994, it was demonstrated that affected members of some kindreds with familial CMM harbor germline mutations in the *CDKN2A* gene on chromosome 9p21 (37,38). Remarkably, the *CDKN2A* gene encodes two unrelated proteins; both are tumor suppressors and play key roles in cell-cycle regulation [(Fig. 3); reviewed in (39)]. Thus, the p19INK4 protein is encoded by exons 1α, 2, and 3 and negatively regulates cell-cycle progression by inhibiting the cyclin-dependent kinases CDK4 and CDK6. Inhibition of the kinases prevents phosphorylation of the retinoblastoma protein pRb and thereby entry into the S-phase of the cell cycle. The second protein is encoded by *CDKN2A* and p14ARF is encoded by splicing of an alternative exon 1β to exon 2. This protein is translated in an alternative reading frame (hence ARF, alternative reading frame) and therefore shows no amino acid homology to p16INK4. p14ARF blocks HDM2-mediated degradation of p53. Mutations in *CDKN2A* thus have the capacity to target negative regulators in two key signaling pathways, the pRb and p53 pathways and both have central roles in cell cycle regulation.

A large number of different germline mutations have been identified in members of kindreds with familial melanoma and also in patients with multiple primary CMM, irrespective of the presence of family history (40–43). Worldwide, it has been estimated that approximately 20% to 40 % of kindreds with familial melanoma are related to germline *CDKN2A* mutations (44). The majority of mutations are missense mutations in exon 1α and exon 2 and they are scattered throughout the gene without any clear hotspots. In some populations, recurrent *CDKN2A* founder mutations have been found (45–48). Depending on whether exon 1 or exon 2 is involved, the mutation affects

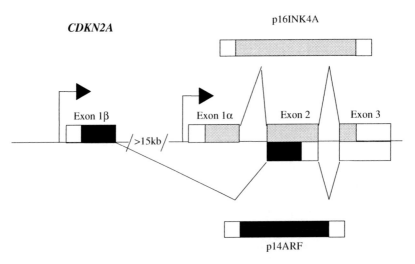

Figure 3 The *CDKN2A* locus on chromosome 9p21. This gene encodes two different proteins: p16INK4A and p14ARF, respectively. The protein p16INK4A is encoded by exons 1α, 2, and 3, whereas the p14ARF protein is encoded by alternative splicing of an alternative exon 1β to exon 2. The two proteins have quite different amino acid sequences as they are translated in different reading frames.

either the p16INK4 protein alone or both p16INK4 and p14ARF, respectively. In addition to the mutations in the coding sequences, mutations have also been described in the 5′ untranslated regions, which affect initiation of translation, and in introns, which affect splicing. Moreover, a small number of families, some of which exhibit a combination of CMM and other tumors, including neural system tumors, show germline alterations in exon 1β, which thus target p14ARF exclusively, demonstrating a role for p16ARF in melanoma development (49–51).

The probability of finding a germline *CDKN2A* mutation in a melanoma family increases with the number of affected individuals with melanoma. For genetic counseling, it is of importance to obtain an estimate of the penetrance of a certain germline gene mutation, that is, the risk of developing the disease among the carriers of the gene mutation. The penetrance of germline *CDKN2A* mutations for melanoma development in kindreds with familial melanoma has been the subject of a large collaborative study by GenoMEL. In this study, members of 80 kindreds with familial melanoma from different parts of the world were investigated. A total of 402 melanoma patients of which 320 were tested for *CDKN2A* mutations and 291 were mutation carriers as well as 713 mutation-tested relatives among which 194 were *CDKN2A* mutation carriers. Overall, *CDKN2A* mutation penetrance was estimated to be 0.30 [95% confidence interval (CI) = 0.12–0.62] by age 50 and 0.67 (95% CI = 0.31–0.96) by age 80. Penetrance was not statistically significantly modified by gender or by whether the *CDKN2A* mutation altered the p14ARF protein. However, there was a statistically significant effect of residing in a location with a high population incidence rate of melanoma ($P = 0.003$). By age 50, *CDKN2A* mutation penetrance reached 0.13 in Europe, 0.50 in the United States, and 0.32 in Australia; by age 80, it was 0.58 in Europe, 0.76 in the United States, and 0.91 in Australia. Thus, the same factors that affect population incidence of melanoma may also modulate *CDKN2A* penetrance.

However, the risk of melanoma in carriers of germline *CDKN2A* mutations in the general population is likely to be much lower, as reported in a recent publication from the Genes Environment and Melanoma study (52). This investigation was based on the analyses of 3550 population-based melanoma patients and 23,485 of their first-degree relatives. The risk of melanoma in carriers of germline *CDKN2A* mutations was 14% (95% CI = 8–22%) by age 50, 24% (95% CI = 15–34%) by age 70, and 28% (95% CI = 18–40%) by age 80. Thus, carriers of *CDKN2A* germline mutations in the general population have a much lower melanoma risk than those that belong to kindreds with familial melanoma. This is most likely due to the influence of other, unknown melanoma-predisposing factors in melanoma kindreds, which interact with and increase the penetrance of *CDKN2A* mutations.

Apart from cutaneous melanoma, an increased risk for pancreatic carcinoma has been documented in several families (45,53–55). The pathogenic mechanisms whereby germline *CDKN2A* mutations predispose to melanoma remain unclear. It has previously been reported that members of some kindreds with familial melanoma and DNS exhibit a genetic instability associated with UV-hypermutability. This defect has however not been linked to *CDKN2A* mutations. In accordance with this, it has been reported that CMM arising in the members of melanoma kindreds with *CDKN2A* mutations exhibit a high frequency of UV-inducible codon 61 mutations in the proto-oncogene NRAS (56). Recently, it has been suggested that p16INK4 normally causes senescence in nevi containing activating *BRAF* proto-oncogene mutations (57). Germline loss of one *CDKN2A* allele would thus weaken this protective mechanism against melanoma development.

Other Predisposing Genes and Candidate Loci for Familial Cutaneous Malignant Melanoma

CDK4

Worldwide only seven families with familial CMM and germline mutations in the *CDK4* gene have been described [reviewed in (39)]. In all cases, the mutations occur in exon 2 and affect codon 24, which is essential for binding to p16INK4A. The phenotype of these families seems to be very similar to those with *CDKN2A* mutations.

Candidate Loci for Novel Genes Predisposing to Familial Cutaneous Malignant Melanoma

GenoMEL has preformed a genome wide screen of 414 microsatellite markers in 82 melanoma families, most of who were from Australia. This yielded a significant linkage to a marker (D1S2779) on chromosome 1p22 (58). A maximum LOD score of 4.19 was obtained in a subset of nine families with early onset melanoma. While loss of heterozygosity (LOH) studies indicate that a tumor-suppressor gene may be present at this locus, so far no susceptibility gene has been identified, despite considerable efforts (59).

Recently, a linkage analysis of three Danish kindreds with both ocular and cutaneous melanoma has yielded a suggested linkage to markers on chromosome 9q21.32, but the putative gene responsible for the syndrome has not been identified (60).

Low Penetrance Risk-Modifying Genes

MC1R

The melanocortin 1 receptor gene, *MC1R*, encodes the membrane receptor for α-melanocyte-stimulating hormone (α-MSH). Upon binding of α-MSH to the receptor, the levels of cyclic adenosine monophosphate (cAMP) increase, which, in turn, results in a shift from pheomelanin to eumelanin synthesis (61). Several variants, single nucleotide polymorphisms (SNPs), have been described in the *MC1R* gene, and some of these may alter the function of the receptor, thereby shifting melanin synthesis from eumelanin towards pheomelanin (62–64) Such variants, which are common in the Caucasian population, are associated with red hair, fair skin, and freckling. Certain SNPs, so-called red hair color (RHC) alleles are associated with a significant, although modest (approximately, two-fold) increased risk of CMM (these include D84E, R151C, R160W, and D294H) (65). Other frequent, non-RHC, alleles are not associated with significantly increased CMM risk. An independent association between some *MC1R* SNPs and melanoma risk after adjustment for phenotype has also been reported (63,66). This suggests that that the α-MSH receptor may have functions apart from its role in pigment metabolism. There are reports that α-MSH, through the receptor, may affect the growth of melanocytic cells and also may have immunomodulatory and anti-inflammatory effects, although the role, if any, of such effects for CMM risk remains to be established (67–70). Although each RHC-allele is associated with an approximately two-fold risk for CMM, each individual may carry two or more RHC SNPs, which will further increase the CMM risk (63).

Other Syndromes Associated with Increased Risk for Cutaneous Malignant Melanoma

Familial Retinoblastoma

This condition, which is caused by a germline mutation in the *RB1* gene, is characterized by a very high risk for retinoblastoma, which is frequently bilateral and occurs at an early age. In reported series of retinoblastoma patients, there is an elevated risk for melanoma (71–75). It is likely that the risk of melanoma in *RB1* mutation carriers is considerably elevated; however, the estimates of risk are uncertain due to the low absolute number of cases.

Li-Fraumeni Syndrome

The Li-Fraumeni syndrome as well as a similar condition, the Li-Fraumeni-like syndrome, are both characterized by an increased risk of several tumor types, which include sarcomas, brain tumors, adenocarcinomas, and childhood tumors (76). A large proportion of such families carry germline mutations in the *TP53* tumor-suppressor gene (76). An association with CMM has been reported in some (77–79), but not in other (80,81) Li-Fraumeni kindreds. Thus, the association with CMM remains controversial.

Neurofibromatosis Type I

This condition is caused by germline mutations in the *NF1* gene and is characterized by alterations of cells of neural crest origin. The clinical manifestations are variable but include neurofibromas, café-au-lait spots, freckling in non-sun-exposed areas, and bone lesions. An increased incidence of tumors has been reported. In some affected kindreds, CMM has been reported and, in addition, there are also reports of extracutaneous melanomas such as ocular and mucosal melanomas (82). The occurrence of melanomas is not unexpected as they represent tumors of neural crest-derived cells.

Xeroderma Pigmentosum

Xeroderma pigmentosum (XP) is a rare autosomal recessive syndrome associated with hypersensitivity to ultraviolet light due to defects in DNA repair. Classical XP is subclassified in seven different genetic complementation groups, XPA–XPG, each associated with defects in separate genes involved in nucleotide excision repair (NER) (83). In addition, there is a mild form called XP variant, which is associated with a defect in postreplication repair, due to mutations in the *POLH* gene-encoding DNA polymerase eta (83). Classical XP is the early occurrence of UV-induced skin lesions due to the NER defects and in some types also neurological abnormalities, although the severity of the phenotype varies among complementation groups with XPA being the most severe form. XP patients have an over 1000-fold increased risk of developing skin cancers, predominantly nonmelanoma skin cancers such as BCC and SCC, which occur early in life. CMM is diagnosed in approximately 5% to 20% of XP patients (83). Interestingly, a large proportion of melanomas in XP patients are lentigo maligna melanomas (LMM), which occur on chronically sun-exposed sites, indicating that chronic, rather than intermittent, UV-damage is the major cause of melanoma in XP.

Werner Syndrome

The Werner syndrome is caused by a defect in the *WRN* gene encoding a DNA helicase with a putative role in DNA repair. The syndrome is characterized by premature aging and increased cancer incidence, including CMM. In a Japanese study, there was a large number of acral lentiginous and mucosal melanomas (84).

BRCA2-Associated Familial Breast/Ovarian Carcinoma

Kindreds with germline *BRCA2* mutations are characterized by greatly increased risk of breast- and ovarian carcinoma. Some of these families have also been reported to have a modestly increased risk of CMM (84), while other groups of families have not (85–87).

MANAGEMENT OF INDIVIDUALS WITH A HIGH RISK OF CUTANEOUS MALIGNANT MELANOMA

There is a consensus that high-risk individuals for CMM, such as the members of families with familial CMM and individuals with multiple primary CMM, should be invited to participate in preventive programs (88) and a consensus statement on the management and counseling of such individuals has been published by GenoMEL (89). Genetic testing of high-risk individuals for germline *CDKN2A* or *CDK4* mutations outside of defined research protocols is not recommended by GenoMEL for several reasons, including the lack of identified mutations in the majority of high-risk individuals and the insufficient information regarding the penetrance of mutations with respect to risk of melanoma and other cancers (89,90).

The recommendations for management given by GenoMEL are summarized below (89). In the absence of data from randomized, controlled clinical trials, the evidence for each of these measures is level IV.

In the case of familial CMM, a careful extended pedigree of the family should be established in collaboration between the healthcare provider and the proband of the family. Verification of diagnoses of CMM and other cancers, preferably through histopathology reports, as well as age at diagnosis should be documented. The pedigree should be revised annually.

As part of primary prevention, education of high-risk individuals regarding the need for sun protection is essential. In particular, parents should be educated about sun-protective measures for infants and children (88,91), including the use of sun-protective clothing, hats and sunglasses, avoidance of sun exposure during peak UV conditions, and absolute avoidance of sunburns. The issue of use of sunscreens remains controversial, but may be considered as a complement to other sun-protective measures. If used, it must be ensured that sunscreens have a sufficient level of broad-spectrum protection for both UVA and UVB (92).

Commencing at puberty, members of kindreds with familial CMM should have a baseline whole-skin examination with characterization of moles. The skin examination must include examination of the scalp and the external genitals. The examination should focus on detecting and characterization of nevi. Overview photographs of the entire skin as well as close-up pictures of DN are very useful for future follow-up. Individuals should be taught about routine self-examination of the skin, and may be provided with their own copies of photographs and be instructed how to use them in self-examination. Information regarding the significance of change in shape and size of pigmented lesions should be given and instruction on the ABCD rules may be useful (93). However, it should be noted that these criteria do not apply to all melanomas, as considerable fraction of early melanomas have a diameter less than 6 mm (94). Moreover, as a proportion of CMM tumors arise apparently de novo and not by progression of a precursor lesion, the individuals must also be informed to be watchful regarding novel skin lesions (95). A monthly self-examination or examination by parent, partner, or other family member is recommended.

Apart from self-examinations, high-risk individuals should also be followed by an appropriately trained healthcare provider with skin examinations every six months, at least until the nevi are stable and the person is judged competent in self-surveillance. Subsequently, the individual should be examined annually or have prompt access to the health provider, as necessary. Individuals with large numbers of clinically DN and with unstable and rapidly changing nevi may require more frequent skin examinations. This may also be necessary for instance during pregnancy when nevi may be particularly unstable. Skin-surface microscopy (epiluminescence microscopy) using conventional dermatoscopes or digital equipment is helpful during skin examinations (96,97).

Any changing nevus should be considered for excision for histopathologic diagnosis. There is however no justification for prophylactic removal of nevi, as the probability of progression to melanoma is low for every individual lesion and over time many nevi will mature and disappear. Furthermore, as melanomas may occur on previously normal skin, removal of nevi would not change the guidelines on skin surveillance by the patient or healthcare provider (95).

As no prospective studies of the outcome of preventive programs in high-risk groups for CMM have been reported, the benefit remains unproven. There is, however, reports which indicate that preventive activities may result in early diagnosis of CMM, as indicated by a low tumor thickness of tumors detected during follow-up (98–100). In a more recent report on long-term follow-up of 844 members of 33 kindreds with familial melanoma, 19 had germline mutations in either *CDKN2A* or *CDK4*, 86 new CMMs were identified (101). Of these, 72 were classified as T1a lesions (tumor thickness ≤1.0 mm, Clark level ≤3, no ulceration) with an average thickness of 0.3 mm. Similarly, in an analysis of 2,080 family members of 280 Swedish familial CMM kindreds who were followed between 1987 and 2001, 41 CMM tumors were detected during follow-up. Of these, 15 (37%) were in situ tumors and among the 26 invasive CMMs 22 were T1a tumors. Overall, 27 of the 41 CMM tumors (66%) lacked vertical growth phase and thus, by definition lacked metastatic capacity (102; submitted for publication). Thus, the existing data support the hypothesis that preventive programs as described earlier can efficiently reduce the risk of potentially metastatic CMMs in high-risk groups.

NONMELANOMA SKIN CANCER

The Gorlin Syndrome and Familial Basal Cell Carcinoma

The Gorlin syndrome is a rare inherited condition which is also called the basal cell nevus syndrome or the nevoid basal cell carcinoma syndrome (103,104). The syndrome, which was described by Gorlin and Goltz in 1960, is an autosomal dominant disorder characterized by the development of multiple BCCs in the skin from an early age, odontogenic keratocysts of the jaw, skeletal abnormalities such as bifid ribs and an increased risk of medulloblastoma. The syndrome is due to mutations in the *PTCH* gene on chromosome 9q22, which encodes the patched protein, a membrane receptor for the hedgehog signaling protein (105). The central importance for the hedgehog signaling pathway is also demonstrated by the frequent occurrence of *PTCH* mutations in sporadic BCC (106). Members of kindreds with the Gorlin syndrome need close and lifelong monitoring of their skin and appropriate therapy for their multiple BCCs.

IMMUNOSUPPRESSION AND ELEVATED RISK FOR NONMELANOMA SKIN CANCER

It has been shown in numerous studies that the incidence of skin tumors is considerably increased in individuals with pronounced and prolonged immunosuppression. The most striking example is represented by transplant recipients who frequently receive prolonged therapy with immunosuppressive drugs. Nonmelanoma skin cancers are the predominant tumors in transplanted patients and the incidence of SCC and BCC as well as actinic keratoses, which can be considered as precursor lesions to SCC (107–111). Moreover, these skin cancers tend to have a more aggressive behavior in transplant recipients, with rapid development and a higher capacity to metastasize (112).

The risk of SCC is particularly increased in transplanted patients, thus in a large study of 2561 kidney and heart transplant patients, the risk of SCC was estimated to be 65-fold increase over the general population (113). In a prospective study of 174 kidney transplant recipients in Spain, with a median follow-up of 72 months, 25% developed skin cancer with a BCC/SCC ratio of 1.4:1. The cumulative incidence of skin cancer was 13% at three years, 28% at six years and 48% at 10 years. In contrast, incidence estimates from Northern European countries tend to be lower with cumulative incidences at 10 years between 5% and 16% (114–118). A recent national Swedish cohort study of 5931 organ-transplanted patients has shown that the relative risk of nonmelanoma skin cancer was 56.2-fold increased (95% CI 49.8–63.2) (119).

The higher incidence of skin cancer in populations with high environmental sun exposure supports an important role for sunlight as a risk factor in these immunosuppressed individuals. The mechanism(s) causing the increased nonmelanoma skin cancer risk in immunosuppressed individuals is unclear, but may in part be due to a higher incidence of human papilloma virus (HPV) infection. In accordance with this viral, warts are common in such patients and, moreover, experimental results indicate that HPV and UVB may be synergistic in skin cancer induction (120).

It is controversial whether the risk of melanoma is increased in transplant recipients. It has been reported that melanocytic nevi (121–123), including clinically atypical nevi (124) are increased in number in transplanted patients, but these reports have not been confirmed in other studies (125,126). There are several reports of an increased risk of melanoma in transplant recipients, with estimated two- to 10-fold increased risks (115,127–129). In the large Swedish national cohort study, there was a 1.6-fold relative risk for melanoma, which was not statistically significant (130).

In conclusion, the available data firmly indicate that nonmelanoma skin cancer, mainly SCC, is greatly increased in transplanted patients and that this necessitates close monitoring of the skin of these individuals as part of lifelong preventive programs.

CONCLUSIONS

At present, high-risk groups for skin cancer, CMM in particular, can be identified mainly through personal or family history of skin cancer. Thus far, progress in understanding of the molecular genetics of CMM has not made a major impact on our ability do identify melanoma risk-groups for preventive programs. The reason for this is that the identified high-penetrance CMM-associated genes, *CDKN2A* and *CDK4*, contribute only to a minor proportion of melanomas at the population level. While *MC1R* variants are well-established as low-risk melanoma genes, the risk increase associated with these variants is too low to be useful for the identification of risk groups for prevention. Therefore, further investigations into the underlying molecular genetics of skin cancer in general, and CMM in particular, should have high priority. This involves both the identification of novel high-risk genes associated with familial CMM as well as lower risk genes that can be used to define a moderate risk profile, which will enable us to select a larger set of risk-individuals for prevention. Such investigations will benefit from international collaboration, exemplified by the research collaboration in the GenoMEL consortium.

In addition, further evaluations of the efficacy, including the cost-effectiveness of preventive programs addressing the known risk groups for skin cancer, are necessary. In order to improve surveillance of risk individuals, novel tools to identify precursor lesions, as well early CMM tumors, need to be developed and validated. Such tools may include novel imaging techniques coupled with computerized image analysis systems. The rational use of novel knowledge and new diagnostic tools in prevention will require the establishment of national or international prevention program, focussing on well-defined risk groups.

REFERENCES

1. Berwick M. WMA epidemiology: current trends. In: Han Balch CM, Sober AJ, Soong S-J, eds. Cutaneous Melanoma. St. Louis, Missouri: Quality Medical Publishing, Inc, 2003:15–23.
2. Elwood JM, Gallagher RP, Hill GB, et al. Pigmentation and skin reaction to sun as risk factors for cutaneous melanoma: Western Canada Melanoma Study. Br Med J (Clin Res Ed), 1984; 288(6411):99–102.
3. Bliss JM, Ford D, Swerdlow AJ, et al. Risk of cutaneous melanoma associated with pigmentation characteristics and freckling: systematic overview of 10 case-control studies. The International Melanoma Analysis Group (IMAGE). Int J Cancer, 1995; 62(4):367–376.
4. Naldi L, Lorenzo Imberti G, Parazzini F, et al. Pigmentary traits, modalities of sun reaction, history of sunburns, and melanocytic nevi as risk factors for cutaneous malignant melanoma in the Italian population: results of a collaborative case-control study. Cancer 2000; 88(12):2703–2710.
5. Tabenkin H, Tamir A, Sperber AD, et al. A case-control study of malignant melanoma in Israeli kibbutzim. Isr Med Assoc J 1999; 1(3):154–157.

6. Garbe C, Buttner P, Weiss J, et al. Risk factors for developing cutaneous melanoma and criteria for identifying persons at risk: multicenter case-control study of the Central Malignant Melanoma Registry of the German Dermatological Society. J Invest Dermatol 1994; 102(5):695–699.
7. Marrett LD, King WD, Walter SD, et al. Use of host factors to identify people at high risk for cutaneous malignant melanoma. CMAJ 1992; 147(4):445–453.
8. MacKie RM, English J, Aitchison TC, et al. The number and distribution of benign pigmented moles (melanocytic naevi) in a healthy British population. Br J Dermatol 1985; 113(2):167–174.
9. Nicholls, EM. Development and elimination of pigmented moles, and the anatomical distribution of primary malignant melanoma. Cancer 1973; 32(1):191–195.
10. Gallagher RP, McLean DI, Yang CP, et al. Anatomic distribution of acquired melanocytic nevi in white children. A comparison with melanoma: the Vancouver Mole Study. Arch Dermatol, 1990; 126(4):466–471.
11. Wachsmuth RC, Gaut RM, Barrett JH, et al. Heritability and gene-environment interactions for melanocytic nevus density examined in a U.K. adolescent twin study. J Invest Dermatol 2001; 117(2):348–352.
12. Swerdlow AJ, English J, MacKie RM, et al. Benign melanocytic naevi as a risk factor for malignant melanoma. Br Med J (Clin Res Ed), 1986; 292(6535):1555–1559.
13. Holly EA, Kelly JW, Shpall SN, et al. Number of melanocytic nevi as a major risk factor for malignant melanoma. J Am Acad Dermatol 1987; 17(3):459–468.
14. Garbe C, Kruger S, Stadler R, et al. Markers and relative risk in a German population for developing malignant melanoma. Int J Dermatol 1989; 28(8):517–523.
15. Augustsson A, Stierner U, Suurkula M, et al. Prevalence of common and dysplastic naevi in a Swedish population. Br J Dermatol 1991; 124(2):152–156.
16. Friedman RJ, Rigel DS, Kopf, AW. Early detection of malignant melanoma: the role of physician examination and self-examination of the skin. CA Cancer J Clin 1985; 35(3):130–151.
17. Garbe C, Buttner P, Weiss J, et al. Associated factors in the prevalence of more than 50 common melanocytic nevi, atypical melanocytic nevi, and actinic lentigines: multicenter case-control study of the Central Malignant Melanoma Registry of the German Dermatological Society. J Invest Dermatol, 1994; 102(5):700–705.
18. Bataille V, Bishop JA, Sasieni P, et al. Risk of cutaneous melanoma in relation to the numbers, types and sites of naevi: a case-control study. Br J Cancer 1996; 73(12):1605–1611.
19. Nordlund JJ, Kirkwood J, Forget BM, et al. Demographic study of clinically atypical (dysplastic) nevi in patients with melanoma and comparison subjects. Cancer Res 1985; 45(4):1855–1861.
20. Grob JJ, Gouvernet J, Aymar D, et al. Count of benign melanocytic nevi as a major indicator of risk for nonfamilial nodular and superficial spreading melanoma. Cancer, 1990; 66(2):387–395.
21. Carli P, Biggeri A, Giannotti B. Malignant melanoma in Italy: risks associated with common and clinically atypical melanocytic nevi. J Am Acad Dermatol 1995; 32(5 Pt 1):734–739.
22. Grulich AE, Bataille V, Swerdlow AJ, et al. Naevi and pigmentary characteristics as risk factors for melanoma in a high-risk population: a case-control study in New South Wales, Australia. Int J Cancer 1996; 67(4):485–491.

23. Marks R, Dorevitch AP, Mason G. Do all melanomas come from "moles"? A study of the histological association between melanocytic naevi and melanoma. Australas J Dermatol 1990; 31(2):77–80.

24. Wassberg C, Thorn M, Yuen J, et al. Second primary cancers in patients with cutaneous malignant melanoma: a population-based study in Sweden. Br J Cancer 1996; 73(2):255–259.

25. Wassberg C, Thorn M, Yuen J, et al. Cancer risk in patients with earlier diagnosis of cutaneous melanoma in situ. Int J Cancer 1999; 83(3):314–317.

26. Platz A, Ringborg, U and Hansson, J Hereditary cutaneous melanoma. Semin Cancer Biol 2000; 10(4):319–326.

27. Ford D, Bliss JM, Swerdlow AJ, et al. Risk of cutaneous melanoma associated with a family history of the disease. The International Melanoma Analysis Group (IMAGE). Int J Cancer 1995; 62(4):377–381.

28. Greene MH, Clark WH Jr, Tucker MA, et al. Precursor naevi in cutaneous malignant melanoma: a proposed nomenclature. Lancet 1980; 2(8202):1024.

29. Norris W. Case of fungoid disease. Edinburgh Med Surg J 1820; 16:562–565.

30. Clark WH Jr, Reimer RR, Greene M, et al. Origin of familial malignant melanomas from heritable melanocytic lesions: 'the B-K mole syndrome'. Arch Dermatol 1978; 114(5):732–738.

31. Lynch HT, Frichot BC 3rd, Lynch JF. Familial atypical multiple mole-melanoma syndrome. J Med Genet 1978; 15(5):352–356.

32. Newton Bishop JA, Bataille V, Pinney E, et al. Family studies in melanoma: identification of the atypical mole syndrome (AMS) phenotype. Melanoma Res 1994; 4(4):199–206.

33. Greene MH, Clark WH Jr, Tucker MA, et al. High risk of malignant melanoma in melanoma-prone families with dysplastic nevi. Ann Intern Med 1985; 102(4):458–465.

34. Kraemer KH, Greene MH, Tarone R, et al. Dysplastic naevi and cutaneous melanoma risk. Lancet 1983; 2(8358):1076–1077.

35. Tucker MA, Fraser MC, Goldstein AM, et al. Risk of melanoma and other cancers in melanoma-prone families. J Invest Dermatol 1993; 100(3):350S–355S.

36. http://www.genomel.org.

37. Hussussian CJ, Struewing JP, Goldstein AM, et al. Germline p16 mutations in familial melanoma. Nat Genet 1994; 8(1):15–21.

38. Kamb A, Gruis NA, Weaver-Feldhaus J, et al. A cell cycle regulator potentially involved in genesis of many tumor types. Science 1994; 264(5157): 436–440.

39. de Snoo FA, Hayward NK. Cutaneous melanoma susceptibility and progression genes. Cancer Lett 2005; 230(2):153–186.

40. Monzon J, Liu L, Brill H, et al. CDKN2A mutations in multiple primary melanomas. N Engl J Med 1998; 338(13):879–887.

41. MacKie RM, Andrew N, Lanyon WG, et al. CDKN2A germline mutations in U.K. patients with familial melanoma and multiple primary melanomas. J Invest Dermatol 1998; 111(2):269–272.

42. Hashemi J, Platz A, Ueno T, et al. CDKN2A germ-line mutations in individuals with multiple cutaneous melanomas. Cancer Res 2000; 60(24):6864–6867.

43. Auroy S, Avril MF, Chompret A, et al. Sporadic multiple primary melanoma cases: CDKN2A germline mutations with a founder effect. Genes Chromosomes Cancer 2001; 32(3):195–202.

44. Hayward NK. Genetics of melanoma predisposition. Oncogene 2003; 22(20): 3053–3062.
45. Gruis NA, Sandkuijl LA, van der Velden PA, et al. CDKN2 explains part of the clinical phenotype in Dutch familial atypical multiple-mole melanoma (FAMMM) syndrome families. Melanoma Res 1995; 5(3):169–177.
46. Hashemi J, Bendahl PO, Sandberg T, et al. Haplotype analysis and age estimation of the 113insR CDKN2A founder mutation in Swedish melanoma families. Genes Chromosomes Cancer, 2001; 31(2):107–116.
47. Ciotti P, Struewing JP, Mantelli M, et al. A single genetic origin for the G101W CDKN2A mutation in 20 melanoma-prone families. Am J Hum Genet 2000; 67(2):311–319.
48. Goldstein AM, Liu L, Shennan MG, et al. A common founder for the V126D CDKN2A mutation in seven North American melanoma-prone families. Br J Cancer 2001; 85(4):527–530.
49. Randerson-Moor JA, Harland M, Williams S, et al. A germline deletion of p14(ARF) but not CDKN2A in a melanoma-neural system tumour syndrome family. Hum Mol Genet 2001; 10(1):55–62.
50. Rizos H, Puig S, Badenas C, et al. A melanoma-associated germline mutation in exon 1beta inactivates p14ARF. Oncogene 2001; 20(39):5543–5547.
51. Hewitt C, Lee Wu C, Evans G, et al. Germline mutation of ARF in a melanoma kindred. Hum Mol Genet 2002; 11(11):1273–1279.
52. Begg CB, Orlow I, Hummer AJ, et al. Lifetime risk of melanoma in CDKN2A mutation carriers in a population-based sample. J Natl Cancer Inst 2005; 97(20):1507–1515.
53. Goldstein AM, Fraser MC, Struewing JP, et al. Increased risk of pancreatic cancer in melanoma-prone kindreds with p16INK4 mutations. N Engl J Med 1995; 333(15):970–974.
54. Borg A, Sandberg T, Nilsson K, et al. High frequency of multiple melanomas and breast and pancreas carcinomas in CDKN2A mutation-positive melanoma families. J Natl Cancer Inst, 2000; 92(15):1260–1266.
55. Goldstein AM, Struewing JP, Fraser MC, et al. Prospective risk of cancer in CDKN2A germline mutation carriers. J Med Genet 2004; 41(6):421–424.
56. Eskandarpour M, Hashemi J, Kanter L, et al. Frequency of UV-inducible NRAS mutations in melanomas of patients with germline CDKN2A mutations. J Natl Cancer Inst 2003; 95(11):790–798.
57. Michaloglou C, Vredeveld LC, Soengas MS, et al. BRAFE600-associated senescence-like cell cycle arrest of human naevi. Nature 2005; 436(7051):720–724.
58. Gillanders E, Juo SH, Holland EA, et al. Localization of a novel melanoma suscep-tibility locus to 1p22. Am J Hum Genet 2003; 73(2):301–313.
59. Walker GJ, Indsto JO, Sood R, et al. Deletion mapping suggests that the 1p22 melanoma susceptibility gene is a tumor suppressor localized to a 9-Mb interval. Genes Chromosomes Cancer 2004; 41(1):56–64.
60. Jonsson G, Bendahl PO, Sandberg T, et al. Mapping of a novel ocular and cutaneous malignant melanoma susceptibility locus to chromosome 9q21.32. J Natl Cancer Inst 2005; 97(18):1377–1382.
61. Salazar-Onfray F, Lopez M, Lundqvist A, et al. Tissue distribution and differential expression of melanocortin 1 receptor, a malignant melanoma marker. Br J Cancer 2002; 87(4):414–422.

62. Kennedy C, ter Huurne J, Berkhout M, et al. Melanocortin 1 receptor (MC1R) gene variants are associated with an increased risk for cutaneous melanoma which is largely independent of skin type and hair color. J Invest Dermatol 2001; 117(2):294–300.

63. Palmer JS, Duffy DL, Box NF, et al. Melanocortin-1 receptor polymorphisms and risk of melanoma: is the association explained solely by pigmentation phenotype? Am J Hum Genet 2000; 66(1):176–186.

64. Valverde P, Healy E, Sikkink S, et al. The Asp84Glu variant of the melanocortin 1 receptor (MC1R) is associated with melanoma. Hum Mol Genet 1996; 5(10): 1663–1666.

65. Sturm RA, Duffy DL, Box NF, et al. The role of melanocortin-1 receptor polymorphism in skin cancer risk phenotypes. Pigment Cell Res 2003; 16(3):266–272.

66. Matichard E, Verpillat P, Meziani R, et al. Melanocortin 1 receptor (MC1R) gene variants may increase the risk of melanoma in France independently of clinical risk factors and UV exposure. J Med Genet 2004; 41(2):e13.

67. Abdel-Malek Z, Swope VB, Suzuki I, et al. Mitogenic and melanogenic stimulation of normal human melanocytes by melanotropic peptides. Proc Natl Acad Sci USA 1995; 92(5):1789–1793.

68. Suzuki I, Cone RD, Im S, et al. Binding of melanotropic hormones to the melanocortin receptor MC1R on human melanocytes stimulates proliferation and melanogenesis. Endocrinology 1996; 137(5):1627–1633.

69. Haycock JW, Rowe SJ, Cartledge S, et al. Alpha-melanocyte-stimulating hormone reduces impact of proinflammatory cytokine and peroxide-generated oxidative stress on keratinocyte and melanoma cell lines. J Biol Chem 2000; 275(21):15629–15636.

70. Luger TA, Scholzen T, Brzoska T, et al. Cutaneous immunomodulation and coordination of skin stress responses by alpha-melanocyte-stimulating hormone. Ann N Y Acad Sci 1998; 840:381–394.

71. Traboulsi EI, Zimmerman LE, Manz, HJ. Cutaneous malignant melanoma in survivors of heritable retinoblastoma. Arch Ophthalmol 1988; 106(8):1059–1061.

72. Eng C, Li FP, Abramson DH, et al. Mortality from second tumors among long-term survivors of retinoblastoma. J Natl Cancer Inst 1993; 85(14):1121–1128.

73. Moll AC, Imhof SM, Bouter LM, et al. Second primary tumors in patients with hereditary retinoblastoma: a register-based follow-up study, 1945–1994. Int J Cancer 1996; 67(4):515–519.

74. Sanders BM, Jay M, Draper GJ, et al. Non-ocular cancer in relatives of retinoblastoma patients. Br J Cancer 1989; 60(3):358–365.

75. Albert LS, Sober AJ, Rhodes, AR. Cutaneous melanoma and bilateral retinoblastoma. J Am Acad Dermatol 1990; 23(5 Pt 2):1001–1004.

76. Malkin D, Li FP, Strong LC, et al. Germ line p53 mutations in a familial syndrome of breast cancer, sarcomas, and other neoplasms. Science 1990; 250(4985):1233–1238.

77. Hisada M, Garber JE, Fung CY, et al. Multiple primary cancers in families with Li-Fraumeni syndrome. J Natl Cancer Inst 1998; 90(8):606–611.

78. Nichols KE, Malkin D, Garber JE, et al. Germ-line p53 mutations predispose to a wide spectrum of early-onset cancers. Cancer Epidemiol Biomarkers Prev 2001; 10(2):83–87.

79. Birch JM, Alston RD, McNally RJ, et al. Relative frequency and morphology of cancers in carriers of germline TP53 mutations. Oncogene 2001; 20(34):4621–4628.

80. Frebourg T, Barbier N, Yan YX, et al. Germ-line p53 mutations in 15 families with Li-Fraumeni syndrome. Am J Hum Genet 1995; 56(3):608–615.

81. Birch JM, Blair V, Kelsey AM, et al. Cancer phenotype correlates with constitutional TP53 genotype in families with the Li-Fraumeni syndrome. Oncogene 1998; 17(9):1061–1068.

82. Guillot B, Dalac S, Delaunay M, et al. Cutaneous malignant melanoma and neuro-fibromatosis type 1. Melanoma Res 2004; 14(2):159–163.

83. Cleaver JE. Cancer in xeroderma pigmentosum and related disorders of DNA repair. Nat Rev Cancer 2005; 5(7):564–573.

84. Goto M, Miller RW, Ishikawa Y, et al. Excess of rare cancers in Werner syndrome (adult progeria). Cancer Epidemiol Biomarkers Prev 1996; 5(4):239–246.

85. Cancer risks in BRCA2 mutation carriers. The Breast Cancer Linkage Consortium. J Natl Cancer Inst 1999; 91(15):1310–1316.

86. Thorlacius S, Olafsdottir G, Tryggvadottir L, et al. A single BRCA2 mutation in male and female breast cancer families from Iceland with varied cancer phenotypes. Nat Genet 1996; 13(1):117–119.

87. Phelan CM, Lancaster JM, Tonin P, et al. Mutation analysis of the BRCA2 gene in 49 site-specific breast cancer families. Nat Genet 1996; 13(1):120–122.

88. National Institutes of Health Consensus Development Conference statement on diagnosis and treatment of early melanoma, January 27–29, 1992. Am J Dermatopathol 1993; 15(1):34–43; discussion 46–51.

89. Kefford RF, Newton Bishop JA, Bergman W, et al. Counseling and DNA testing for individuals perceived to be genetically predisposed to melanoma: a consensus statement of the Melanoma Genetics Consortium. J Clin Oncol 1999; 17(10):3245–3251.

90. Kefford R, Bishop JN, Tucker M, et al. Genetic testing for melanoma. Lancet Oncol 2002; 3(11):653–654.

91. Ferrini RL, Perlman M, Hill L. American College of Preventive Medicine practice policy statement: skin protection from ultraviolet light exposure. The American College of Preventive Medicine. Am J Prev Med 1998; 14(1):83–86.

92. Krien PM, Moyal D. Sunscreens with broad-spectrum absorption decrease the trans to cis photoisomerization of urocanic acid in the human stratum corneum after multiple UV light exposures. Photochem Photobiol 1994; 60(3):280–287.

93. McGovern TW, Litaker MS. Clinical predictors of malignant pigmented lesions. A comparison of the Glasgow seven-point checklist and the American Cancer Society's ABCDs of pigmented lesions. J Dermatol Surg Oncol 1992; 18(1):22–26.

94. Shaw HM, McCarthy WH. Small-diameter malignant melanoma: a common diagnosis in New South Wales, Australia. J Am Acad Dermatol 1992; 27(5 Pt 1):679–682.

95. Kelly JW, Yeatman JM, Regalia C, et al. A high incidence of melanoma found in patients with multiple dysplastic naevi by photographic surveillance. Med J Aust 1997; 167(4):191–194.

96. Kenet RO, Kang S, Kenet BJ, et al. Clinical diagnosis of pigmented lesions using digital epiluminescence microscopy: grading protocol and atlas. Arch Dermatol 1993; 129(2):157–174.

97. Menzies SW, Ingvar C, McCarthy WH. A sensitivity and specificity analysis of the surface microscopy features of invasive melanoma. Melanoma Res 1996; 6(1):55–62.

98. Rhodes AR. Intervention strategy to prevent lethal cutaneous melanoma: use of dermatologic photography to aid surveillance of high-risk persons. J Am Acad Dermatol 1998; 39(2 Pt 1):262–267.

99. Masri GD, Clark WH Jr, Guerry Dt, et al. Screening and surveillance of patients at high risk for malignant melanoma result in detection of earlier disease. J Am Acad Dermatol 1990; 22(6 Pt 1):1042–1048.

100. MacKie RM, McHenry P, Hole D. Accelerated detection with prospective surveillance for cutaneous malignant melanoma in high-risk groups. Lancet 1993; 341(8861):1618–1620.

101. Tucker MA, Fraser MC, Goldstein AM, et al. A natural history of melanomas and dysplastic nevi:an atlas of lesions in melanoma-prone families. Cancer 2002; 94(12):3192–3209.

102. Hansson J. Manuscript submitted for publication, 2006.

103. Gorlin RJ. Nevoid basal cell carcinoma (Gorlin) syndrome. Genet Med 2004; 6(6):530–539.

104. High A, Zedan W. Basal cell nevus syndrome. Curr Opin Oncol 2005; 17(2):160–166.

105. Ingham PW, Hedgehog signaling: a tale of two lipids. Science 2001; 294(5548): 1879–1881.

106. Unden AB, Holmberg E, Lundh-Rozell B, et al. Mutations in the human homologue of Drosophila patched (PTCH) in basal cell carcinomas and the Gorlin syndrome: different in vivo mechanisms of PTCH inactivation. Cancer Res 1996; 56(20):4562–4565.

107. Caforio AL, Fortina AB, Piaserico S, et al. Skin cancer in heart transplant recipients: risk factor analysis and relevance of immunosuppressive therapy. Circulation 2000; 102(19 suppl 3):III222–III227.

108. Espana A, Martinez-Gonzalez MA, Garcia-Granero M, et al. A prospective study of incident nonmelanoma skin cancer in heart transplant recipients. J Invest Dermatol 2000; 115(6):1158–1160.

109. Ramsay HM, Fryer AA, Reece S, et al. Clinical risk factors associated with nonmelanoma skin cancer in renal transplant recipients. Am J Kidney Dis 2000; 36(1):167–176.

110. Otley CC, Pittelkow, MR. Skin cancer in liver transplant recipients. Liver Transpl 2000; 6(3):253–262.

111. Ulrich C, Schmook T, Nindl I, et al. Cutaneous precancers in organ transplant recipients: an old enemy in a new surrounding. Br J Dermatol 2003; 149(suppl 66):40–42.

112. Veness MJ, Quinn DI, Ong CS, et al. Aggressive cutaneous malignancies following cardiothoracic transplantation: the Australian experience. Cancer 1999; 85(8): 1758–1764.

113. Fuente MJ, Sabat M, Roca J, et al. A prospective study of the incidence of skin cancer and its risk factors in a Spanish Mediterranean population of kidney transplant recipients. Br J Dermatol 2003; 149(6):1221–1226.

114. Naldi L, Fortina AB, Lovati S, et al. Risk of nonmelanoma skin cancer in Italian organ transplant recipients. A registry-based study. Transplantation 2000; 70(10):1479–1484.

115. Hartevelt MM, Bavinck JN, Kootte AM, et al. Incidence of skin cancer after renal transplantation in The Netherlands. Transplantation 1990; 49(3):506–509.

116. Gaya SB, Rees AJ, Lechler RI, et al. Malignant disease in patients with long-term renal transplants. Transplantation 1995; 59(12):1705–1709.

117. Webb MC, Compton F, Andrews PA, et al. Skin tumours posttransplantation: a retrospective analysis of 28 years' experience at a single centre. Transplant Proc 1997; 29(1–2):828–830.

118. Behrend M, Kolditz M, Kliem V, et al. Malignancies in patients under long-term immunosuppression after kidney transplantation. Transplant Proc 1997; 29(1–2):834–835.
119. Adami J, Gabel H, Lindelof B, et al. Cancer risk following organ transplantation: a nationwide cohort study in Sweden. Br J Cancer 2003; 89(7):1221–1227.
120. Jackson S, Harwood C, Thomas M, et al. Role of Bak in UV-induced apoptosis in skin cancer and abrogation by HPV E6 proteins. Genes Dev 2000; 14(23): 3065–3073.
121. Szepietowski J, Wasik F, Szepietowski T, et al. Excess benign melanocytic naevi in renal transplant recipients. Dermatology 1997; 194(1):17–19.
122. McGregor JM, Barker JN, MacDonald DM. The development of excess numbers of melanocytic naevi in an immunosuppressed identical twin. Clin Exp Dermatol 1991; 16(2):131–132.
123. Smith CH, McGregor JM, Barker JN, et al. Excess melanocytic nevi in children with renal allografts. J Am Acad Dermatol 1993; 28(1):51–55.
124. Barker JN, MacDonald DM. Eruptive dysplastic naevi following renal transplantation. Clin Exp Dermatol 1988; 13(2):123–125.
125. Gulec AT, Seckin D, Saray Y, et al. Number of acquired melanocytic nevi in renal transplant recipients as a risk factor for melanoma. Transplant Proc 2002; 34(6):2136–2138.
126. Andreani V, Richard MA, Blaise D, et al. Naevi in allogeneic bone marrow transplantation recipients: the effect of graft-versus-host disease on naevi. Br J Dermatol 2002; 147(3):433–441.
127. Bouwes Bavinck JN, Hardie DR, Green A, et al. The risk of skin cancer in renal transplant recipients in Queensland, Australia: a follow-up study. Transplantation 1996; 61(5):715–721.
128. Greene MH, Young TI, Clark WH Jr. Malignant melanoma in renal-transplant recipients. Lancet 1981; 1(8231):1196–1199.
129. Leveque L, Dalac S, Dompmartin A, et al. Melanoma in organ transplant patients. Ann Dermatol Venereol 2000; 127(2):160–165.
130. Lindelof B, Sigurgeirsson B, Gabel H, et al. Incidence of skin cancer in 5356 patients following organ transplantation. Br J Dermatol 2000; 143(3):513–519.

15

Behavioral Aspects of Prevention and Early Detection

Richard Bränström

Department of Oncology-Pathology, Karolinska Institute, Stockholm, Sweden

INTRODUCTION

The rapid and steady increase in skin cancer incidence observed worldwide is most likely a result of several factors, but, in particular, an increased exposure to ultraviolet (UV) light and earlier detection of skin cancer. Exposure to ultraviolet radiation (UVR) is considered the most important preventable risk factor for skin cancer, as it increases the risk of all three major forms of skin cancer (1). Skin cancer risk can therefore theoretically be reduced by decreasing exposure to UV light. Outdoor sunbathing, outdoor activities involving sun exposure, vacations to sunny resorts, sunbed use, and sun protection behavior are all behaviors related to the exposure of UV light. Skin self-examination, screening attendance, and early detection of malignant melanoma are also relevant for preventing skin cancer, as early detection is associated with better prognosis (2). Theories and methods developed within the behavioral and social sciences can make valuable contributions to our understanding of these behaviors, and give valuable guidance on how interventions should be constructed to promote behavior change. Firstly, in this chapter, a few of the most frequently used models of individual health behavior are briefly described. Secondly, a review of the results from studies of determinants for skin cancer relevant behaviors is presented, along with models trying to explain these behaviors. Lastly, some recommendations for future preventive efforts in the field are given.

THEORIES OF HEALTH BEHAVIOR AND HEALTH BEHAVIOR CHANGE

A number of social–psychological theories have been developed to describe and explain the health behavior of people. Some of the most widely applied theories relevant for sun-related behaviors are presented here. Studies of skin cancer prevention, as well as studies in many other public health areas, have mainly focussed on identifying attitudes, beliefs, and personality characteristics of high-risk individuals compared with low-risk individuals (3–5). These studies are important for finding groups that should be targeted with interventions. General attitudes and personality are, however, difficult to change with educational campaigns, and thus, more applicable models for behavior change need to be used. During recent years, several attempts have been made to produce comprehensive models of sun-related behaviors. These models have been based on one or several of the theories presented subsequently. Our understanding of the complex way in which behavior and environment interact and influence each other offers an important insight into how health-related behavior can be modified through health promotion interventions, and highlights the obstacles in prevention (6).

Health-Belief Model

Health-belief model (HBM) is the most well-known and used theory designed to explain health behavior by beliefs about health. The HBM has been applied to a variety of health-related issues such as screening behaviors, preventive actions, and illness behavior, as well as sick-role behaviors. HBM was initially developed in the 1950s in an effort to explain why people failed to participate in programs to prevent and detect disease (7). Since then, the model has been transformed and expanded, and its constructs have been clarified. In short, the theory postulates that individuals will take action if they believe themselves to be susceptible to the condition, or that the condition to have potentially serious consequences (severity), or that a course of action available will be beneficial in reducing either the susceptibility or the severity of the condition, or that the anticipated barriers to taking the action outweigh its benefits. Later refinement of the model has added cues for action, for example, public campaign, personal characteristics, and social circumstances (7). To increase the model's predictive power, the concept of self-efficacy was also added, that is, a person's perceived competence to take appropriate action (7). A summary of the major constructs in the model is presented in Figure 1.

Protection-Motivation Theory

Protection-motivation theory (PMT) is an extension of the HBM that was developed by Ronald Rogers in the seventies (8,9). The major factors included in this theory are: severity (e.g., skin cancer is a serious disease), vulnerability (e.g., I am at risk of getting skin cancer), response effectiveness (e.g., avoiding

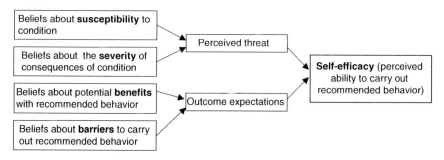

Figure 1 Major constructs included in health-belief model.

extensive sun exposure would lessen my risk of getting skin cancer), self-efficacy (e.g., I am confident that I can avoid getting sunburnt), and fear (e.g., I get worried when reading about skin cancer in the newspapers). A model of the PMT is presented in Figure 2. According to PMT, two types of information sources influence the factors in the model: environmental information (e.g., verbal persuasion, observational learning) and intrapersonal information (e.g., prior experience) (9).

Theory of Planned Behavior

According to the theory of planned behavior (TPB), developed by Martin Fishbein and Icak Ajzen, human behavior can be predicted by a person's beliefs about behavior and thoughts about the consequences of that behavior (behavioral beliefs), beliefs about the normative expectations of others and motivation to comply with these norms (normative beliefs), and perceptions about the presence of factors that may facilitate or impede the performance of the behavior and the perceived power of these factors (control beliefs) (10). Together, these three factors or behavioral belief constructs, attitudes toward the behavior, subjective norms, and perceived behavioral control lead to an

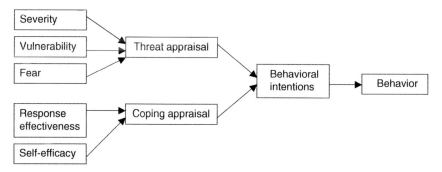

Figure 2 Major constructs of protection-motivation theory.

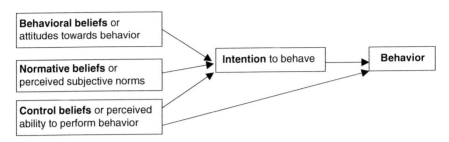

Figure 3 Major constructs of theory of planned behavior.

intention to behave (Fig. 3). If enough actual degree of control exists, the intention is expected to lead to actual behavior. The theory is supported in a meta-analysis in which 185 studies were included (11). In that study, the theory seemed to explain between 27% and 39% of the variance in behavior and behavioral intention. The theory has been applied to a wide variety of health-related behaviors.

Transtheoretical Model and Stages of Change

A problem in many public health projects is that people have different needs for education and information. One way to meet the differing need of different persons is suggested by Prochaska and DiClemente, who have constructed the transtheoretical model (TTM). The model has been applied to a wide variety of health-related behaviors and is based on knowledge derived from interviews with spontaneous behavior changers (12). The model is based on the assumption that everyone passes through several stages on their way toward a new behavior. From a stage where behavior change is not considered necessary (precontemplation), into a stage where a change might be considered (contemplation), further into a stage where you prepare for a behavior change (preparation), and next into a stage where a behavior change is initiated (action), and finally into a stage where the new behavior is established (maintenance). The model also describes a number of processes that people use to succeed in their behavior change. The processes differ depending on the stage of change (Fig. 4). By the use of stages and processes, tailored interventions to people with differing levels of motivation can be constructed (12).

BEHAVIORS RELATED TO PREVENTION AND EARLY DETECTION

There are a large number of behaviors related to skin cancer prevention, for example, outdoor sunbathing, outdoor activities involving sun exposure, vacations to sunny resorts, sunbed use, sun-protection behavior, skin self-examination, and screening attendance. Successful skin cancer prevention should include strategies for changing several different behaviors, for example, when

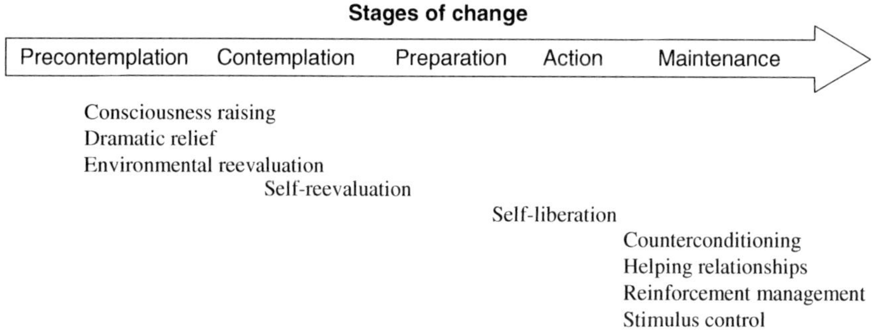

Stages of change

Precontemplation	Contemplation	Preparation	Action	Maintenance

Consciousness raising
Dramatic relief
Environmental reevaluation
          Self-reevaluation
                    Self-liberation
                         Counterconditioning
                         Helping relationships
                         Reinforcement management
                         Stimulus control

Figure 4 Major constructs of the transtheoretical model and stages of change. *Source:* Adapted from Ref. 13.

and where people spend time outdoors, what they are wearing, whether they properly use sunscreens, and whether they carry out regular self-skin-examinations. A majority of the studies on frequency, by which people engage in sun-related behaviors, have been conducted in countries with high levels of ambient UVR, and among inhabitants with white and sun-sensitive skin. However, many countries around the world are beginning to acknowledge the increasing importance of skin-cancer preventive efforts. The behaviors and their frequency vary considerably between countries, and they are affected by a number of factors, for example, latitude, climate, and geography, but also cultural norms and habits. No frequencies of prevalence of these behaviors will be presented in this section as more research is needed, and standardized measurements of these behaviors need to be developed for international comparisons. The purpose of the following section is to summarize the findings concerning factors associated with skin-cancer relevant behaviors.

Outdoor Sunbathing

Sunbathing often refers to an intentional stay in the sun with the purpose of obtaining a tan. This type of behavior has become more frequent in Western society since the shift in the meaning of tanned skin in the early 1900s. Before the Industrial Revolution, a pale complexion was prized as an indication of status, demonstrating that the individual was not a laborer who needed to work outside. With industrialization, the working class left the fields for the factories. This included a change in lifestyle and a re-evaluation of the meaning of tanned skin. The year-round tan became associated with status and wealth, as it indicated that the person could afford to spend time in the sun and travel to sunny resorts (14). Since then, people have enjoyed sunbathing and tanning during leisure time, and studies of people's attitudes have indicated that, for many, a suntan means physical and emotional health and attractiveness (14–16). A large number of studies have been conducted with the aim of finding relevant factors associated with sunbathing. However, the studies use a wide variety of questions measuring both behaviors and associated factors making comparisons difficult. Some broad conclusion about characteristics is nevertheless possible to make. Gender seems to be the most important factor relevant to sun exposure through intentional tanning. Numerous studies have found that women sunbathe to a greater extent than men (3,5,17–22). However, considering gender differences in UV exposure, it is very important to distinguish between sunbathing with the intention to tan and outdoor activities that lead to sun exposure. When sun exposure is measured as a combination of intentional and unintentional exposure, women do not receive a higher UV dose. On the contrary, it has been found that men's exposure to the sun is greater than women's (4,23,24). Several studies have examined the relationship between age and sunbathing (3,5,25). Most studies indicate that intentional tanning peaks in the late adolescence (21). Studies of younger children's often find a steady increase of sun exposure with age (26). Skin sun-sensitivity or the ability to tan and the risk of burning when exposed to solar radiation are associated with sunbathing frequency. Studies have generally shown that those with sensitive skin sunbathe less frequently than those with less sun-sensitive skin (3,5). However, some studies have found no difference in sunbathing between skin types (4,27). These studies, however, categorized people as sun-sensitive or not sun-sensitive instead of using a more differentiated skin type classification. Some studies have found that higher socio-economic status, higher educational level, and high school grades are associated with higher frequency of sunbathing (5,26), but other studies have found no relationship (28). Several studies indicate a positive association between a high level of *knowledge* about the risks of sunbathing, knowledge of solar radiation and risk factors for skin cancers and sunbathing frequency (3,29,30). A possible explanation is that people who like sunbathing and tanning are more inclined to search for information about it. Other studies have found no relation between knowledge and sunbathing (24,31,32). The most obvious motivator for sunbathing seems to be the positive effects of sunbathing on appearance (20,25,31,33). People generally judge themselves and others as more attractive if they are tanned. Another reported reason to sunbathe is that people experience sunbathing as relaxing (25,31). Positive effects of sun exposure on certain skin conditions such as psoriasis and acne have also been documented (34,35). Perceptions of susceptibility and severity of skin cancer are related to sunbathing as those who believe that they are more susceptible to skin cancer and those that consider skin cancer to be a serious disease are less likely to sunbathe (4,5,20,27,31,36). Perceptions of other people's sunbathing and the prevailing social norms are also important predictors of sunbathing (5,24,36,37). Tolerating norms and other people's frequent sunbathing are related to one's own sunbathing. People belonging to health clubs and those spending more hours exercising are more likely to sunbathe, according to a U.S. study (24). A study in France found children's sun exposure to be related to mothers' sun-protective habits (33). Mothers with good sun-protective habits were more restrictive in exposing their children to the sun. One study of Swedish adolescents showed associations between sunbathing and self-image (25). Boys who were satisfied with themselves and girls who were not satisfied with themselves sunbathed the most. It has also been suggested that people with a higher degree of appearance motivation engage more in sunbathing (14,38,39). A few studies have shown an increased frequency of sunbathing among people who have a general positive attitude toward risk taking and low need for achievement (24,40). In one study, excessive tanning was positively related to obsessive-compulsive tendencies (39). Frequent sunbathing has been found to be associated with other health-risk behaviors such as tobacco smoking (5) and a less frequent use of car seatbelts (24). A study in the United States showed that people residing in areas with a lower number of sunny days were more likely to sunbathe intentionally (19).

Two studies using the TPB (27,36) have shown that attitudes toward sunbathing, for example, enhancing appearance, positive mental and physical reinforcements, were the most important predictors of intentions to sunbathe and actual sunbathing. Perceived susceptibility to skin cancer and photo aging were highly predictive of intentions to sunbathe less. Social norms positive to sunbathing also significantly contributed to the prediction of sunbathing behavior. The sun-related behavior of friends and important others seemed more important than norms from the fashion and movie industries. Perceived behavioral control moderated the effects of attitudes on intentions to sunbathe. The relationship between attitude and intention was weaker for those who perceived themselves to have low degree of control over their behavior.

Jaccard (1981) has described a theory of alternative behaviors as a model for explaining decision-making (41). A study using his theory was conducted on a sample of university students. It showed that being appearance-oriented, having friends that sunbathe, liking outdoor life, believing that everyone sunbathes at some time in their life, and not being health-oriented all contributed to the attitude toward sunbathing. Actual sunbathing was predicted by attitudes toward alternative concurrent behaviors such as shopping, working out, and going to the cinema.

Outdoor Activities Involving Sun Exposure

Sailing, fishing, canoeing, outdoor sports, hiking, gardening, and so on are all activities that include some degree of sun exposure. This type of exposure can include intermittent as well as cumulative or total sun exposure and thus probably contribute to the incidence of all forms of skin cancer. The frequency of people's participation in them has so far been less extensively investigated than intentional tanning. When sun exposure is measured as a combination of intentional and unintentional exposure, for example, as hours spent outside, no gender differences have been found. Studies indicate that men are more exposed to the sun than women (4,24,42,43). In one study, "having a tan last summer" was more common among men than women even though sunbathing was not (17). Time spent in the sun seems also to increase during adolescence (42) and peak at early adulthood (28). Skin sun-sensitivity does not seem to be connected to time spent outside (4,42). A negative association has been found for knowledge about skin cancer and hours spent outside (24). A positive social norm for sunbathing, positive attitudes toward having a tan and sunbathing have been found to be related to time spent in the sun at peak hours (28).

Occupational Exposure to Ultraviolet Light

Outdoor workers expose themselves to a large amount of UVR, and outdoor work has been found to be associated with an increased risk of nonmelanoma skin cancers (44). Studies of Canadian adults and U.S. adolescents found that men were much more likely to work outside than women (23,42). In another U.S. study, occupational exposure was positively associated with lower education and male gender (43).

Vacations at Sunny Resorts

Since the sixties and seventies, vacations at sunny resorts abroad have become increasingly popular among the population in many Western societies. The increase of international tourism has been suggested as one of the major factors for the high increase in skin cancer incidence (45). The increase of family holidays to sunny destinations might be especially worrisome as excessive sun exposure and severe sunburn during childhood might be an important risk factor for future skin cancer development (46). In a Swedish study, there was no apparent gender difference in the frequency of vacations spent at sunny resorts (21). Adolescents and young adults seem to be somewhat more likely to travel abroad than older persons are. As expected, the number of lifetime vacations to sunny resorts increased with age. In another study, there was no difference in the frequency of travel depending on educational level (28). Skin sun-sensitivity or skin types were related to the frequency of vacations abroad, with those with less sensitive skin being more likely to have traveled (28). A positive social norm for sunbathing and positive attitudes toward having a tan and sunbathing have been found to be related to the frequency of vacations (28).

Indoor Tanning

Since the seventies, people have added to their amount of exposure to UV light by using sunbeds. Even though the detrimental effects of exposure to UV light in sunbeds is still not fully understood, studies indicate an increased risk of skin cancer from their use (47–49). There are gender differences in sunbed use with women using them more frequently (18,21,25,50–53). Sunbed use seems to increase during adolescence (53). Both men and women seem to use sunbeds the most in early adulthood (21). Skin sun-sensitivity is related to sunbed use as skin type III (sometimes burns, always tans) (54) is predominant among sunbed users (55). In a study of Swedish adolescents, respondents with acne/seborrhea, eczema, or psoriasis used sunbeds more than those without skin diseases (55). Appreciation of a tan and the belief that sunbed use relieves acne problems are positively associated with sunbed use (50,53). Indifference to a tan is negatively linked to sunbed use. The belief that tanning in a sunbed is safer than outdoor sunbathing is positively associated with sunbed use (51). The belief that a tan improves appearance and contributes to feelings of healthiness is positively related to sunbed use (51,52). Being more knowledgeable about the long-term effects of UV exposure has been found to be positively associated with sunbed use (18). Having a family history of skin cancer is negatively associated with sunbed use (51). One study found single persons to be more likely to use sunbeds (52). Studies of Swedish adolescents showed associations between sunbed use and self-image or perceived physical attractiveness (25,50). Adolescents who were not satisfied with themselves used sunbeds the most. Adolescents with friends and family who use sunbed are more likely to use them (53). The frequency of sunbed use is much higher in countries with a lower degree of ambient solar radiation. A study conducted in the European Union in 1996 revealed a much higher use of sunbeds in northern Europe compared with countries in southern Europe, for example, Italy, France, Greece, and Spain (56). Frequent sunbed use has been found to be associated with other health risk behaviors such as excessive exposure to natural sun and tobacco smoking (30,50,51,57).

A study using appearance motivation, self-monitoring, and the TPB has been conducted among university students in the United States to explain the use of sunbeds (58). This study showed that the most influential predictor of sunbed use was the intention to use a sunbed and perceived behavioral control. Intention was predicted by attitudes, social norms, and perceived behavioral control. Appearance motivation had no direct or interaction effect on sunbed intention but predicted attitudes favorable to sunbed use. Self-monitoring, defined as the tendency to be guided in life predominantly by situational cues, interacted with subjective norms in the prediction of intention to use sunbeds. High self-monitors presented a stronger relationship between subjective norms and intention to use sunbeds than did low self-monitors.

Getting Sunburned

Sunburn or sun-induced erythema is the result of excessive exposure to UV light and it is considered to be a good proxy of too much exposure to UV light. There are various definitions of sunburn in the literature and no superior definition has yet been constructed. However, in 1998, a group of public health practitioners and researchers in Canada developed several recommendations on measuring self-reported sunburn (59). They concluded that sunburn was an indirect measure of sun exposure and protection, important in the etiology of melanoma and basal cell carcinoma, and a relatively memorable and distinct event. Thus, sunburn was identified as the most important outcome to assess in surveys and intervention program evaluations. One important aspect of sunburn is severity. As most data in skin cancer research are based on self-reports, the public's own definition of sunburn is of major importance. In one study, people were asked to report the degree of their sunburn (28). Thirty-one percent reported redness without pain, 12% reported severe redness without pain, 53% reported redness and pain, and 4% reported severe burns with blisters (60). These results indicate that, when sunburn is self-reported, a majority of the responders have experienced severe erythema, and that "sunburn" has to be clearly defined in each survey. Some studies have found that men become sunburned more often than women (19,22,61,62). However, other studies have found that women sunburn more frequently (21,42,63). In a Swedish study, there was a curvilinear relationship between sunburn and age regarding both sunburn in Sweden and sunburn abroad, with sunburn frequency peaking during late adolescence and early adulthood (21). Children's sunburn has also been found positively related to parents sunburn, and negatively to parent's protective behavior (64). Not surprisingly, skin sun-sensitivity is associated with sunburn as those with sensitive skin are more likely to become sunburned (22,29,30,42,61,63,65). Sunburn has been found to be related to time spent outside in the sun and to an intention to acquire a tan (22,42). As expected, higher desirability of a tan is positively related to sunburn among both adolescents and adults (22,42). Having the opinion that it is worth becoming burned to tan is more common among those who become sunburned frequently (63). Having a preference for natural or paler skin is negatively related to sunburn (63). Having many friends who sunbathe is positively related to sunburn (63).

Use of Sun Protection

One major concern in primary prevention of skin cancer is how to persuade people to protect themselves from sun exposure. The most important messages for sun-protection are: wear sun-protective clothing (including a hat) when in the sun, avoid the sun during peak hours between 10 a.m. and 4 p.m., avoid artificial sources of UV light, and use sunscreen with a high sun-protection factor (SPF), that is, SPF ≥ 15. Further recommendations are that children under the age of one should not stay in the sun at all. Even though sunscreens are recommended as a protection from UV light, they are not always used as protection. Several studies have found a positive association between sunscreen use and time spent in the sun (66–68). Instead of using sunscreen as a complement to other means of avoiding excessive sun exposure, sunscreens are used to make it possible to spend more time in the sun. Some studies have also found an increased risk of skin cancer among sunscreen users (69), although the overall epidemiological data do not support such an association (70). In studies of predictors of sun protection, a differentiation between sunscreen use and use of other ways to protect is not always done. This makes the analysis of predictors of sun-protective behavior very complicated as people use sunscreen for different reasons. Measuring sunscreen use is also difficult as it involves a number of different issues such as amount of sunscreen applied, SPF number, and the frequency of application.

Several studies have found gender differences in sun-protective behavior. Women seem to protect themselves more than males (3–5,18,65,71,72). Subsequently, use of sunscreen is related to gender; women seem to use it more. Studies of U.S. and Australian children, and adolescents have found a decreasing frequency of sunscreen use with age (63,73). After adolescence, sun-protective behavior seems to increase somewhat. A study of white adults in the United States found that people between 26 and 40 years of age used sunscreen more than persons aged between 16 and 25 (74). Skin sun-sensitivity is related to use of sunscreen. Those who burn easily are more likely to use sunscreen (4,5,18,28,63,65,75). Educational level has also been found to be associated with sunscreen use, that is, the higher the level of education the greater the use of sunscreen (65,74).

Many studies have found a relationship between *age* and sun-protective behavior. Most studies find a decreasing use of sun protection with age, that is, from childhood up to young adulthood (3,26,72,76), and a later positive relationship with age (77). A positive linear relationship was found between sun-protective behavior and skin sun-sensitivity in a study of Swedish adolescents (3). Those with blond or red hair color have been found to be somewhat keener on engaging in protective behavior than people with dark hair (23). Those playing down the risk of sunbathing or those who think that it is worth becoming burned to obtain a tan used less sunscreen (5,63). In contrast, adolescents with better knowledge and a higher awareness about skin cancer, and those who perceive themselves as being at risk of contracting skin cancer are more inclined to use sunscreen and other sun-protection measures (4,78). Common reasons not to use sunscreen are that its application is time-consuming and that it prevents tanning (79). People with positive attitudes toward sun-protective behavior and less negative attitudes toward using sunscreen are more likely to use sunscreen (31). Among women, those with more knowledge of sunscreens and those not experiencing sunbathing as relaxing are more likely to use a sunscreen with a high SPF (31). In a study of Swedish university students, no association was found between sun protection and knowledge about the risks of sunbathing, knowledge of solar radiation, and the risk factors for skin cancers (30). Children and adolescents preferring a natural or light skin color are more inclined to use sunscreen (63). Knowledge about skin cancer and knowing someone who has had skin cancer were associated with sunscreen use in one study (24). Adolescents who believe that they can avoid developing skin cancer are more likely to take sun-protective action (73). Measurements of perceived behavioral control and self-efficacy have been linked to sun-protective behavior (27,36). Other people's use of sunscreen seems important as the number of friends who usually use sunscreen is positively associated with sunscreen use (5) as well as best friend's use of sunscreen (75). Also, *parental insistence* on the use of sunscreen increases its use among teenagers (75). Other people's use of sun protection, for example, parent's use of sun protection and parental tanning behaviors, is associated with children's sun-protective behavior (76). A study in Norway showed a negative association between latitude and use of sunscreen, probably due to weaker sun in the north (5). The same study found a positive association between the frequency of sunbathing and vacations at sunny resorts and sunscreen use.

The HBM has been used in one study to predict sun-protective behavior (71). This study showed inconsistent support for the HBM in explaining sun protection behavior. Susceptibility to skin cancer was negatively associated with sun protection use among males, contrary to theoretical expectations, and no association was found between susceptibility and sun protection among women. However, perceived benefits with sun protection and perceived barriers to sun protection were connected with actual sun protection. The complexity of sun protection, that is, if it is used to be able to stay longer in the sun or if it is used as real protection, may account for the inconsistent support for the model.

A study of Dutch adolescents, using a behavior change model that integrated several different theories of behavior change, for example, TPB, HBM, and TTM, showed that sunscreen was the most frequently used way of protection from the sun (80). The use of sunscreen was predicted by positive attitudes toward using sunscreen, support from family and friends, and perceived risk of getting skin cancer. Wearing protective clothing was predicted by support for parents and friends, a positive attitude toward using clothes as protection, seeking shade, high level of self-efficacy, low exposure to the sun, and being male. Using shade as protection was most strongly related to positive attitudes toward seeking shade, support from parents and friends, using protective clothing, high self-efficacy, a negative attitude toward tanning and perceived skin cancer risk.

Screening Attendance, Skin Self-Examinations, and Early Detection

Early detection and treatment of malignant skin lesions have the potential to increase survival and decrease medical costs associated with skin cancer (81). Even though there is little scientific evidence supporting the effectiveness of screening as a way to reduce mortality and decrease health costs at a population level, various forms of screening have been carried out (82). Early detection, by skin self-examination or having someone else check one's skin for suspicious lesions, is another potential way to improve secondary prevention of melanoma. The benefits of skin self-examination have not been established, however, one case-control study suggested that it is possible to reduce mortality from melanoma by 63% through self-examination of the skin (83). Today, approximately half of the reported cases of malignant melanoma are detected by the patients themselves (84,85).

A U.S. study of skin-cancer screening attendance between 1992 and 2000 found a general low frequency of skin examination (between 14% and 21% had ever had their skin examined) (86). White non-Hispanics were screened more often, as was older persons, those with a family history of melanoma, those with a higher education, and those with a regular place for healthcare. A Swedish study comparing screening attendees with the general population found attendees to be more concerned about nevi, having more often been in contact with physicians about skin lesions (87). Attendees were better informed about risk factors for skin cancer and were more knowledgeable of melanoma. Another study comparing attendees and non-attendees found no difference in knowledge of risk factors for melanoma, but non-attendees scored lower on perceived susceptibility to melanoma (88). Most of the recommended improvements for increasing screening attendance suggested by the non-attendees concerned reduction of practical barriers. Decreased barriers were also found to be related to total skin examination among relatives of patients with malignant melanoma (89). Other factors related to examination among this group were, in particular, physician recommendation, and also knowledge about malignant melanoma and knowledge about risk factors for melanoma (89).

A telephone survey in the United States in 1996 found skin self-examination to be correlated to gender, age, educational level, perceived own risk of developing melanoma or other skin cancer, own history of skin cancer, and discussions with physician or nurse about sun protection (90). Older women, with a high level of education, who perceived themselves at greater risk of developing melanoma, who had a personal history of skin cancer, and who recalled a discussion with a physician or nurse about sun protection were more likely to perform skin self-examinations. Another study from the United States analyzed factors related to self-examination separately for men and women. Men were more likely to perform self-examinations if they had a family history of skin cancer, had a physician examine their skin, or had changed their diet to decrease their cancer risk (91). Women were more likely to perform skin self-examination if they previously had removed pigmented nevi, had an abnormal mole, or had light hair color. Several studies have found an increase in skin self-examination among those who had been advised to conduct examinations by their healthcare provider (89,92,93). A study of Gold Coast residents in Australia found a positive association between skin self-examinations and individual primary preventive behavior (94).

SKIN CANCER PREVENTION USING BEHAVIORAL PROFILES

There is a large variety in the types of skin cancer preventive interventions, which makes classification of interventions difficult. However, in a recent review of effective skin cancer preventive strategies, Saraiya et al. (95) have suggested a classification of interventions into four broad groups, that is, individual-directed strategies, environmental and policy interventions, media campaigns, and multicomponent programs and comprehensive community-wide interventions. Further, individual-directed interventions can be classified according to setting i.e., childcare, primary school, secondary school, and college, recreational and tourism sites, occupational, and healthcare settings. In the review, Saraiya et al. (95) concludes that education and policy approaches to increase sun-protection behaviors were effective when implemented in primary schools and in recreational and tourism settings. However, they found insufficient evidence of effectiveness of educational and policy approaches in other settings, for example, childcare centers, secondary schools and colleges, and in occupational settings. Further, they found insufficient evidence of the effectiveness of preventive activities targeting healthcare settings and providers, media campaigns alone, interventions oriented to parents, and community-wide multicomponent interventions. The review highlights the need for more well-evaluated studies of skin-cancer preventive interventions.

One way to use theories of individual health behavior in prevention is to use them to identify individuals or groups with specific needs for information or preventive interventions. A successful assessment of groups with differing need for interventions enables tailoring or targeting of preventive strategies toward these groups. Assessing and targeting people with different sun-exposure profiles, is one way to match differing needs with appropriate intervention. Below, a categorization of people into sun-exposure profile is presented on the basis of the underlying motive for exposure.

Sun-Exposure Profiles

As skin-cancer prevention involves multiple behaviors that are associated with somewhat different factors, there is a need to develop an easier categorization of these behaviors. Based on the studies of the predictors of sun-related behaviors, some typical sun-exposure profiles can be identified. These profiles have different motives for being exposed to UV light or to protect from the sun and they have different behavioral patters, and thus, different preventive strategies are needed to change their behavior. The profiles are ordered on a dimension of volition from profiles characterized by intentional tanning, through profiles more characterized by incidental tanning, and finally profiles inevitably exposed to UVR. These profiles are not mutually exclusive, and each individual can probably identify with several of these profiles at different times, and might behave differently in different situation. Even though these profiles need to be empirically validated, they can serve as basis for the development of preventive interventions. The characteristics and typical behavior pattern of the profiles are presented in Table 1, and they are subsequently explained in more detail.

Compulsive sunbathers love being in the sun and they spend as much time as possible sunbathing. They enjoy traveling to sunny resorts and have no or few thoughts about a potential risk with excessive sun exposure. This group of people

Table 1 Sun-Exposure Profiles and Their Different Characteristics and Typical Behavior, with Recommendations for Interventions Targeting These Profiles

	Characteristics	Behavior	Example	Preventive strategy
Compulsive sunbathers	Like to sunbathe Desire a tan See no or few risks Do not want to change	Tan frequently Do not use protection Do not seek information	Travelers to sunny vacation resorts	Provide information about risk Change the positive attitude toward having a tan Educational and policy interventions toward travel industry
Professional tanners	Like to sunbathe Desire a tan See some risks with tanning Do not want to stop sunbathing	Tan frequently Use sunscreen but not other ways to protect Seek information	Travelers to sunny vacation resorts Sunbed users	Inform about the preferable use of other ways to protect than using sunscreens Change the positive attitude toward having a tan
Incidental tanners	Do not necessarily like to sunbathe Might desire a tan See some risks with tanning Do not want to change	Spend time in the sun Do not protect from the sun Do not seek information	People who spend time on outdoor activities e.g., gardening, sailing, golfing	Set straight myth about less risk with incidental tanning Information about adequate ways to protect Provide safe environments
Inevitably sun-exposed	Might like to sunbathe Do not necessarily desire a tan Might be unconscious of risks	Spend a lot of time in the sun Do not protect from the sun Do not seek information	Outdoor workers	Provide safe environments Sun protective clothing Information about risks Educational and policy interventions
Unprotected children	Do not like to sunbathe Do not desire a tan Are unconscious of risks	Spend time in the sun Are not sufficiently protected Do not seek information	Young children on shade-less beach	Provide safe environments Sun-protective clothing Educational and policy interventions

needs to be motivated to change behavior and learn how to protect properly from UV light. This group is most easily located at recreational and tourist settings and might be targeted at these arenas. Interventions should include information about skin-cancer risk and proper sun-safe behaviors, activities to change attitudes, and norms concerning sunbathing and having a tan, but should also include policy and environmental approaches, that is, provision of shade at recreational settings and at beaches. Some studies have shown effects of educational and policy interventions at recreational and tourist settings on adult sun-protective behavior. Effects on the number of sunburns have, however, not been shown so far (95). One strategy for progress is to promote the responsibilities of travel companies for tourist sun-safety (45).

The second group are the *professional tanners*. Even though professional tanners are highly motivated and eager to get a tan, they are also somewhat concerned with the negative effects of excessive sun exposure. Professional tanners want a safe and nice-looking tan, and as a result, get themselves well-informed about sunscreens, sun protection, and skin cancer. Those belonging to this profile spend a lot of time exposing themselves to UVR, and they prefer to use sunscreens to prolong their stay in the sun. An interview study in Canada, examining adolescents' development toward becoming a sun tanner found that many intentional tanners used sunscreen judiciously to achieve the right tan, that is, not too dark and not too light (96). Strategies to promote sun-safe practices among this group should resemble those used for the compulsive sunbathers. However, the professional tanner is more concerned about skin-cancer risk and more knowledgeable about how to protect. The professional tanners are convinced that they can acquire a "safe tan" without increasing their risk of getting skin cancer. Even though people in this group might avoid getting severely sunburned, they are exposed to a large amount of UV light and increase their risk of nonmelanoma skin cancer. This group are receptive for information and should be targeted with information about the detrimental effects of solar and artificial radiation to their skin, and be informed about the preferable use of other ways of protection than the use of sunscreens. Appearance-based prevention strategies should also be suitable for this group. Some studies have found positive effects of appearance-based intervention on sunbathing frequency and sunbed use (97,98). For this group, messages emphasizing the negative consequences of sun exposure for appearance might be more effective than messages concerning negative health effects.

Many people are exposed to the sun without the explicit motive to acquire a tan. This group of people could be identified as *incidental tanners*. They are engaged in an outdoor activity other than lying in the sun, and their goal for the stay is not to be tanned, even though it might be a positive by-product. The incidental tanners often describe the sun exposure and tanning as an inevitable result, and incidental tanning is often considered healthier that intentional tanning (96). However, there is no reason to believe that unintentional exposure to the sun should be less damaging than intentional, and thus, interventions targeting incidental tanning should be developed. In addition to information about proper protection from the sun, it is important to set straight common myths about sun exposure, for example, that incidental tanning is less harmful than intentional. Other interventions appropriate to target this group are policy and environmental strategies at recreational settings and sporting organizations.

The inevitably sun exposed are most likely outdoor workers that spend a lot of time in the sun because they have to. The inevitably sun exposed might or might not be aware of the risks with excessive sun exposure, and their underlying motive for being in the sun is that they need to be. Intervention strategies targeting this group should include programs in outdoor occupational settings and the development of worksite policies, provision of protective clothing (hats, T-shirts etc.) by employers, and interventions aiming at altering norms among these workers regarding "dress code" and UV protection. Even though outdoor occupational settings are an ideal site for skin-cancer preventing, so far there is no evidence of effects from this type of prevention strategy (95).

One group of special concern for prevention is unprotected children. Some studies indicate that severe sun exposure during childhood might be linked to an increased risk of skin cancer and therefore sun-safe practice is particularly important for children. Further, as it seems that a large proportion of lifetime sun exposure occurs during childhood (95), strategy to minimize children's exposure to UV light might include provision of information to children and activities to change children's behavior, education of teachers, parents, or other caregivers, and environmental and policy approaches to increase sun-safety. There are yet too few studies and insufficient evidence of the effectiveness of educational, environmental, and policy interventions in childcare settings or intervention targeted at parents and caregivers (95). However, educational and policy interventions in primary schools seem to be effective.

CONCLUSIONS

Several behaviors are relevant for skin-cancer prevention such as wearing protective clothing, avoiding the sun at sun-peak hours, use of sunscreen, and self skin-examination. Factors that motivate and promote these behaviors are complex and vary in different settings and populations. Assessment of local information concerning skin-cancer relevant factors is important for the planning of preventive action. A valuable tool in such assessments would be standardized measures for skin-cancer relevant factors.

Reviews of evidence-based intervention methods to promote primary prevention of skin cancer reveal the need for more well-evaluated prevention activities. Thus, more theory-based and evidence-based intervention methods need to be developed. Interventions need to be evaluated thoroughly and proper outcome variables should be measured. However, there are sufficient evidence to recommend intervention activities in primary schools and at recreational or tourist settings. Nevertheless, new prevention strategies need to be developed for other settings and toward other target groups, and they should preferably be guided by the models of behavior change, and our present knowledge about predictors of skin-cancer relevant behaviors.

Even though more knowledge is needed about why people avoid sun-protective behaviors, interventions should target populations with different motives for their exposure to UV light. Assessing and targeting people with different sun-exposure profiles, is one way to match differing needs with appropriate intervention. In particular, interventions should target unintentional sun exposure as well as intentional tanning. Appearance-based intervention is a promising strategy, targeting intentional tanners, along with information about the preferable use of other strategies to protect from the sun than the use of sunscreens. Unintentional tanners might be targeted with educational, environmental, and policy interventions at appropriate settings.

Self-skin-examination could be a potential way to promote early detection of malignant melanoma. Even though there are some hopeful examples (99,100), more studies on how self skin-examinations can be encouraged need to be conducted and properly evaluated.

REFERENCES

1. Armstrong BK, Kricker A. The epidemiology of UV-induced skin cancer. J Photochem Photobiol B 2001; 63(1–3):8–18.
2. Sahin S, Rao B, Kopf AW, et al. Predicting ten-year survival of patients with primary cutaneous melanoma: corroboration of a prognostic model. Cancer 1997; 80(8):1426–1431.
3. Bränström R, Brandberg Y, Holm L-E, et al. Beliefs, knowledge and attitudes as predictors of sunbathing habits and use of sun protection among Swedish adolescents. Eur J Cancer Prev 2001; 10:337–345.
4. Mermelstein RJ, Riesenberg LA. Changing knowledge and attitudes about skin cancer risk factors in adolescents. Health Psychol 1992; 11:371–376.
5. Wichstrøm L. Predictors of Norwegian adolescents' sunbathing and use of suncreen. Health Psychol 1994; 13:412–420.
6. Bandura A. Social Learning Theory. Englewood Cliffs: Prentice-Hall, 1977.
7. Glanz K, Lewis FM, Rimer BK. Health Behaviour and Health Education. 3rd ed. San Francisco: Jossey-Bass, 2001.
8. Rodgers RW. A protection motivation theory of fear appeals and attitude change. J Psychol 1975; 91:93–114.
9. Ogden J. Health beliefs. In Health Beliefs. Buckingham: Open University Press, 1996.
10. Ajzen I. Percieved behavioral control, self-efficacy, locus of control, and the theory of planned behaviour. J Appl Soc Psychol 2002; 32(4):665–683.
11. Armitage C, Conner M. Efficacy of the Theory of Planned Behaviour: a meta-analytic review. Br J Soc Psychol 2001; 40(4):471–99.
12. Prochaska JO, Norcross JC, Diclemente CC. Changing for Good. New York: Harper Collins Publisher, 1994.

13. Prochaska JJ, Redding CA, Evers KE. The transtheoretical model and stages of change. In: Glanz K, Rimer B, Lewis FM, eds. Health Behaviour and Health Education. San Francisco: Jossey-Bass, 2001.
14. Koblenzer CS. The psychology of sun-exposure and tanning. Clin Dermatol 1998; 16(4):421–428.
15. Borland R, Marks R, Noy S. Public knowledge about characteristics of moles and melanomas. Aust J Publ Health 1992; 16:370–375.
16. Broadstock M, Borland R, Gason R. Effects of suntan on judgements of healthiness and attractiveness by adolescents. J Appl Soc Psychol 1992; 22:157–172.
17. McGee R, Williams S. Adolescence and sun protection. N Z Med J 1992; 105:401–403.
18. Mawn VB, Fleischer AB, Jr. A survey of attitudes, beliefs, and behavior regarding tanning bed use, sunbathing, and sunscreen use. J Am Acad Dermatol 1993; 29(6):959–962.
19. Robinson JK, Rigel DS, Amonette RA. Trends in sun exposure knowledge, attitudes, and behaviors: 1986 to 1996. J Am Acad Dermatol 1997; 37(2 Pt 1):179–186.
20. Vail-Smith K, Felts WM. Sunbathing: college students' knowledge, attitudes, and perceptions of risks. Coll Health 1993; 42:21–26.
21. Boldeman C, Bränström R, Dal H, et al. Tanning habits and sunburn in a Swedish population aged 13–50 years. Eur J Cancer 2001; 37:2441–2448.
22. Stott MA. Tanning and sunburn: knowledge, attitudes and behaviour of people in Great Britain. J Public Health Med 1999; 21(4):377–384.
23. Campbell HS, Birdsell JM. Knowledge, beliefs, and sun protection behaviors of Alberta Adults. Prev Med 1994; 23:160–166.
24. Keesling B, Friedman HS. Psychosocial factors in sunbathing and suncreen use. Health Psychol 1987; 6:477–493.
25. Brandberg Y, Ullén H, Sjöberg L, et al. Sunbathing and sunbed use related to self-image in a randomized sample of Swedish adolescents. Eur J Cancer Prev 1998; 7(4):321–329.
26. Severi G, Cattaruzza MS, Baglietto L, et al. Sun exposure and sun protection in young European children: an EORTC multicentric study. Eur J Cancer 2002; 38(6):820–826.
27. Hillhouse JJ, Adler CM, Drinnon J, et al. Application of Ajzen's theory of planned behavior to predict sunbathing, tanning salon use, and sunscreen use intentions and behaviors. J Behav Med 1997; 20(4):365–378.
28. Branstrom R, Ullen H, Brandberg Y. Attitudes, subjective norms and perception of behavioural control as predictors of sun-related behaviour in Swedish adults. Prev Med 2004; 39(5):992–999.
29. Broadstock M, Borland R, Hill D. Knowledge, attitudes and reported behaviours relevant to sun protection and sun tanning in adolescents. Psychol Health 1996; 11:527–539.
30. Jerkegren E, Sandrieser L, Brandberg Y, et al. Sun-related behaviour and melanoma awareness among Swedish university students. Eur J Cancer Prev 1999; 8(1):27–34.
31. Hillhouse JJ, Stair AW 3rd, Adler CM. Predictors of sunbathing and sunscreen use in college undergraduates. J Behav Med 1996; 19(6):543–561.
32. Arthey S, Clarke VA. Suntanning and sun protection: a review of the psychological literature. Soc Sci Med 1995; 40:265–274.

33. Grob JJ, Guglielmina C, Gouvernet J, et al. Study of sunbathing habits in children and adolescents: application to the prevention of melanoma. Dermatology 1993; 186(2):94–98.
34. Wharton JR, Cockerell CJ. The sun: a friend and enemy. Clin Dermatol 1998; 16:415–419.
35. Horio T. Skin disorders that improve by exposure to sunlight. Clin Dermatol 1998; 16(1):59–65.
36. Jackson KM, Aiken LS. A psychosocial model of sun protection and sunbathing in young women: the impact of health beliefs, attitudes, norms, and self-efficacy for sun protection. Health Psychol 2000; 19(5):469–478.
37. Miller AG, Ashton WA, McHoskey JW, et al. What price attractiveness? stereotype and risk factors in suntanning behavior. J Appl Social Psychol 1990; 20:1272–1300.
38. Jones JL, Leary MR. Effects of appearance-based admonitions against sun exposure on tanning intentions in young adults. Health Psychol 1994; 13(1):86–90.
39. Leary MR, Saltzman JL, Georgeson JC. Appearence motivation, obsessive-compulsive tendencies and exessive suntanning in a community sample. J Health Psychol 1997; 2(4):493–499.
40. Beech JR, Sheehan E, Barraclough S. Attitudes towards health risks and sunbathing behavior. J Psychol 1996; 130(6):669–677.
41. Turrisi R, Hillhouse J, Gebert C, et al. Examination of cognitive variables relevant to sunscreen use. J Behav Med 1999; 22(5):493–509.
42. Davis KJ, Cokkinides VE, Weinstock MA, et al. Summer sunburn and sun exposure among US youths ages 11 to 18: national prevalence and associated factors. Pediatrics 2002; 110(1 Pt 1):27–35.
43. Robinson JK, Rademaker AW, Sylvester JA, et al. Summer sun exposure: knowledge, attitudes, and behaviors of Midwest adolescents. Prev Med 1997; 26(3):364–372.
44. Koh HK, Lew RA. Skin cancer: prevention and control. In: Greenwald, Kramer, Weed, eds. Cancer Prevention and Control. New York: Dekker, 1995:611–640.
45. Peattie S, Clarke P, Peattie K. Risk and responsibility in tourism: promoting sun-safety. Tourism Manage 2005; 26:399–408.
46. Østerlind A. Epidemiology on malignant melanoma in Europe. Acta Oncol 1992; 31(8):903–908.
47. Chen YT, Dubrow R, Zheng T, et al. Sunlamp use and the risk of cutaneous malignant melanoma: a population-based case-control study in connecticut, USA. Int J Epidemiology 1998; 27(5):758–765.
48. Swerdlow AJ, Weinstock MA. Do tanning lamps cause melanoma? An epidemiologic assessment. J Am Acad Dermatol 1998; 38(1):89–98.
49. Westerdahl J, Ingvar C, Masback A, et al. Risk of cutaneous malignant melanoma in relation to use of sunbeds: further evidence for UV-A carcinogenicity. Brit J Cancer 2000; 82(9):1593–1599.
50. Boldeman C, Jansson B, Nilsson B, et al. Sunbed use in Swedish urban adolescents related to behavioral characteristics. Prev Med 1997; 26(1):114–119.
51. Amir Z, Wright A, Kernohan EE, et al. Attitudes, beliefs and behaviour regarding the use of sunbeds amongst healthcare workers in Bradford. Eur J Cancer Care 2000; 9(2):76–79.
52. Rhainds M, De Guire L, Claveau J. A population-based survey on the use of artificial tanning devices in the province of Qubec, Canada. J Am Acad Dermatol 1999; 40(4):572–576.

53. Lazovich D, Forster J. Indoor tanning by adolescents: prevalence, practices and policies. Eur J Cancer 2005; 41(1):20–27.
54. Fitzpatrick TB. The validity and practicality of sun-reactive skin types I through VI. Arch Dermatol 1988; 124(6):869–871.
55. Boldeman C, Beitner H, Jansson B, et al. Sunbed use in relation to phenotype, erythema, sunscreen use and skin diseases. A questionnaire survey among Swedish adolescents. Brit J Dermatol 1996; 135:712–716.
56. INRA (EUROPE) European Coordination Office. Eurobarometre 46.0-Les Européens et le Soleil. Brussels; 1997.
57. Brandberg Y, Sjoden PO, Rosdahl I. Assessment of sun-related behaviour in individuals with dysplastic naevus syndrome: a comparison between diary recordings and questionnaire responses. Melanoma Res 1997; 7(4):347–351.
58. Hillhouse JJ, Turrisi R, Kastner M. Modeling tanning salon behavioral tendencies using appearance motivation, self-monitoring and the theory of planned behavior. Health Edu Res 2000; 15(4):405–414.
59. Shoveller JA, Lovato CY. Measuring self-reported sunburn: challenges and recommendations. Chronic Dis Canada 2001; 22(3/4):83–98.
60. Bränström R. Skin Cancer Prevention—Behaviours Related to Sun Exposure and Early Detection. Stockholm: Karolinska Institutet, 2003.
61. Hill D, White V, Marks R, et al. Melanoma prevention: behavioral and nonbehavioral factors in sunburn among an Australian urban population. Prev Med 1992; 21(5):654–669.
62. Saraiya M, Hall HI, Uhler RJ. Sunburn prevalence among adults in the United States, 1999. Am J Prev Med 2002; 23(2):91–97.
63. Geller AC, Colditz G, Oliveria S, et al. Use of sunscreen, sunburning rates, and tanning bed use among more than 10 000 US children and adolescents. Pediatrics 2002; 109(6):1009–1014.
64. O'Riordan DL, Geller AC, Brooks DR, et al. Sunburn reduction through parental role modeling and sunscreen vigilance. J Pediatr 2003; 142(1):67–72.
65. Cardinez CJ, Cokkinides VE, Weinstock MA, et al. Sun protective behaviors and sunburn experiences in parents of youth ages 11 to 18. Prev Med 2005; 41(1):108–117.
66. McCarthy EM, Ethridge KP, Wagner RF. Beach holiday sunburn: the sunscreen paradox and gender differences. Cutis 1999; 64:37–42.
67. Autier P, Doré J-F, Négrier S, et al. Sunscreen use and duration of sun exposure: a double-blind, randomized trial. J Natl Cancer Inst 1999; 91(15):1304–1309.
68. Autier P, Doré J-F, Reis AC, et al. Sunscreen use and intentional exposure to ultraviolet A and B radiation: a double blind randomized trial using personal dosimeters. Brit J Cancer 2000; 83(9):1243–1248.
69. Westerdahl J, Ingvar C, Masback A, et al. Sunscreen use and malignant melanoma. Int J Cancer 2000; 87(1):145–150.
70. Huncharek M, Kupelnick B. Use of topical sunscreens and the risk of malignant melanoma: a meta-analysis of 9067 patients from 11 case-control studies. Am. J Public Health 2002; 92(7):1173–1177.
71. Cockburn J, Hennrikus D, Scott R, et al. Adolecents use of sun-protection measures. Med J Aust 1989; 151(3):136–140.
72. Coogan PF, Geller A, Adams M, et al. Sun protection practices in preadolescents and adolescents: a school-based survey of almost 25,000 connecticut schoolchildren. J Am Acad Dermatol 2001; 44(3):512–519.

73. Lowe JB, Borland R, Stanton WR, et al. Sun-safe behaviour among secondary school students in Australia. Health Educ Res 2000; 15(3):271–281.

74. Koh HK, Bak SM, Geller AC, et al. Sunbathing habits and sunscreen use among white adults: results of a national survey. Am J Public Health 1997; 87(7):1214–1217.

75. Banks BA, Silverman RA, Schwartz RH, et al. Attitudes of teenagers towards sun exposure and sunscreen use. Pediatrics 1992; 89(1):40–42.

76. Balanda KP, Stanton WR, Lowe JB, et al. Predictors of sun protective behaviors among school students. Behav Med 1999; 25:28–35.

77. Santmyire BR, Feldman SR, Fleischer AB. Lifestyle high-risk behaviors and demografics may predict the level of participation in sun-protection behaviors and skin cancer prevention in the United States. Cancer 2001; 92(5):1315–1324.

78. Grunfeld EA. What influences university students' intentions to practice safe sun exposure behaviors? J Adolesc Health 2004; 35(6):486–492.

79. Harth Y, Schemer A, Friedman-Birnbaum R. Awarness to photodamage versus the actual use of sun protection methods by young adults. J Eur Acad Dermatol Venereol 1995; 4:260–266.

80. de Vries H, Lezwijn J, Hol M, et al. Skin cancer prevention: behaviour and motives of Dutch adolescents. Eur J Cancer Prev 2005; 14(1):39–50.

81. Weinstock MA. Early detection of melanoma. JAMA 2000; 284(7):886–889.

82. Edman RL, Klaus SN. Is routine screening for melanoma a benign practice? JAMA 2000; 284(7):883–886.

83. Berwick M, Begg CB, Fine JA, et al. Screening for cutaneous melanoma by skin self-examination. J Natl Cancer Inst 1996; 88(1):17–23.

84. Koh HK, Miller DR, Geller AC, et al. Who discovers melanoma? Patterns from a population-based survey. J Am Acad Dermatol 1992; 26(6):914–919.

85. Brady MS, Oliveria SA, Christos PJ, et al. Patterns of detection in patients with cutaneous melanoma. Cancer 2000; 89(2):342–347.

86. Saraiya M, Hall HI, Thompson T, et al. Skin cancer screening among U.S. adults from 1992, 1998, and 2000 national health interview surveys. Prev Med 2004; 39(2):308–314.

87. Brandberg Y, Bolund C, Michelson H, et al. Perceived susceptibility to and knowledge of malignant melanoma: screening participants vs the general population. Prev Med 1996; 25:170–177.

88. Bergenmar M, Törnberg S, Brandberg Y. Factors related to non-attendance in a population-based melanoma screening program. Psycho-oncology 1997; 6:218–226.

89. Manne S, Fasanella N, Connors J, et al. Sun protection and skin surveillance practices among relatives of patients with malignant melanoma: prevalence and predictors. Prev Med 2004; 39(1):36–47.

90. Robinson JK, Rigel DS, Amonette RA. What promotes skin self-examination? J Am Acad Dermatol 1998; 38(5 Pt 1):752–757.

91. Oliveria SA, Christos PJ, Halpern AC, et al. Evaluation of factors associated with skin self-examination. Cancer Epidemiol Biomarkers Prev 1999; 8(11):971–978.

92. Weinstock MA, Martin RA, Risica PM, et al. Thorough skin examination for the early detection of melanoma. Am J Prev Med 1999; 17(3):169–175.

93. Borland R, Meehan JW. Skin examination for signs of cancer. Aust J Public Health 1995; 19(1):85–88.

94. Anderson PJ, Lowe JB, Stanton WR, et al. Skin cancer prevention: a link between primary prevention and early detection? Aust J Public Health 1994; 18(4):417–420.
95. Saraiya M, Glanz K, Briss PA, et al. Interventions to prevent skin cancer by reducing exposure to ultraviolet radiation: a systematic review. Am J Prev Med 2004; 27(5):422–466.
96. Shoveller JA, Lovato CY, Young RA, et al. Exploring the development of sun-tanning behavior: a grounded theory study of adolescents' decision-making experiences with becoming a sun tanner. Int J Behav Med 2003; 10(4):299–314.
97. Mahler HI, Kulik JA, Harrell J, et al. Effects of UV photographs, photoaging information, and use of sunless tanning lotion on sun protection behaviors. Arch Dermatol 2005; 141(3):373–380.
98. Mahler HI, Kulik JA, Gibbons FX, et al. Effects of appearance-based interventions on sun protection intentions and self-reported behaviors. Health Psychol 2003; 22(2):199–209.
99. Oliveria SA, Dusza SW, Phelan DL, et al. Patient adherence to skin self-examination: effect of nurse intervention with photographs. Am J Prev Med 2004; 26(2):152–155.
100. Robinson JD, Silk KJ, Parrott RL, et al. Healthcare providers' sun-protection promotion and at-risk clients' skin-cancer-prevention outcomes. Prev Med 2004; 38(3):251–257.

16

Periods-of-Life Program

Continuous Primary Prevention of Skin Cancer in Certain Age Groups

Rudiger Greinert and B. Volkmer
Center of Dermatology, Elbe Kliniken, Klinikum Buxtehude, Buxtehude, Germany

S. Welz
Commentum Public Relations, Hamburg, Germany

Eckhard W. Breitbart
Center of Dermatology, Elbe Kliniken, Klinikum Buxtehude, Buxtehude, Germany

INTRODUCTION

Nonmelanoma skin cancer (NMSC; basal cell carcinoma, BCC; squamous cell carcinoma, SCC) and malignant melanoma (MM) of the skin represent the most common type of cancer in the white population worldwide (1,2). Skin cancer incidence is still increasing and reaches epidemic proportions (1). In Europe, the United States, Canada, and Australia, the average increase in NMSC has been published to be in the range of 3% to 8% per year since the 1960s (1,3,4). Standardized European incidence rates of MM for different European countries are in the range of 3–17/100,000 cases per year. Therefore, in 2000, approximately, 26,000 males and 33,000 females have been diagnosed with melanomas in Europe, and around 8300 males and 7600 females died of their disease. As for NMSC, incidence of MM is still increasing (5). Cutaneous malignant melanoma is the most rapidly increasing cancer in white populations with estimated doubling of rates every 10 to 20 years. A cumulative lifetime risk for melanoma has been estimated to be in the order of 1:25 and around 1:75 in Australia and in the United States by the year 2000 (1,6,7). MM is much more fatal (20–25% mortality) than NMSC. However, due to the high incidence of NMSC, these types of skin cancer also induce a high burden in health systems because of the increasing human and economic costs. On the other hand, skin cancer should be highly preventable, because the main risk factor, UV radiation, is known and exposure (to artificial and solar UV) can be reduced by means of primary prevention, which can give liable information to reduce the risk (UV exposure) in order to stay healthy.

UV AND SKIN CANCER

There is no doubt anymore that UV radiation is the main risk factor for the induction (and promotion as well as progression) of NMSC and MM (e.g., 2, 8, 9). Intermittent UV exposure, sun burns in childhood and youth, and acquired nevi are known to be the main risk factors for the development of MM. SCC development depends on cumulative UV dose, whereas BCCs have been shown to develop after intermittent and/or cumulative UV exposure (8,9). Different genetic pathways are involved including a variety of tumor-suppressor genes like *p53* (SCC), *ptch* (BCC) and $p16^{INk4A}$ (MM) (2,10,11). UV-induced (signature-) mutations have been found in the genes of these pathways (e.g., 12,13), furthermore increasing evidence that UV radiation is the main risk factor in the etiology of skin cancer.

PERIODS-OF-LIFE PROGRAM

The prominent role of UV radiation renders skin cancer most suitable for primary prevention, because the main risk factor can easily be avoided by sticking to simple rules for the behavior in the sun or under artificial UV (e.g., sunbeds).

However, because UV exposure cannot and should not be avoided totally, recommendations and information for the public should be as clear and as weighted as possible. It is, furthermore, of special importance to reach different age groups of the public, which show different attitudes, behavior, and skin sensitivity, continuously with age-specific intervention programs in primary prevention. Especially any advice to avoid UV exposure at a certain age should not introduce any deficits in the possible beneficial health effects of UV radiation (e.g., vitamin D_3 production).

In order to achieve these goals, the Association of German Dermatologists (ADP) introduced a "periods-of-life program" (POLP) at a WHO workshop ("Children's Sun Protection Education"), held at the second EUROSKIN conference "Children under the Sun," 2001, in Orvieto, Italy. POLP defines certain target groups for age-specific education levels in the population. This target grouping starts with parents of unborns (lasting from fertilization to birth),

Periods-of-Life Program

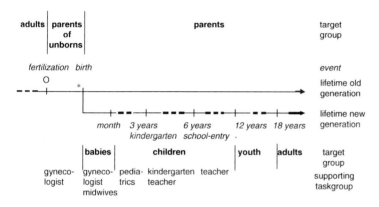

Figure 1 Schematic representation of the periods-of-life program (for further explanation, see text).

followed by babies (up to 12 month), children (1–6 years of age), youth (12–17 years of age), adults (≥18 years of age), and parents (Fig. 1). As can be seen from Figure 1, the target group of children can be further subdivided into three groups: children at the age of 1 to 3 years, kindergarten children (3–6 years of age), children at the age after (ground-) school entry (6–11 years of age).

For all the target groups, certain caretakers in the health and education system were identified, and special information and education material were developed and distributed to them. This was done in order to integrate their help as important members of supporting target groups. These include gynecologists, midwives, pediatrics, kindergarten teachers, teachers at schools, and (always) parents (Fig. 1).

In 2002, the ADP started in Germany a POLP with the target group of babies and their parents. This was followed in 2003 by an intervention campaign targeting kindergarten children. In 2004, children entering (ground-) school represented the next target group. This campaign closely followed WHO's sun protection programs in schools (14). Materials have been developed and distributed to more than 16,000 ground schools in Germany, containing information and materials for pupils as well as for their teachers. These education materials were supported by a special CD of a German songwriter who composed a number of "sun-songs," which were easily learned, adopted, and often sung by pupils at school. The 2005 campaign tried to reach the teens (12–17 years of age). For this age, group prizes were awarded for the best video clips produced by

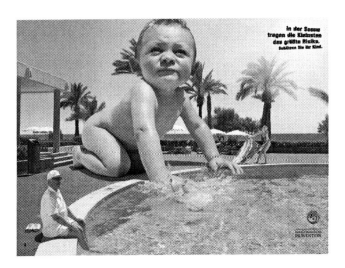

Figure 2 Example of a poster (eye-opener) used in the German POLP (target group: babies and their parents). The German text in the upper right corner translates to: "In the sun, babies carry the higher risk. Save your child."

groups at school, conveying sun-protection and sun-behavior messages like "seek shade," "use textile protection," "use sunscreens," and so on.

All interventions in the context of a POLP since 2002 have been accompanied by huge efforts in public relations, including press conferences,

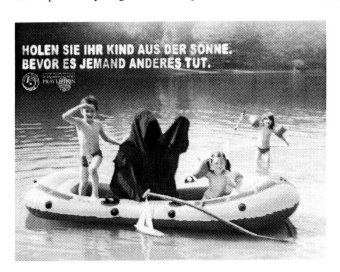

Figure 3 Example of a poster (eye-opener) used in the German POLP (target group: kindergarten children). The German text in the poster translates to: "Take your kids out of the sun, before someone else is doing it."

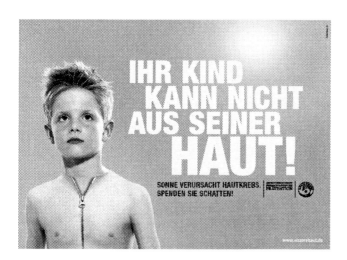

Figure 4 Example of a poster (eye-opener) used in the German POLP (target group: school ground children). The German text in the poster translates to: "Your child is not able to escape its skin! Sun causes skin cancer. Please donate shade."

spots for TV, and in cinemas, as well as by nation wide bill-posting of so called "eye-openers" to awake interest in the public. Some examples are shown in Figures 2–4. All the efforts have been financially supported by the German Cancer Aid.

So far, all campaigns in the framework of a POLP in Germany have been very successful by means of acceptance and response in the target groups and supporting target groups. It is expected that the future evaluation of various rounds of POLP will show that this continuous program will vigorously change the behavior of the target groups and the public as a whole concerning solar and artificial UV exposure. This will then contribute to the aim of decreasing morbidity and mortality of skin cancer.

REFERENCES

1. Diepgen TL, Mahler V. The epidemiology of skin cancer. Br J Dermatol 2002; 146(suppl 61):1–6.
2. Cleaver JE, Crowley E. UV damage, DNA repair and skin carcinogenesis. Front Biosci 2002; 7:d1024–d1043.
3. Green A. Changing patterns in incidence of nonmelanoma skin cancer. Epithelial Cell Biol 1992; 1:47–51.
4. Glass AG, Hoover RN. The emerging epidemic of melanoma and squamous cell skin cancer. JAMA 1989; 262:2097–2100.
5. deVries E, Coebergh JW. Cutaneous malignant melanoma in Europe. Eur J Cancer 2004; 40:2355–2366.

6. Giles G, Thursfield V. Trends in skin cancer in Australia. Cancer Forum 1996; 20:188–191.
7. Rigel DS. The gender-related issues in malignant melanoma. Hawaii Med J 1993; 52:124–146.
8. Armstrong BK, Kricker A. The epidemiology of UV-induced skin cancer. J Photochem Photobiol B 2001; 63:8–18.
9. Dulon M, Weichenthal M, Blettner M, et al. Sun exposure and number of nevi in 5- to 6-year old European children. J Clin Epidemiol 2002; 55:1075–1081.
10. Brellier F, Marionnet C, Chevallier-Lagente O, et al. Ultraviolet irradiation represses patched gene transcription in human epidermal keratinocytes through an activator protein-1-dependent process. Cancer Res 2004; 64:2699–2704.
11. Chin L. The genetics of malignant melanoma: lessons from mouse and man. Nat Rev Cancer 2003; 3:559–570.
12. Daja-Grosjean L, Sarasin A. UV-specific mutations of the human patched gene in basal cell carcinomas from normal individuals and xeroderma pigmentosum patients. Mutat Res 2000; 450:193–199.
13. Kim MY, Park HJ, Baek SC, et al. Mutations of the *p53* and *PTCH* gene in basal cell carcinoma: UV mutation signature and strand bias. J Dermatol Sci 2002; 29:1–9.
14. http://www.who.int/phe/uv.

17

Aims of Primary Prevention of Skin Cancer

Karen Glanz

Department of Behavioral Sciences and Health Education, Rollins School of Public Health, Emory University, Atlanta, Georgia, U.S.A.

INTRODUCTION

Skin cancer is a significant and, in many parts of the world, growing health problem (1). Although skin cancer is among the most common cancers, it is also one of the most preventable. Recommendations for primary prevention of skin cancer aim to reduce exposure to ultraviolet radiation (UVR)—both outdoor sun exposure and exposure to artificial ultraviolet light. The most common recommended behavioral strategies for reducing UVR exposure include: limit time spent in the sun, avoid the sun during peak hours, use a broad spectrum sunscreen when outside, wear protective clothing (hats, shirts, pants) and sunglasses, seek shade when outdoors, and avoid indoor tanning (or solaria) (2,3).

Using a general public health approach to primary prevention suggests focusing on the classic public health model that emphasizes three main factors: host, agent, and environment. In the case of primary prevention of skin cancer, the "host" is the person or population that is at risk for the disease—in terms of risk factors such as skin, hair and eye color, and tendency to sunburn, or according to age group or occupational exposure. The most important "agent" of disease causation, in the simplest terms, is excess UVR; in turn, prevention involves avoidance of the agent through individual behaviors and environmental/organizational change. Finally, the "environment": while diverse environmental situations can lead to greater risk (e.g., sunnier climates and higher elevations), the social settings where people come together provide a structure and vehicle for primary prevention.

This chapter uses this framework to introduce the aims of primary prevention of skin cancer, several of which will be discussed in greater detail in the chapters that follow in this section. The first section reviews the target outcomes for primary prevention, ranging from primary behavioral targets to their determinants, environmental changes, and reductions in cancer and precancerous lesions. This is followed by a discussion of key population targets and settings. A broad typology of primary prevention strategies and discussion of international considerations then set the stage for the consideration of behavioral and communication intervention programs.

TARGET OUTCOMES FOR PRIMARY PREVENTION

Analytic Framework

A conceptual model or analytic framework can be helpful to illustrate the hypothesized relationship of primary prevention strategies to relevant intermediate outcomes (e.g., knowledge, attitudes, intentions regarding sun-protective behaviors) and to behaviors and reduction in skin cancer incidence (4). The framework developed for the *Guide to Community Preventive Services* is shown in Figure 1. Key outcome targets identified in the framework include increases in knowledge, attitudes, and intentions to reduce UV exposure or increase solar protection, changes in exposure and protection, reduction of sunburn, and changes in policies and environments to reduce exposure (e.g., limiting exposure during peak sun hours, increasing shade, providing sunscreen, etc.). Although most prevention research does not measure decreased incidence of precancer, nevi, or photodamage or decreased incidence of skin cancer, the analytic framework and the epidemiologic literature suggest that significant behavioral changes and reduction of sunburn, if found, can lead to lower rates of cancer (5).

Knowledge, Attitudes, and Intentions

Historically, health educators considered behaviors to be determined by rational beliefs, opinions about behaviors, and also to be easily articulated in terms of behavioral intentions (6). It is now recognized that knowledge is necessary, but not sufficient for healthful behavior; that attitudes can influence and be affected by behavior; and that nonvoluntary factors can intervene between behavioral intentions and the practice of health-protective behavior. Nevertheless, at a minimum, people need to know the instrumental steps required for adequate sun protection, have the skills and resources to engage in sun-safety behaviors, and make skin cancer prevention a routine in their daily lives. The current view is that these prevention targets are important, but that effective prevention

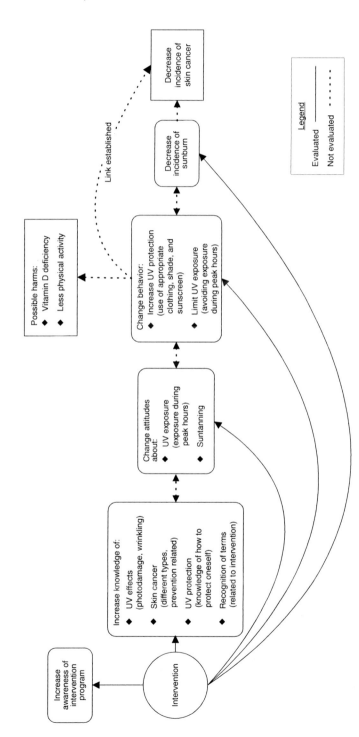

Figure 1 A conceptual approach to prevention of skin cancer through interventions to reduce UV light exposure. *Note:* Improvements in sunscreen use alone do not result in a recommendation outcome (see full MMWR report).

programs must aim improvements in knowledge, attitudes, and intentions as foundations for disease prevention and not as final endpoints.

Behavioral Targets of Primary Prevention

The central targets of primary prevention are behaviors that increase or decrease the risk of developing skin cancer by UVR exposure: sun exposure behaviors, sun protection, and indoor tanning or use of solaria.

Sun Exposure

Sun exposure has several dimensions that all reflect time spent outdoors in the sun and people may be distinct in terms of their behavioral determinants, and thus require different prevention approaches. The first is "incidental sun exposure," that is, time spent outdoors on sunny days for the purpose of travel and/or routine activities of daily living. The second is "recreational sun exposure," which occurs when people are enjoying recreational and/or sports activities outdoors in the sun; for example, swimming, cycling, skiing, fishing, or playing. The third type of sun exposure is "occupational sun exposure," which may be prolonged for certain occupations ranging from postal and maintenance workers to lifeguards. Finally, the fourth type of sun exposure is "intentional sun exposure," taken for the purpose of sunbathing or getting a suntan. Further, sun exposure typically varies between weekdays and weekends (7), with all types of exposure other than occupational exposure being higher on weekend days.

These types of sun exposure tend to differ in terms of their associations with skin cancer risk, the populations most affected, and promising approaches to prevention. For example, protective clothing and work rules may significantly reduce outdoor workers' UVR exposure. However, intentional sunbathers may be much more resistant to information and persuasive appeals regarding skin cancer prevention.

Sun Protection

Sun-protection behaviors (SPBs) are multidimensional, most often described in three main categories: using sunscreen, covering up (wearing hats and protective clothing), and seeking shade. The use of sunglasses is also often included in this category. Sunscreen is the most often-practiced prevention behavior, though its role in preventing melanoma has not been unequivocally shown and remains complex (8,9). (The chapter by Dore addresses the use and usefulness of sunscreens in greater detail.) Ideal covering-up behaviors are considered to include wearing a wide-brim hat, long sleeves, and long pants; though the wearing of a hat with any brim and at least clothing covering the torso may also be preferred to minimal body covering. Shade-seeking including using an umbrella or moving "under cover" when out in the sun is a proactive practice for reducing UVR exposure and one that can be encouraged by environmental supports (discussed subsequently).

Indoor Tanning

The use of indoor tanning, mainly solaria, is widespread in the United States and Europe (10). Even though there is increased evidence of the dangers of artificial UVR, the popularity of indoor tanning has been growing in recent years. Reduced use of solaria is an important behavioral target of primary prevention for certain population groups, particularly adolescents and young women. (See also the chapter by Cesarini for more details.)

Environmental Changes

Environmental changes are important outcomes of primary prevention strategies to reduce UVR exposure. These can include a variety of changes in sun-safety environments and policies, such as increasing available shade, providing sunscreen, and posting skin cancer prevention information (11). They can contribute directly to behavior changes, for example, by reducing UVR exposure by providing shade, and can even affect health outcomes without modifying individuals' knowledge and attitudes. The two main categories of environmental change are: (*i*) environmental supports—mainly increasing shade, offering sunscreen, and posting information about sun protection; and (*ii*) sun-protection policies, including organizational policies to require or recommend covering-up with hats and/or shirts, scheduling activities to avoid peak sun times and comprehensive sun-protection policies (12,13). A more thorough discussion of environmental and policy intervention strategies is found later in this chapter.

Nevi, Precancerous Lesions, and Reductions in Skin Cancer

A reduction in disease is the ultimate ideal aim of primary prevention programs and strategies. A few studies of primary prevention agents have examined outcomes such as reduced numbers of moles (i.e., nevi); however, these have been mainly controlled trials of selected volunteers rather than the evaluations of population-based prevention strategies (13). Only one community-based study to date, in Australia, has used mole counts as an endpoint for a skin cancer prevention program, although no significant differences between treatment and control groups were found in that case (14). Nevertheless, it is generally accepted that successful primary prevention efforts that reduce UVR exposure can result in reductions in the incidence of skin cancer.

POPULATION TARGETS AND SETTINGS FOR PRIMARY PREVENTION

Population Targets

One of the axioms of health education and promotion is that interventions are most likely to be effective when they are designed specifically for, and with information about, a definable audience (6). Population targets of special interest for primary prevention of skin cancer include those who are at greatest biological risk, for example, persons with fair skin, hair, and eye color that confers phenotypic risk (15), and persons with a family history of skin cancer. Outdoor workers and persons living close to the equator also have increased risk and are important population targets. A third way of defining population targets for prevention involves life stages—beginning with infants, toddlers, children, adolescents, adults, and the elderly. This approach is often central to prevention programming, as people in these ages or life-cycle age groupings tend to share behavioral risks and can often be convened in organizational settings, where prevention strategies can be implemented. (Readers should refer to the chapter by Greinert that further describes the "periods-of-life program" approach to primary prevention.)

There is no single, clear-cut way to classify interventions to reduce UVR exposure. Whereas some can be easily identified within a single category (e.g., education for school-age children), many more involve multiple methods or communication strategies. Further, interventions often target multiple audiences, for example, both parents and children, or physicians and patients.

Settings for Primary Prevention

The nature of intervention strategies is also often influenced by their organizational context or setting (11). Parallel to several of the population segments mentioned earlier, important settings for primary prevention include childcare centers, primary schools, secondary schools, and colleges, healthcare settings, occupational settings, and recreational and tourism settings. These settings were key foci of the U.S.-based evidence review of primary prevention programs (4). In that review, three other categories focussed on a target population—children's parents and caregivers, broad types of interventions, media campaigns and community-wide multicomponent interventions.

BROAD TYPOLOGY OF PRIMARY PREVENTION STRATEGIES

Bearing in mind the complexities of delineating population and setting targets for prevention, it is useful to provide a broad typology of four types of interventions that readers may use to group various strategies and studies: (*i*) individual-directed strategies; (*ii*) environmental, policy, and structural interventions; (*iii*) media campaigns; and (*iv*) community-wide multi-component interventions (11). Each type of intervention is briefly characterized here.

Individual-Directed Strategies

Individual-directed strategies include informational and behavioral interventions aimed primarily at individuals or groups. These interventions usually occur within organizational contexts, such as schools, recreation programs, or healthcare settings. They aim to teach and motivate individuals by improving knowledge, attitudes, and behavioral skills for skin-cancer prevention. They include the use of small media (brochures, pamphlets, printed materials, etc.), didactic programs (e.g., classroom lessons, lectures), interactive activities (games, multimedia programs), and skill development (role play, teaching sunscreen application, etc.). These strategies can be directed toward any age, occupational, or risk group and are often combined with other strategies.

Environmental, Policy, and Structural Interventions

Environmental, policy, and structural interventions aim to provide and/or maintain a physical, social, and/or information environment that supports sun protection and sun-safety practices. These interventions aim to improve the sun-protective conditions for all people in a defined population (school, community setting, etc.), and not just for those who are most motivated. They reach populations by passively reducing UVR exposure, providing sun-protection resources, and broadening the accessibility and reach of skin cancer prevention information. Examples include increasing shade areas, supplying sunscreen, providing environmental sources of information and/or prompts, and many other possible strategies. Policies establish formal rules or standards for organizational actions or legal requirements or restrictions related to skin cancer prevention measures. Policies may be developed by a school, school board, or community organization, or by other legal entities such as municipal, state, and federal governments. Environmental strategies involve providing supportive resources for skin cancer prevention in the physical, social, and/or information environment. They may be based on, and restricted or assisted by, policies. However, environmental supports can also be undertaken in the absence of a formal policy.

Media Campaigns

Media campaigns use mass media channels such as print (newspaper, magazines) and broadcast media (radio, television), and the Internet to disseminate information and behavioral guidance to a wide audience. They may be aimed at specific types of target audiences, but are typically characterized by broad distribution channels. Media campaigns have some of the characteristics of individual-directed interventions, but without the face-to-face interpersonal interaction and "captive audience" in a defined organizational setting. Media campaigns tend to have a public health orientation and often seek to raise the levels of awareness or concern, and to help shape the policy agenda that drives other interventions. (Chapter 19 of this book discusses key communication strategies in greater detail.)

Community-Wide Multicomponent Interventions

Community-wide multicomponent interventions, often called population-wide programs or campaigns, seek to combine elements of the three other types of strategies into an integrated effort in a defined geographic area (city, state/province, or country). They often include individual-directed strategies, environmental and policy changes, media campaigns, and a variety of setting-specific strategies delivered with a defined theme, name/logo, and set of messages (4,11). One of the earliest such programs, and the one with the longest continuous activity over 20 years, is the SunSmart program established in the state of Victoria in Australia (16).

There is a wide range of target audiences, settings, and types of applicable interventions to reduce UVR exposure. Most efforts cut across categories and can be informative about more than a single audience, setting, and/or strategy.

INTERNATIONAL CONSIDERATIONS

International approaches to skin cancer prevention are shaped by the patterns of disease and risk, recognition of trends in disease prevalence and mortality, competing priorities in public health and cancer prevention, and the resources and actions of clinicians, scientists, and advocates in different regions of the world.

For example, in the United States, skin cancer prevention activities are marked by their diversity and efforts coming from many organizations. These strategies are sponsored by multiple funding agencies with modest funding, and education for youth occurs in the context of decentralized school systems and school health curricula. There are many providers of healthcare who distribute public health information: a very robust mass media, and few consistently assessed outcome measures.

In the United States, there are several key challenges to progress in skin cancer prevention. They include competing educational agendas; the tendency to want to "educate in a sound bite"; and a modest research foundation. Coordination of public education with advocacy for skin cancer prevention legislative policies and efforts to influence social norms will continue to be a focus of U.S. prevention activities (17).

In Europe, there are many countries with different languages, political leadership, and cultures. There is also great variation in skin cancer rates across Europe: northern countries generally have higher rates of melanoma, and while more women are diagnosed with melanoma, more men die of the disease (18). Rates of melanoma and nonmelanoma skin cancers are increasing in Europe, and mortality rates have been nearly constant over the last decade (18). The EUROSKIN organization was founded to coordinate efforts to reduce the toll of disease and death from skin cancer in Europe. Over the past five years, EUROSKIN's main activities have focussed on harmonization of skin cancer prevention in Europe, sun protection education for children, identification and management of risk factors for skin cancer, and the role of skin cancer screening (19). Currently, primary prevention of skin cancer in Europe is progressing. Keys to continuing progress are the use of harmonized strategies, ongoing use of available interventions, and attention to the need for new interventions that are intense enough to change difficult behaviors such as solarium use.

Australia has very high rates of skin-cancer morbidity and mortality. In Australia, primary prevention efforts aim to reduce incidence and mortality by attitude change, behavior change, and structural and organizational changes. The elements of comprehensive prevention efforts include mass media, sponsorship of sporting organizations, resource development and dissemination, professional education, advocacy of policy development, and research and evaluation. Educational efforts began more than 20 years ago, with media campaigns focusing on protecting children, using surf lifeguards as role models, and more recently using fear-arousing communications to draw attention to the negative consequences of skin cancer (16).

Evaluation of intermediate endpoints of skin cancer prevention campaigns in Australia has been continuous since the 1980s, particularly in the Australian state of Victoria. Extensive program evaluation information is available in a series of reports and publications (20). Mean time spent outside during peak UV hours of 11 a.m. to 3 p.m. declined between 1988 and 2001, and most forms of weekend sun protection increased during that period. During the 1990s, there was a trend toward more male youths spending most of the peak sun hours indoors, with females reporting steady rates. However, 80% reported a painful sunburn in the previous summer in 1999; and only 21% of males and 15% of female youths usually wore clothing covering most of their bodies. The Centre for Behavioral Research on Cancer at the Cancer Council Victoria is currently analyzing data on trends in sunburn and sun protection in the state of Victoria: national surveys of children, adolescents, and adults and the relationship between advertising and sun protection.

In Australia, skin cancer prevention and control are key national health priorities; trends in incidence and mortality of melanoma in Australia are considered to be the most important indicators of progress in primary prevention. The data present an optimistic picture: mortality is stable, and increases in incidence appear to be slowing. There have been no increases in people under 45 years of age; thick melanoma rates are stable in younger persons; and in-situ and thin invasive melanomas are still increasing, but more slowly. To put this in perspective, it is important to remember that primary prevention (i.e., sun protection) should lower the incidence of skin cancers, and increased detection should increase the detection of thin and in-situ melanomas and lower the incidence of thicker melanomas. With its long history of comprehensive primary prevention efforts, positive progress in Australia appears to be significant and encouraging. The Australian experience illustrates the enormous potential of prevention when it is supported by resources, political will, and scientific grounding.

Experiences in primary prevention of skin cancer in different parts of the world are different because of unique trends in morbidity and mortality, population characteristics, policy trends, and the extent and efforts of advocacy and activism. An important step toward long-term success is the sharing of experiences, learning from each other, and collective review of the evidence for progress in primary prevention of skin cancer.

DISCUSSION

Importance of Population Targets and Settings

As described in this chapter, many primary prevention programs and most published studies have reported interventions located within specific organizational settings. These venues provide useful ways to reach important audiences like children and high-risk patients. They can also increase the relevance of the intervention, as with programs in outdoor recreation, outdoor workplaces, and healthcare settings. Organizational settings also provide clear opportunities for policy and structural supports to complement educational efforts. Thus, population targets and organizational and community settings should be considered together in planning primary prevention programs.

With regard to specific settings for which larger numbers of studies have been published, we can draw additional conclusions. Schools appear to provide a good foundation for sun-safety education for children and youth, but have been limited in their success at influencing long-term behavioral changes. Most likely, they should link with other community organizations and with families, to achieve transfer to those occasions when children are selecting sun-protective products and spending time outdoors. Healthcare settings appear to be appropriate and feasible places to teach healthcare providers (including pharmacists) better skin cancer prevention-counseling skills. The salience of prevention messages in healthcare settings is likely to be high. However, attendance at provider education programs has been a limitation, and skin cancer prevention (like other types of primary prevention) is likely to compete with other priorities for the attention of doctors and nurses.

Increasing the Success of Primary Prevention

Ideally, intervention strategies to reduce UVR exposure should be coordinated, sustained, community-wide approaches that combine education, mass media, and environmental and structural changes. The longest established and most studied of these programs, SunSmart in the state of Victoria in Australia, has reduced several skin cancer risk behaviors by roughly one-half, although some subgroups and behaviors present continuing challenges (16). Because SunSmart (with its predecessor Slip! Slap! Slop!) appears to have achieved society-wide normative changes, it has good prospects for continuing to build on this success. What is less clear is whether this type of effect can be accomplished in areas with lower skin cancer rates, larger populations, or more ethnically-mixed populations. There will always be a need to adapt both intervention programs and expectations to a specific country, audience, and epidemiologic profile.

Promise of Environmental, Policy, and Structural Interventions

It is generally agreed nowadays that environmental and structural changes are necessary components of successful skin cancer prevention efforts. In fact, a recent review of the literature found that environmental supports, policy changes, and/or structural interventions have been part of carefully evaluated prevention programs in virtually all types of settings, although their impact has not been specifically studied in school programs (4). In preschool settings, policies regarding hats and sunscreen have been most prominent. Outdoor recreation settings have used free or discounted sunscreen, shade supports, environmental prompts (signs, posters), and free hats or reduced-price hats. Supply of protective gear and sunscreen, as well as regulations, has been used in workplace settings. A broad range of structural changes have been used in comprehensive community-wide programs (11).

Despite the wide inclusion of environmental, policy and structural changes in health-promotion efforts, the research reveals some limitations to their efficacy. Adoption of sun-protection policies is often a strategy for change and an outcome in itself. Some studies have found that changes in the adoption of policies are not necessarily accompanied by changes in the "clients"—children, patients, and/or workers. Other studies have not measured changes in the intended beneficiaries of prevention strategies. Another complication in some regions, for example, in the United States, is that the increasing public demand for supportive sun-safety items can make it difficult to separate their influence from educational programs.

When do environmental and structural supports make a difference? They may take longer than individual-directed strategies to make a difference. They may need to be stronger or more intense than they have been in reported programs. And finally, some supports (e.g., free sunscreen, hats) may be effective mainly by reducing obstacles to action for already-motivated people, rather than changing behaviors or exposures of those who are unmotivated.

Research Methodology: Outcomes, Design, and Measurement

Of all outcomes measured, increase in knowledge is the most often reported. Among behavioral outcomes, the use of sunscreen is the main outcome for which success is reported. Increased sunscreen use also seems to account for much of the increase in composites SPBs in many reports. Some studies have found increases in hat use or general covering-up, but this has been less common.

Information on primary prevention of skin cancer is recorded in the available research literature. We analyzed the research reported in the Guide to Community Preventive Services evidence review (4) to examine the type of study designs and measures that were used (13). Of the studies reviewed, about half used experimental designs and many involved group-randomized trials. Most of the randomized controlled trials were studies of individuals or setting-specific strategies, but the majority of evaluations of mass media and community-wide interventions used other designs. Some studies have used repeat cross-sectional or time-series designs. The remainder of the studies has used various non-experimental designs. These designs make causal inference more difficult, but can reduce problems with internal validity, such as contamination. The importance of experimental designs is illustrated by some studies that found improvements in the control groups and experimental groups. Others found negative trends in control groups, again drawing attention to the importance of studying appropriate controls (11).

Duration of interventions and length of follow-up are other limitations to our knowledge of strategies for reducing UVR exposure. About two-thirds of the interventions had a duration of less than six weeks, and more than half the evaluations followed subjects for less than three months. The trend toward longer intervention and follow-up periods is an important advancement, though the commitment of research resources may constrain longer-term programs and evaluations.

There is also substantial variability in the rigor of data analytic methods, and many studies do not include statistical controls for relevant confounders such as risk levels and weather conditions. An important research question that is not usually examined is whether the hypothesized "active ingredients" or mediating factors changed, and whether changes in these factors are associated with behavior change. Few studies in the solar protection area have reported on mediator's analysis up to now.

Measurement of UVR exposure behaviors seems simple and straightforward, but this aspect of the research actually faces important challenges in conceptualizing and operationalizing the main behavioral outcomes of interest. UVR exposure behaviors are both habitual and contingent, multidimensional, and not necessarily additive (e.g., staying indoors may make wearing sunscreen or a hat unnecessary). The interactions among different SPBs have seldom been studied (13). Also, the distinction between intentional and incidental sun exposure has not been well studied. Only, recently have behavioral scientists begun to focus on better understanding behavioral outcome measures and their functioning (21).

Most studies rely on self-report of behaviors and their presumed determinants. A current effort to develop core measures of skin cancer prevention behaviors addresses outdoor UVR exposure and sun-protection practices, as well as solaria use; the recommended core measures are expected to be published some time in 2006. There is also a need for further development of measures of environmental and policy-change strategies for sun safety.

This chapter has offered a conceptualization and broad overview of the aims of primary prevention of skin cancer, the main strategies, international issues, and some of the important themes and challenges to research in this area.

ACKNOWLEDGMENT

The preparation of this chapter was completed in part with support from a Distinguished Scholar Award to Glanz from the Georgia Cancer Coalition.

REFERENCES

1. Howe HL, Wingo PA, Thun MJ, et al. Annual report to the nation on the status of cancer (1973 through 1998), featuring cancers with recent increasing trends. J Natl Cancer Inst 2001; 93:824–842.

2. Diffey BL. What can be done to reduce personal ultraviolet radiation exposure? In: Hill D, Elwood JM, English DR, eds. Prevention of Skin Cancer. Dordrecht: Kluwer Academic Publishers, 2004:241–258.
3. U.S. Department of Health and Human Services. Healthy people 2010, 2nd ed. U.S. Government Printing Office: Washington D.C., 2000.
4. Saraiya M, Glanz K, Briss PA, et al. Interventions to prevent skin cancer by reducing exposure to ultraviolet radiation: a systematic review. Am J Prev Med 2004; 27(5):422–466.
5. Ries LA, Wingo PA, Miller DS, et al. The annual report to the nation on the status of cancer, 1973–1997, with a special section on colorectal cancer. Cancer 2000; 88:2398–2424.
6. Glanz K, Rimer BK, Lewis, FM, eds. Health Behavior and Health Education: Theory, Research, and Practice, 3rd ed. San Francisco: Jossey-Bass Inc. Publishers, 2002.
7. Glanz K, Silverio R, Farmer A. Diary reveals sun protective practices. Skin Cancer Found J 1996; 14:27–28.
8. IARC Working Group on the Evaluation of Cancer Preventive Agents. IARC Handbooks of Cancer Prevention. In: Vainio H, Bianchini F, eds. Sunscreens. Vol. 5. Lyon, France: International Agency for Research on Cancer, 2001.
9. Dennis LK, Beane Freeman LE, VanBeek MJ. Sunscreen use and the risk for melanoma: a quantitative review. Ann Int Med 2003; 139:966–978.
10. Lazovich D, Forster J. Indoor tanning by adolescents: prevalence, practices, and policies. Eur J Cancer 2005; 41(1):20–27.
11. Glanz K, Saraiya M, Briss PA. Impact of intervention strategies to reduce UVR exposure. In: Hill D, Elwood JM, English DR, eds. Prevention of Skin Cancer. Dordrecht: Kluwer Academic Publishers, 2004:259–293.
12. Glanz K, Saraiya M, Wechsler H. Guidelines for school programs to prevent skin cancer. MMWR Morb Mortal Wkly Rep 2002; 51:1–18.
13. Glanz K, Mayer JA. Reducing ultraviolet exposure to prevent skin cancer: methodology and measurement. Am J Prev Med 2005; 29(2):131–142.
14. Milne E, Johnston R, Cross D, et al. Effect of a school-based sun-protection intervention on the development of melanocytic nevi in children. Am J Epidemiol 2002; 155:739–745.
15. Weinstock MA. Assessment of sun sensitivity by questionnaire: validity of items and formulation of a predictive rule. J Clin Epidemiol 1992; 45(5):547–552.
16. Montague M, Borland R, Sinclair C. Slip! Slap! Slop! and SunSmart, 1980–2000: skin cancer control and 20 years of population-based campaigning. Health Educ Behav 2001; 28(3):290–305.
17. Glanz K, Greinert R, English D, Halpern AC. Primary prevention of melanoma: update from the United States, Europe, and Australia. Skin Cancer Found J 2006; 14:59–61.
18. Severi G, English DR. Descriptive epidemiology of skin cancer. In: Hill D, Elwood JM, English DR, eds. Prevention of Skin Cancer. Dordrecht: Kluwer Academic Publishers, 2004:73–88.
19. http://www.euroskin.info/ (accessed December 2005).
20. http://www.sunsmart.com.au/ (accessed December 2005).
21. Steffen AD, Glanz K, Wilkens LR. Dimensionality, Reliability, and Differential Item Functioning for Two Measures of 'Usual Sun Protection Practices'. At Developing Consensus Measures of Skin Cancer Prevention Behaviors: An Investigators' Workshop. Atlanta: NCI/Emory University, December 2005.

18

Screening for Melanoma

Alan C. Geller

Department of Dermatology, School of Medicine,
School of Public Health, Boston University, Boston, Massachusetts, U.S.A.

INTRODUCTION

Incidence and mortality rates for melanoma are rising faster than for nearly all other cancers (1). Occurring in nearly 60,000 Americans each year (2), invasive melanoma is a potentially fatal malignancy for which cure depends critically on early diagnosis (3). Typically, screening and early diagnosis are greatly facilitated by the tumor's visibility from its onset, its highly characteristic clinical features, and the existence of a minimally invasive, definitive diagnostic test (skin biopsy) (3). Visual examination by a qualified healthcare provider should improve early detection (3,4).

In the absence of population-based screening recommendations, targeting screening to those at greatest risk of advanced melanoma warrants public health attention. Of particular relevance to mortality rates, during the past decade, the incidence of thick tumors (>4 mm) increased significantly only in males aged 60 and older (5). Nearly, 50% of all melanoma deaths in the United States are in white men aged 50 and above (6). It is well documented that men particularly those aged over 50 have higher incidence and mortality rates for melanoma (7–8). Among this group, screening yield could be further enhanced by physician and patient's awareness of changing moles or skin type.

In this chapter, we discuss the rationale and definition of melanoma screening, identify high-risk populations and appropriate venues for screening and education, and propose strategies and steps needed to instigate and promote discussion.

RATIONALE AND DEFINITIONS FOR MELANOMA SCREENING

Screening and early detection programs could save many lives otherwise lost by melanoma. This cancer is external and visible, readily discernible risk factors are well established, and screening tests are safe and acceptable to the public. Furthermore, early melanoma can be cured by simple surgical excision. Melanoma screening runs the gamut from an average-risk person conducting casual self-examination to high-risk persons (without disease) undergoing careful, regular, and systematic monthly examination of the entire skin by a skin-cancer specialist (8–10).

However, without randomized trials testing the efficacy of screening for melanoma, recent evidence-based guidelines have not endorsed routine screening.

APPLICATIONS OF SCREENING DEFINITIONS TO MELANOMA

Distinguishing screening from early detection, education, and case finding can be challenging in this visible tumor. However, this might be simply a semantic exercise and have little bearing or relevance. Precise definitions of the word "screening" could apply to any process of visually examining the skin for early detection: a narrower use would distinguish screening from "surveillance," "case-finding" (when searching for cancer within a routine physical examination by a physician), "early detection," and "opportunistic surveillance." Furthermore, screening can take place in a variety of settings: within the physician examination at his or her office, at health fairs, workplaces, or in mass efforts where persons select themselves to attend (8–11).

Trying to apply standard textbook definitions of cancer screening to melanoma underscores the difficulties of making rigid distinctions between screening and education. As an external tumor, melanoma should be more readily discovered than other types of cancer—"melanoma writes its message in the skin with its own ink and is there for all to see" (12). Education can alert the public about the ways to recognize melanoma, especially stressing the Asymmetry, Border irregularity, Color, and Diameter (ABCD) or Asymmetry, Border, Color, Diameter, Evolution (ABCDE) rule of melanoma (13–14). Publicity should also promote awareness of risk factors, prompt medical attention for suspect lesions, and improve skin self-examination rates for high-risk persons. Because patients may be unaware of melanoma on the back and other areas that are difficult for self-inspection, visual examinations by physicians, nurses, family members, and others could aid early detection. Professional education can be facilitated by melanoma's unique visual nature and teaching through pictorial displays, digital photographs, and Web-based education.

THEORETICAL ASPECTS OF MELANOMA SCREENING

Cancer screening helps most when (*i*) the disease is highly prevalent and causes considerable morbidity and mortality, (*ii*) the natural history of the disease is known, (*iii*) early treatment can prevent morbidity and mortality, and (*iv*) an acceptable, safe, and a relatively inexpensive screening test exists (11).

Using these criteria, many cancer-control experts would agree that cutaneous melanoma screening has theoretic appeal, but has a number of barriers as well (Table 1). In the United States, the disease is increasingly prevalent, with rising incidence and mortality rates (although plateauing in the past 10 years) (1,6). Surgical treatment of early thin melanoma can lead to cure, whereas metastatic melanoma remains generally incurable. The screening examination (a visual examination by a qualified observer) can take only a few minutes, is safe and acceptable, and is regarded by many as reliable in diagnostic situations. Such examinations could detect melanoma on the back and posterior legs (which cannot be viewed easily by the person with the lesion). Moreover, skin-screening examinations also offer opportunities for personalized health education at a teachable moment (3,15).

Some biologic and clinical considerations, however, may diminish the effect of screening, most notably (*i*) a fraction of melanomas may be amelanotic, or clinically unrecognizable, reducing the sensitivity of skin examinations, (*ii*) the radial growth phase in some melanomas may be absent (e.g., nodular melanoma) or of too short duration for detection by periodic screening, (*iii*) a significant minority of melanoma might arise de novo with a brief or even non-existent "window" for earlier detection, and (*iv*) screening can introduce a host of biases, such as lead-time bias or length bias, or uncover "pseudodisease" (thin non-metastasizing form of melanoma) (16–19). Future studies should consider the benefits, including potential cost reductions of diagnosing unsuspected nonmelanoma skin cancer within the context of a screen for melanoma.

Table 1 Facilitators and Barriers for Melanoma Screening

Facilitators
  Natural history of the disease is well known for most invasive melanoma
  Rising incidence and mortality rates
  Easily identifiable risk factors
  Many at-risk individuals currently in healthcare system
  Physicians can examine hard-to-see areas
Barriers
  Lack of randomized clinical trial
  Prohibitive costs for screening trial
  Lack of fully trained medical force
  Issues of melanoma thickness as key outcome variable

DEFINING CRITERIA FOR SUCCESSFUL CONTROL PROGRAMS

Finding a reduction in melanoma mortality rates within a screened versus unscreened population is the major goal for melanoma control. With the apparent cessation of the screening trial in Australia, it should be noted that no randomized trial or definitive data about mortality reduction from screening exists; therefore, current recommendations for skin-cancer screening vary greatly. Launching such a study would pose significant logistical challenges, requiring screening and follow-up of nearly a million persons for years (and perhaps even a decade or more), costing millions of dollars, and training a large medical force (8,10).

Intermediate endpoints other than mortality rates may include documenting fewer late-stage or thick lesions in a defined population. Trials must be able to accurately monitor such measures; national Surveillance, Epidemiology, and End Result Registry (SEER) registries would need to be used, as some state-based registries still do not record tumor thickness more than 10 years after an initial report (20–21). Still other evaluations tracking intermediate outcome measures (after initiating screening or education) provide initial data but require careful interpretation in light of possible biases. In an analysis of trends in Australia and New Zealand, Burton and Armstrong emphasized the importance of measuring the reduction of thick tumors, as there has been a large increase in the incidence of very thin melanomas (16).

Other types of studies offer initial data to evaluate screening programs. Case-control studies, such as Berwick et al.'s (22) study on self-screening for melanoma, can provide critical information. Surveillance studies following the establishment of community pigmented lesion clinics is another approach (23).

Economic savings represent yet another potential measure of evaluating a skin-cancer control program. Tsao et al. (24) provided a baseline estimate of melanoma-related costs in the United States. The annual direct cost of treating newly diagnosed melanoma in 1997 was estimated to be $563 million. Stage I and II disease, each comprised about 5% of the total cost; stage III and IV disease consumed 34% and 55% of the total cost, respectively. About 90% of the total annual direct cost of treating melanoma in 1997 was attributable to <20% of patients with advanced disease (24).

SCREENING RECOMMENDATIONS FOR MELANOMA

Herein, we review recommendations (1989–2001) from many influential organizations. No randomized trials have examined the efficacy of different strategies for the early detection of melanoma, although a promising randomized trial had successfully recruited numerous Queensland communities before its recent cessation (25). Recommendations from the early 1990s to mid-decade were diverse, but more recent recommendations have not endorsed population-based screening. It is worth noting that increased attention to evidence-based recommendations has resulted in changes in the United States Preventive Services

Task Force (USPSTF) series of three recommendations from 1989 to 2001. The 1989 report recommended screening for high-risk populations (family or personal history of skin cancer, clinical evidence of precursor lesions, and those with increased occupational or recreational exposure to sunlight). The 1996 USPSTF found insufficient evidence to recommend for or against either routine screening for skin cancer by primary care providers. Most recently, the Third United States Preventive Services Task Force (2001) concluded, "evidence is lacking that the skin examination by clinicians is effective in reducing mortality or morbidity from skin cancer" (26–27).

The Institute of Medicine report (2000) concluded that there is "insufficient evidence to support positive or negative conclusions about the adoption of a new program of clinical screening of asymptomatic Medicare beneficiaries" (28). However, since the publication of these recommendations, there has been no federal initiative to improve risk assessment, screening, or education to this high-risk group.

IDENTIFICATION OF HIGH-RISK POPULATIONS AND APPROPRIATE VENUES FOR SCREENING AND EDUCATION

With evidence pointing away from endorsement of new population-based screening programs, an important challenge to national programs for skin cancer education and screening is the identification of individuals who are at greater than average risk of developing melanoma and who therefore might benefit most from screening. Because it will allow effective targeting, this identification process would improve the success and acceptability of skin cancer education and screening programs, while decreasing the societal cost.

Men 50 Years of Age and Above

It is well documented that men particularly those aged over 50 have higher incidence and mortality rates for melanoma (29–34) and a recent population-based study using the Florida Tumor Registry found males to be more than twice as likely to have late-stage melanoma (35). Birth-cohort adjusted incidence rates show even more striking differences between men and women (36). This may reflect less prudent lifetime sun exposure, less sun protection, or exposure of a larger proportion of the body among men, although as yet unrecognized biologic factors may also contribute. In the future, as the population ages and melanoma rates continue to increase in the "baby boomer generation," the relatively high morbidity and mortality of older men is expected to be even more striking (36). Likewise, 50% of deaths from melanoma in New South Wales, Australia occur in males over 50 (37) prompting a call for improved opportunistic screening by Australian general practitioners at the time of medical visits for other reasons (38). In Australia, the mortality for men aged 60 and over has also increased, with a plateau in the rest of the population (37).

Hospital-based studies also indicate that men had thicker lesions (median 1.4 mm vs. 1.0 mm), as well as more ulcerated and fewer extremity lesions than did women (39). In particular, men with back lesions had worse survival rates as compared with women ($P = 0.163$). Another retrospective study of 674 patients in a tertiary referral center in New South Wales, Australia found that men were more likely than women to be diagnosed with thick lesions (exceeding 3.00 mm) (40).

Social Class

Melanoma incidence rates correlate with higher social class status, attributed by some to recreational sun exposure. However, five studies have found disproportionate mortality among persons of lower socioeconomic status (SES) (41–44). One study of melanoma cases and deaths in Massachusetts found case-fatality rates to be 50% higher in persons of low SES (44).

Data from more than 28,000 cancer patients in Florida found that the uninsured were more likely than persons with insurance to be diagnosed with late stage melanoma OR = 2.59, $P = 0.004$. Patients insured by Medicaid compared with commercial indemnity insurance were more likely diagnosed at a late stage of melanoma (OR = 4.69, $P < 0.001$) (45).

Special screenings of World War II veterans, particularly those from specific regions, may have some merit as it has been suggested that exposure to high levels of solar radiation in young adulthood, in the World War II Pacific and European theaters, was associated with a higher risk of melanoma mortality (46).

CURRENT VENUES IN MELANOMA SCREENING AND EDUCATION

Dermatologist-Delivered Skin Cancer Screening (United States)

The annual American Academy of Dermatology (AAD) screening programs have provided free screening and education to more than one million Americans, with 1.2 million screenings being performed since 1985 (47). In the spring of each year, local and national media publicize the risk factors and the warning signs for melanoma/skin cancer (48).

The yield and predictive value of confirmed melanoma according to demographics and risk factors recorded during screening have been demonstrated. Middle-aged and older men (≥ 50 years) comprised 25.2% of AAD screenees but 44.4% of confirmed cases. The overall yield of melanoma (number of confirmed cases per number of screenees) was 1.5/1000 (363/242, 374) in contrast to 2.6/1000 among men ≥ 50 years. The yield was further improved for men ≥ 50 years who reported either a changing mole (4.6/1000) or skin type I/II (3.8/1000). The predictive value of a screening diagnosis of melanoma was more than twice as high for men ≥ 50 years, with either a changing mole or skin type I/II compared with all other participants (49).

AAD programs have detected thinner lesions than have been recorded in population-based registries, however, these programs are conducted among self-selected populations, and subject to bias (48). More than 98% of confirmed melanomas in AAD screenings (1992–1994) were localized and more than 90% were in situ or thin lesions. The 8.3% of AAD cases with advanced melanoma is a lower proportion than that reported by the 1990 SEER (48). Of persons with a confirmed melanoma, 39% indicated that without the free program, they would not have considered having a physician examine their skin.

Evaluation of AAD programs found that the predictive value positive of a visual examination by a dermatologist for melanoma was 27% to 31% in Massachusetts screenings (1986–1989) and 17% in national AAD screenings (1992–1994) (48,50). Rampen et al. (51) linked information on 1551 persons with a negative screening result with population-based registries (during 42 months of follow-up), and they found 15 persons with new skin cancers. Of these, three were present at the 1990 screening, and most likely were missed; 12 were considered to have new lesions. No melanomas were found among the missed cases.

Available data suggest that the cost-effectiveness of such screenings is comparable to that of other cancer screenings, including breast cancer (52). Freedberg et al. (52) found that AAD skin cancer screening increased both life expectancy and quality-adjusted life expectancy. Although the AAD screen could not be directly compared with other cancer-screening cost-effectiveness studies, a one-time skin cancer screening was generally comparable in cost-effectiveness to screening for breast cancer in women aged 55 to 65 (53). There were strong benefits for men 50 years of age and above (52).

A single study of Massachusetts screenees attempted to quantify the educational effect of screenings. In an analysis of 643 Massachusetts residents with positive screening diagnoses, rates of self-screening improved from 60% prior to screening to 84% after screening; physician examinations improved from 39% to 55% (54).

Dermatologist-Delivered Skin-Cancer Screening (International)

In general, international screening efforts have yielded similar results to those found in the United States. Rampen et al. (55) yielded similar findings in a screening of 2564 self-selected participants in the Netherlands. Nine melanomas were pathologically confirmed. Hoffman et al. (56) reported on-screening activities in Bochum, Germany that resulted in 14 melanomas being diagnosed in a screening population of 1467.

Yield in melanoma screening among 520 residents of British Columbia, Canada for the period 1994 and 1995 were virtually identical to U.S. studies (57). A French study in the occupational setting demonstrated the efficiency of this maneuver (58).

Rossi et al. (59) reported on programs with intensive pre-screening outreach in Italy. Screening organizers produced 90,000 leaflets in a population of

243,000, leading to 2050 individuals attending screening programs. The sensitivity and the predictive value of the visual examination were 93% and 7%, respectively (59–61).

SCREENING IN THE PRIMARY CARE SETTING

Screening Data

Despite increased publicity and increased attention to screening during the 1990s, recent Federal data indicate that the proportion of Americans reporting that they had ever received a screening examination remained static at 21% from 1992 to 1998 (62). Screening rates among more than 30,000 people completing the National Health Interview Survey Cancer Control Supplement (1992, 1998) were lowest among younger persons, people with less than a high school degree, and those living close to the poverty line (62).

STRATEGIES TO IMPROVE MELANOMA SCREENING AND EDUCATION

Rationale

Melanoma patients typically have contacts with physicians in the year before diagnosis, suggesting many lesions might be diagnosed earlier. Routine examinations provide an excellent opportunity for melanoma detection.

In one study of 216 melanoma cases, 87% had regular physicians and 63% had seen those physicians in the year prior to diagnosis, but only 24% of patients had examined their own skin prior to diagnosis, and 20% reported physician skin examinations (although data on patient recollection of physician skin examinations may be an underestimate) (63). Fewer than 20% of Americans have a dermatologist (47), whereas approximately 85% see a physician every two years (64). In a single study, physician-detected melanoma compared with patient or family detection was associated with an increase in the probability of detecting thinner (<0.75 mm) melanomas (relative risk, 4.2 95% confidence interval, 1.4–11.1; $P = 0.01$) (65). An Australian study of the cost-effectiveness of every five-year screening for melanoma by family practice physicians for men over the age of 50 found a cost-effectiveness of Aus \$6900/yr of life saved for men (66).

Performance of Physicians in Screening and Education

Early detection by physicians should be exceedingly important, but their ability to detect melanoma has not been well studied. Screening performance has very important implications if physicians are to be involved in randomized trials testing the efficacy of this procedure or if they are to serve as "gatekeepers" in large managed care organizations.

Primary care physicians are in a unique position to perform cancer screenings and to provide prevention counseling, as approximately 40% of office visits to physicians in the United States are to a family practitioner or internist (67). Almost all physician-detected melanoma is discovered by primary care physicians rather than specialists (68). However, while most melanoma patients have at least one primary care visit in the year prior to diagnosis, only 20% report receiving a skin cancer examination (68). While physicians should be attuned to the risk factors of all of their patients, professional education efforts should inform non-dermatologist physicians about the features of early cutaneous melanoma, such as new or changing moles (13–14).

How Can Screening Yield Be Boosted?

Strategies to improve mass screening and education for skin cancer with a particular emphasis on middle-aged and older men emerge from an analysis of more than 200,000 Americans attending the AAD's free national skin cancer screening programs during the 1990s (49). Many current venues exist to optimize screening of these high-risk individuals (Table 2).

First, the melanoma yield and predictive value among middle-aged and older men is nearly double that for any other age and sex group (49). In general, in the absence of mass screening, these men are less likely than women to see a dermatologist, have a regular doctor, or practice self-examination for skin cancer, and presumably at least in part for these reasons tend to present with more advanced melanoma with higher associated case-fatality (29–33). This suggests that in order to optimize benefit from mass skin cancer screening and public education, publicity campaigns should expand outreach to men aged 50 and above. Efforts might center on workplaces and recreational activities frequented by men in this age group.

Second, a person's perception of a changing mole was a strong predictor of melanoma. Over 50% of screenees with confirmed melanoma reported that they had a changing mole. This confirms an earlier report that a persistently changed or changing mole was the strongest prediagnostic indicator for melanoma (69).

Table 2 Venues for Screening and Education for Middle-Aged and Older Men

Physician's offices
Public health clinics
American Academy of Dermatology national screenings
Recreational settings
Workplaces
National media efforts
Family education, via spouse and significant other
Corporate sponsorship, in retail outlets frequented by men
Screenings for other health conditions such as prostate cancer, hypertension

Many of those with a changing mole did not have a dermatologist and reported that they would not have seen a doctor for a skin examination if they had not attended the screening. This suggests that the mass screening provides an important service for these people and that special outreach to those who are aware of a changing mole is appropriate, even if this factor has low specificity. Third, the yield of screening middle-aged persons with another key risk factor, namely, fair skin, also results in a relatively high screening yield.

Steps for Improving Screening Rates for High-Risk Individuals

Improving the rate of screening examinations for melanoma will be best accomplished through a multi-pronged approach. These components include (*i*) health policy revisions, (*ii*) changes at the health plan/insurance level, (*iii*) public education, (*iv*) professional education, and (*v*) legislative efforts.

In the following sections, we outline the major components of a national proposal, recommend steps to monitor the development and implementation of the plan, and review the principal challenges to such a plan. While some of the proposals are better suited to the U.S. healthcare system, we hope that many of the ideas could be applicable to other nations.

The cornerstone of our proposal is that all Caucasian Americans 50 years of age and above receive a baseline skin cancer examination performed by a physician skilled in the examination or having the motivation and ability to triage successfully. This would appear to be the most cost-effective first step, and the evidence from this effort could be used toward planning for at-risk Americans from other age groups, if warranted. Examinations should be paid for by mandated coverage, including federally funded programs. Uninsured people should have opportunities for free or low-cost skin cancer screening such as through annual mass-screening programs. Consensus should be established on issues such as the precise definitions of the high-risk population and optimal time periods for repeat screens, according to findings during the initial (or baseline) screen. As consensus evolves, a prudent policy would call for high-risk individuals, such as those with atypical moles, self-reports of changing moles, or those with prior suspicious biopsy findings, to be actively tracked and followed.

Major Components of a National Plan

Initiate Policy Changes

1. In states where major healthcare plans share and disseminate a common set of practice guidelines to all physicians, adherence to these guidelines should be evaluated. These consortia also provide educational tools, learning opportunities, and strategies to facilitate improvement within and between the organizations. Massachusetts Health Quality Partnership has recently adopted a series of skin cancer screening recommendations (70).

2. Medicaid experiment: States occasionally allow for demonstration projects to evaluate innovative approaches in the provision of health services. In high-incidence states, such as Florida (discussed subsequently), where state legislation has led to more expedient referrals to dermatologists, demonstration programs could experiment with providing the needed service in the Medicaid population.
3. Emphasize the inclusion of melanoma screening in health maintenance organizations (HMOs) with predominantly elderly populations as one third of melanoma deaths are in the Medicare population and mortality rates have increased nearly 100% from 1969 to 1999 among persons aged above 65 (6). Mandated coverage for melanoma screening over age 50 should be explored in HMOs that primarily insure elderly patients, including Medicare.

Seek Changes at the Health Plan Level

1. Educate managed care medical directors and HMO providers about the cost benefits of melanoma screening. Available data suggest that the cost-effectiveness of such screening is generally comparable to that of other cancer screenings (52,71).
2. Bundle services: Include screening or information about melanoma screening and skin self-examinations with other health promotion activities for middle-aged and older people, such as other cancer screenings, flu shots, blood pressure screenings, and diabetes checks.
3. Update medical intake forms to highlight prominent major risks for melanoma, such as family history of melanoma, changing moles, or multiple atypical moles (69,72–73).
4. Enhance follow-up systems to improve screening; computerized tracking should remind patients of the risk factors for melanoma.
5. Implement risk-assessment strategies. Primary care providers should assess risk for melanoma and triage (74) or treat patients at increased melanoma risk: older age with fair complexion, patients with numerous and/or atypical moles, strong family history of melanoma, nonmelanoma skin cancer, excessive sun exposure prior to age 20, or blistering childhood sunburns.

Expand Public Outreach

1. Actively educate health plan members via websites, regular newsletters, targeted mailings, and family educational evenings. Computerized access to specific age and gender groups should promote more selective, tailored educational strategies. Pictures showing the ABCDE (14) warning signs for early melanoma accompanied by messages below can be distributed to health plan members.
2. Skin-cancer advocacy organizations can work with organizations such as the American Association of Retired Persons to notify

Medicare recipients about ways to improve physician screening and attention to abnormal skin lesions. Although Medicare does not cover screening for skin cancer in asymptomatic people, it does cover a physician visit initiated by a concerned patient who has noticed, for example, a change in the color of a mole or a new skin growth (28).

3. AAD screenings generally reach 80,000 individuals per year; among these attendees, 50% have no other source of dermatologic care (75). Special efforts must continue to be made to reach individuals without any access to dermatology care and actively recruit high-risk individuals who have yet to be screened in the AAD-sanctioned and other skin cancer screening programs.

Augment Provider Education

1. Provide practical resources that busy physicians can use most efficiently to get melanoma screening for high-risk patients into routine visits:

    Provide physicians with reminders of high-risk patient profile, stamping charts if necessary as successfully used for tobacco counseling reminders (76).

    Develop waiting-room materials such as wall posters to motivate patients to seek skin evaluation from their primary physician.

    Remind physicians that comprehensive skin examination takes no more than one to three minutes, that it can be highly effective even if performed only once per year, and that it can be focussed on high-risk, but hard-to-see areas, such as the back, where at least a third of melanomas are found in men (77) and sun-exposed areas (head, neck, and arms) for certain melanoma subtypes in older individuals (77).

2. Involve nurse practitioners and physician assistants in preventive screening.

3. Participate in skin cancer educational courses such as the online Basic Skin Cancer Triage curriculum to overcome physician obstacles of lack of training and confidence. This two-hour curriculum has been shown to improve diagnostic and triage skills of clinicians as well as to increase their confidence in both detecting and counseling patients about skin cancer (74).

Advocate for Legislation to Support Increased Melanoma Screening and Education

1. Promote a mandate for a federally funded melanoma screening and education program, with Medicare coverage and Medicaid options for follow-up and treatment services for persons with positive results from melanoma screening.

2. Educate state and federal legislators on the necessity of reserving funding for melanoma-screening programs.
3. Expedite referrals to dermatologists. In 1997, the Florida legislature adopted new legislation that allows for direct access for Florida residents to see a dermatologist. Health services researchers should be charged to determine the effectiveness of the screening process and to evaluate whether higher screening rates and earlier diagnosis are attained in a cost-effective manner.

In conclusion, we suggest that male sex and age over 50 be added to other established risk factors for melanoma. We suggest that improving screening of these middle-aged and older men will boost case finding for melanoma, reduce unnecessary deaths, and result in a more cost-effective screening. Although, the yield of melanoma may be lower in primary care settings than in dermatologist-led mass screening, we propose that generalist physicians examine the skin of their middle-aged and older male patients during visits for other problems. As "melanoma writes its message in the skin with all of us to see," (12) other family members should be alerted to the risk of new moles, changing moles, or unusual moles in this age group. This is of particular importance as men in this age group are less likely than women to examine their own skin for melanoma.

We call on leading cancer advocacy organizations, medical societies, dermatologists, directors of managed health plans, and federal health officials to convene to develop a national five-year plan for boosting screening rates for melanoma, particularly for high-risk middle-aged and older men.

REFERENCES

1. Jemal A, Clegg LX, Ward E, et al. Wingo PA. Annual report to the nation on the status of cancer, 1975–2001, with a special feature regarding survival. Cancer 2004; 101: 3–27, also accessed at www.seer.cancer.gov.
2. Jemal A, Murray T, Ward E, et al. Cancer statistics, 2005. CA Cancer J Clin 2005; 55:10–30.
3. Koh HK. Cutaneous melanoma. N Engl J Med 1991; 325:171–182.
4. Tsao H, Atkins MB, Sober AJ. Management of cutaneous melanoma. N Engl J Med 2004; 351:998–1012.
5. Jemal A, Devesa SS, Hartge P, Tucker MA. Recent trends in cutaneous melanoma: incidence among whites in the United States. J Natl Cancer Inst 2001; 93:678–683.
6. National Center for Health Statistics. Vital statistics mortality data multiple cause of death detail (machine-readable public use data tape). Maryland, U.S.: Bethesda Maryland, 2004.
7. Geller AC, Miller DR, Annas GD, Demierre MF, Gilchrest BA, Koh HK. Melanoma incidence and mortality among U.S. whites, 1969–1999. JAMA 2002; 288: 1719–1720.
8. Koh HK, Geller AC, Miller DR, Grossbart TA, Lew RA. Prevention and early detection strategies for melanoma and skin cancer. Arch Dermatol 1996; 132:436–443.

9. Koh HK, Geller AC, Lew RA. Melanoma. In: Kramer BS, Gohagan JK, Prorok PC, eds. Cancer Screening Theory and Practice. New York-Basel: Marcel Dekker, Inc., 1999:379–408.
10. Geller AC. Issues in melanoma screening. In: Rigel DR, ed. Special Edition on Melanoma and Pigmented Lesions in Dermatologic Clinics of North America. Vol. 20. Philadelphia, PA: WB Saunders Company, 2002:629–641.
11. Miller A. Screening for Cancer. Orlando, Fl: Academic Press, 1985.
12. Davis N. Modern concepts of melanoma and its management. Ann Plast Surg 1978; 1:628–629.
13. Friedman RJ, Rigel DS, Silverman MK, Kopf AW, Vossaert KA. Malignant melanoma in the 1990's: the continued importance of early detection and the role of physician examination and self-examination of the skin. CA Cancer J Clin 1991; 41:201–226.
14. Abbasi NR, Shaw HM, Rigel DS, et al. Early diagnosis of cutaneous melanoma: revisiting the ABCD criteria. JAMA 2004; 292:2771–2776.
15. Rigel DS. Is the ounce of screening and prevention for skin cancer worth the pound of cure? CA Cancer J Clin 1998; 48:236–238.
16. Burton R, Armstrong B. Recent incidence trends imply a nonmetastasizing form of invasive melanoma. Melanoma Res 1994; 4:107–113.
17. Swerlick RA, Chen S. The melanoma epidemic: is increased surveillance the solution or the problem? Arch Dermatol 1996; 132:881–884.
18. Elwood JM. Screening for melanoma and options for its evaluation. J Med Screen 1994; 1:22–38.
19. Andersen WK, Silvers DN. 'Melanoma'? It can't be melanoma: a subset of melanomas that defines clinical recognition. JAMA 1991; 266:3463–3465.
20. Koh HK, Adame N, Geller AC, et al. Cancer registry data on melanomas (letter). N Engl J Med 1990; 323:921–922.
21. Merlino LA, Sullivan KJ, Whitaker DC, Lynch CF. The independent pathology laboratory as a reporting source for cutaneous melanoma incidence in Iowa, 1977–1994. J Am Acad Dermatol 1997; 37:578–585.
22. Berwick M, Begg CB, Fine JA, Roush GC, Barnhill RL. Screening for cutaneous melanoma by skin self-examination. J Natl Cancer Inst 1996; 88:17–23.
23. MacKie RM, Hole D. Audit of public education campaign to encourage earlier detection of malignant melanoma. BMJ 1992; 304:1012–1015.
24. Tsao H, Rogers G, Sober A. An estimate of the annual direct cost of treating cutaneous melanoma. J Am Acad Dermatol 1998; 38:669–680.
25. Aitken JF, Elwood JM, Lowe JB, Firman DW, Balanda KP, Ring IT. A randomised trial of population screening for melanoma. J Med Screen 2002; 9:33–37.
26. US Preventive Services Task Force. Guide to Clinical Preventive Services. 2nd ed. Baltimore: Williams Wilkins, 1996.
27. Helfand M, Mahon SM, Eden KB, Frame PS, Orleans CT. Screening for skin cancer. Am J Prev Med April 2001; 20(3 suppl):47–58.
28. Institute of Medicine. Extending Medicare Coverage for Prevention and Other Services. Washington, D.C.: National Academy Press, 2000.
29. Death rates of malignant melanoma among white men—United States, 1973–1988. MMWR 1992; 41:20–21, 27.
30. Hersey P, Sillar RW, Howe CG, et al. Factors related to the presentation of patients with thick primary melanomas. Med J Aust 1991; 154:583–587.

31. Cooke KR, McNoe BM. Targeting early detection of malignant melanoma of the skin. N Z Med J 1991; 103:551–553.
32. Swetter SM, Geller AC, Kirkwood JM. Melanoma in the older person. Oncology 2004; 18:1187–1196; discussion 1196–1197.
33. Chamberlain AJ, Kelly JW. Nodular melanomas and older men: a major challenge for community surveillance programs. Med J Aust 2004; 180:432.
34. Demierre MF. Thin melanomas and regression, thick melanomas and older men: prognostic implications and perspectives on secondary prevention. Arch Dermatol 2002; 138:678–682.
35. Van Durme DJ, Ferrante JM, Pal N, et al. Demographic predictors of melanoma stage at diagnosis. Arch Fam Med 2000; 9:606–611.
36. Dennis LK. Increasing risk of melanoma with increasing age. JAMA 1999; 282:1037–1038.
37. Hanrahan PF, Hersey P, D'Este CA. Factors involved in presentation of older people with thick melanoma. Med J Aust 1998; 169:410–414.
38. Kelly JW. Melanoma in the elderly: a neglected public health challenge. Med J Aust 1998; 169:403–404.
39. Balch C, Soong S, Shaw H. An analysis of prognostic factors in 8500 patients with cutaneous melanoma. In: Balch C, Houghton A, Milton G, eds. Cutaneous Melanoma. Philadelphia: Lippincott, 1992:165–187.
40. Bonnett A, Roder D, Esterman A. Epidemiological features of melanoma in South Australia: implications for cancer control. Med J Aust 1989; 151:502–509.
41. Geller AC, Miller DR, Lew RA, Clapp RW, Wenneker MB, Koh HK. Cutaneous melanoma mortality among the socioeconomically disadvantaged in Massachusetts. Am J Public Health 1996; 86:538–543.
42. MacKie RM, Hole DJ. Incidence and thickness of primary tumours and survival of patients with cutaneous malignant melanoma in relation to socioeconomic status [see comments]. BMJ 1996; 312:1125–1128.
43. Shaw HM. Cutaneous malignant melanoma: occupation and prognosis. Med J Aust 1981; 1:37–38.
44. Vagero D, Persson G. Risks, survival and trends of malignant melanoma among white and blue collar workers in Sweden. Soc Sci Med 1984; 19:475–478.
45. Roetzheim RG, Pal N, Tennant C, et al. Effects of health insurance and race on early detection of cancer. J Natl Cancer Inst 1999; 91:1409–1415.
46. Page WF, Whiteman D, Murphy M. A comparison of melanoma mortality among WW II veterans of the Pacific and European theaters. Ann Epidemiol 2000; 10:192–195.
47. American Academy of Dermatology, Schaumburg IL.
48. Koh HK, Norton LA, Geller AC, et al. Evaluation of the American Academy of Dermatology's National Skin Cancer Early Detection and Screening Program. J Am Acad Dermatol 1996; 34:971–978.
49. Geller AC, Sober AJ, Zhang Z, et al. Strategies for improving melanoma education and screening for men age 50+ years. Cancer 2002; 95:1554–1561.
50. Koh HK, Geller AC, Miller DR, Caruso A, Gage I, Lew RA. Who is being screened for melanoma/skin cancer? J Am Acad Dermatol 1991; 24:271–277.
51. Rampen FHJ, Casparie-van Velsen IJ, van Huystee BE, et al. False-negative findings in skin cancer and melanoma screening. J Am Acad Dermatol 1995; 33:59–63.
52. Freedberg KA, Geller AC, Miller DR, Lew RA, Koh HK. Screening for malignant melanoma: a cost-effectiveness analysis. J Am Acad Dermatol 1999; 41:738–745.

53. Eddy DR. Screening for breast cancer. Ann Intern Med 1990; 111:389–399.
54. Geller AC, Halpern AC, Sun T, et al. Participant satisfaction and value in American Academy of Dermatology and American Cancer Society Skin Cancer Screening Programs in Massachusetts. J Am Acad Dermatol 1999; 40:563–566.
55. Rampen FHJ, van Huysteee EWL, Kiemeney LALM. Melanoma/skin cancer screening clinics: experience in the Netherlands. J Am Acad Dermatol 1991; 25:776–777.
56. Hoffman K, Dirschka T, Schatz H, et al. A local education campaign on early diagnosis of malignant melanoma. Eur J Epidemiol 1993; 9:591–598.
57. Engleberg D, Gallagher RP, Rivers JK. Follow-up and evaluation of skin cancer screening in British Columbia. J Am Acad Dermatol 1999; 41:37–42.
58. Guibert P, Mollat F, Ligen M, Dreno B. Melanoma screening: report of a survey in occupational medicine. Arch Dermatol 2000; 136:199–202.
59. Rossi CR, Vecchiato A, Bezze G, et al. Early detection of melanoma: an educational campaign in Padova, Italy. Melanoma Res 2000; 10:181–187.
60. Bulliard JL, Levi F, Panizzon RG. The 2003 Solmobile prevention campaign for skin cancers of the Swiss League against cancer: results and stakes. Rev Med Suisse Romande 2004; 124:237–240.
61. Lowe JB, Ball J, Lynch BM, et al. Acceptability and feasibility of a community-based screening program for melanoma in Australia. Health Promot Int 2004; 19:437–444.
62. Santmyire BR, Feldman SR, Fleischer AB Jr. Lifestyle high-risk behaviors and demographics may predict the level of participation in sun-protection behaviors and skin cancer primary prevention in the United States: results of the 1998 National Health Interview Survey. Cancer 2001; 92:1315–1324.
63. Koh HK, Miller DR, Geller AC, Clapp RW, Mercer MG, Lew RA. Who discovers melanoma? Patterns from a population-based survey. J Am Acad Dermatol 1992; 26:914–919.
64. Health, United States. Socioeconomic status and health chartbook. US Department of Health and Human Services, DHHS Publication Number (PHS) 98, 1998
65. Epstein DS, Lange JR, Gruber SB, et al. Is physician detection associated with thinner melanomas? JAMA 1999; 281:640–643.
66. Girgis A, Clarke P, Burton RC, Sanson-Fisher RW. Screening for melanoma by primary health care physicians: a cost-effectiveness analysis. J Med Screen 1996; 3:47–53.
67. Oliveria SA, Christos PJ, Halpern AC. Skin cancer screening and prevention in the primary care setting: national ambulatory medical care survey 1997. J Gen Intern Med 2001; 16:297–301.
68. Geller AC, Koh HK, Miller DR, Mercer MB, Lew RA. Health services before the diagnosis of melanoma. Implications for early detection and screening. J Gen Intern Med 1992; 3:154–158.
69. Rhodes AR, Weinstock MA, Fitzpatrick TB, et al. Risk factors for cutaneous melanoma: a practical method of recognizing predisposed individuals. JAMA 1987; 258:3146–3154.
70. Massachusetts Health Quality Partners, Inc., 2003.
71. Losina E, Walensky RP, GellerAC, Beddingfield FC, Gilchrest BA, Freedberg KA. Screening for malignant melanoma: clinical impact and cost-effectiveness. Arch Dermatol 2006 (in press).

72. Marrett LD, King WD, Walter SD, From S. Use of host factors to identify people at high risk for cutaneous malignant melanoma. Can Med Assoc J 1992; 147:445–453.

73. Ford D, Bliss JM, Swerdlow AJ, et al. Risk of cutaneous melanoma associated with a family history of the disease. The International Melanoma Analysis Group (IMAGE). Int J Cancer 1995; 62:377–381.

74. Mikkilineni R, Weinstock MA, Goldstein MG, Dube CE, Rossi JS. The impact of the basic skin cancer triage curriculum on providers' skills, confidence, and knowledge in skin cancer control. Prev Med 2002; 34:144–152.

75. Geller AC, Zhang Z, Sober AJ, et al. The first 15 years of the American academy of dermatology skin cancer screening programs (1985–1999). J Am Acad Dermatol 2003; 48:34–42.

76. Piper ME, Fiore MC, Smith SS, et al. Use of the vital sign stamp as a systematic screening tool to promote smoking cessation. Mayo Clin Proc 2003; 78:716–722.

77. Balch CM, Soong SJ, Shaw HM, et al. An analysis of prognostic factors in 8500 patients with cutaneous melanoma. In: Balch CM, Houghton AN, Milton GW, Sober AJ, Soong SJ, eds. Cutaneous Melanoma. 2nd ed. Philadelphia: JB Lippincott Company, 1992.

19

Communicating the Incalculable

Gunilla Jarlbro

Media and Communication Studies, Lund University, Lund, Sweden

The phenomenon of risk and its role in contemporary society is one of the questions most avidly debated by sociologists and other social scientific scholars. Three main theoretical perspectives in risk research emerged in the early 1980s and attained widespread acceptance in the 1990s. Anthropologist Mary Douglas (1) is the leading proponent of the first perspective, the social constructivist. In a nutshell, Douglas asserts that all perception of risk is culturally informed. In adopting this perspective, one deflects the objectivist's perspective and can make a distinction between objective and subjective risks. In other words, there is no objective risk to discover "out there" and all risks are socially constructed.

The second perspective is represented mainly by theoreticians Ulrich Beck (2) and Anthony Giddens (3). Beck and Giddens belong to the social constructivist school but differ from Douglas in that they discuss the changed nature of society. According to Beck, the hallmark of the risk society is that it no longer distributes goods like the industrial society; instead, there is a distribution of risks. In Beck's argument, some people are also affected more than others, by which means different risk positions in society arise. Beck also discusses the role of the mass media, insofar that risks are mutable and socially constructed and that these constructions are defined by actors including the media (4). Giddens' thoughts reveal similarities and dissimilarities with Beck's arguments. More so than Beck, Giddens emphasizes that to be able to feel trust, the individual is dependent on expert systems. Beck and Giddens alike, however, assert that modern risk is global rather than personal and invisible and vague rather than visible and predictable.

The third perspective originates with Foucault's writings on governmentality, which discuss how the state and other power systems control the people via risk discourses and strategies (5). The hallmark of these three perspectives is that they all stand in stark contrast to the objectivist's perspective or, if you prefer, the realistic perspective. Unlike the social constructivist, the objectivist's perspective is strongly influenced by technology and science. The fundamental principle is that risk is calculable and risk analysis thus entirely feasible. Risk is thus defined as the probability that an unfavorable event will occur. The difference between objective risk and risk perceived by the individual, subjective risk, is an important element of this perspective. Objective risk is tantamount to an actual risk, one that exists whether we as individuals are aware of it or not. Subjective risk is our perception of the actual risk. This kind of risk research often studies the difference between the risk perception of ordinary citizens and the experts' assessment of a specific risk (6). The accessibility of the risk, that is to say how easily people think about or make associations with it, is a key factor in risk perception. In this context, the media probably play a significant role.

The majority of Nordic research on risk and risk communication has been based on the objectivist's perspective. The social constructivists are highly critical of this use of the concept of risk. Douglas (1) believes that the sense of calculability and science embedded in the concept of risk is very appealing to the modern human being. She also asserts that most people instead imagine "danger" and fear when the concept of risk is presented to them. Beck (2), on the other hand, says that risks exist only in terms of our knowledge about them; if we are not aware of the risk, there is no risk. Without taking a position as to which of the two dominant perspectives may inherently be regarded as the most fruitful in research, we can confirm that the majority of communication research on the subject of risk has taken an objectivist's perspective. The social constructivist's perspective has been developed and used mainly by sociologists and social anthropologists, but media and communication scholars have shown greater interest in the social constructivist's perspective in recent years, with keener interest in studying how the media construct and represent risks.

In this chapter, I will be taking an intermediate position between the two perspectives, although in the minds of doctrinaire social constructivists, the perspective of this chapter would be purely objectivist, as I will be discussing both objective risk and subjective risk perceptions.

THE INDIVIDUAL'S RELATIONSHIP TO THE RISK

In connection with risk communication, it is naturally important to study the individual's relationship to the risk, which determines how the individual will work as an information processor, that is, how she accepts, rejects, processes and preserves the transmitted information. The objective risk for an individual may be high or low, just as the subjective perception of risk may be high or low. In other words, we may have four different relationships to a risk situation. On one side of the equation, we have the individuals at high objective risk who are also aware of it, that is, their subjective perception of risk is also high. This type of individual may be called a realist. On the other side, we have the optimists—individuals who dismiss the risk even though there is high objective risk. Finally, we have the pessimists—individuals whose objective risk is low, but who overestimate their personal risk—and the second type of realists, individuals whose perception of risk is adequate in relation to the objective risk. The primary target groups in connection with information about health risks are thus those who dismiss the risk—optimists—and those who overestimate the risk—pessimists. In one case, the goal is to heighten personal perception of risk and in the other to alleviate unnecessary fear and worry. This begs the question of what factors may conceivably explain why the individual dismisses or overestimates risks.

MEDIA IMPACT ON PEOPLE'S ASSESSMENT OF RISK

Risk perception, or people's ability to assess risk, is a comprehensive field of research. This type of risk studies is based mainly on an objectivist's perspective, and those engaged in it usually study risk perception among ordinary citizens and compare it to objective risk as calculated by experts. There is often a discrepancy between the assessments of the public and the experts. The phenomenon of risk communication comes into the picture in this context. Its purpose is to get the public to perform "accurate" risk assessments, which are meant to help induce individuals to take measures to reduce the risk. Several studies have also shown that the individuals who tend to dismiss risk situations often demonstrate the most reckless behavior. "Risk perception" is a complex and general term that incorporates many aspects. The individual's perception of the magnitude of the risk is a critical element, of course, but emotional aspects such as worry about the risk also seem significant. Jarlbro (7) also emphasizes that American studies do not always ask respondents about perceived magnitude of risk, but rather about concern or worry. In Swedish studies as well, "worry" is sometimes used rather than "perceived risk" or "risk perception" (8). The vagueness of the terminology impedes the interpretation and comparison of research findings, as scholars do not appear to be measuring the same phenomenon. The main interest of this chapter is not risk perception research, however, but rather the research that has studied the impact of the media on public risk perception and how we can communicate about risk.

A significant portion of international research related to media exposure and risk perception has been focussed on various kinds of health risks, and the bulk of that research has taken a quantitative approach. It is not terribly surprising that quantitative research has also had an objectivist's perspective, insofar as that scholars have studied respondents' perceptions of "general risk," that is, what is risky for others and what they consider risky for themselves, or "personal risk." A rather uncontested finding of this research has been that the media influence the public's assessment of general risk, whereas perception of personal risk is instead influenced by interpersonal communication (9). Studies that shed light on respondents' risk assessment in relation to their exposure to media have been based implicitly or explicitly on the agenda-setting theory. Assumptions were thus made that there is an association between high ranking on the media agenda and high ranking on the interpersonal agenda, that is, when certain risks are given widespread media coverage, it influences the public to assess those risks as greater than risks that the media have not covered (10,11). Theoretically, it is thus assumed that it is the media agenda that controls the interpersonal agenda. But Morton and Duck (11) believe that under certain circumstances—when the individual feels the stress, worry, feels exposed to risk, and so on—people may turn to the media for more information or confirmation. Nevertheless, the same authors believe that the relationship between the influence of the media versus the influence of interpersonal communication is more complex than postulated by earlier research. They claim that there is a mutual dependency between mass and interpersonal communication when it comes to what shapes human beliefs regarding health risks.

Research that studies the impact of the media on public risk perception has a hard time, other than at the aggregated level, empirically demonstrating the significance of the media when it comes to proving changes in how people assess risk over time.

Sjöberg (12), on the other hand, asserts that it is widely believed that the media are regarded as directly responsible for public risk perception but that the correlation is highly uncertain. If we study the public, we find that they allow themselves, not entirely uncritically, to be influenced by media coverage of risks. A Norwegian study thus shows that a full 75% of respondents believe that Norwegian newspapers exaggerate when they report risks related to food (13). Similar findings came out of a Swedish study in which three out of four respondents reported that increased media coverage of food-related risks had not increased their worry. The remaining respondents said that media coverage had increased their worry, but only for a short while (14). But Storstad (15) says that when discussing media impact on public perception of risk, one must consider the following: what risk is being discussed, the people's degree of control and volition, and the consequences of the risk.

As the cited research findings have shown, the results are often somewhat confusing when it comes to explaining the impact or significance of the media to people's risk perception. Other researchers are more critical of arguments that the media influence people's perception of risk and believe that media representations of risks have little bearing on people's everyday lives and their genuine concerns (16). Tulloch and Lupton (17) also criticize the arguments surrounding the significance of the media to the construction of the risk society and find instead in their ethnographical studies that people form their perceptions via their everyday experience and in interaction with other people close to them.

In summary, international research on public risk perception, media content and public exposure to the same shows partially contradictory results. Much of the contradiction stems from the use of differing definitions of terms by different studies—sometimes they measure worry about something, other times perception of various risks—and from the use of differing methodological approaches in the cited studies. The quantitative studies seem to find to a greater extent than those more ethnographically oriented that the media have some influence on public risk perception, at least to the extent that risks covered by the media seem also to be present in people's awareness. The more ethnographically oriented studies put emphasis on how recipients react and interpret media texts pertaining to risks in different ways and how those interpretations, combined with other factors, influence and affect people's beliefs about what risks actually are.

This begs the question of how we should explain why people perform the risk assessments they in fact do. One possible explanatory model is that the individual's risk assessment depends first on individual character traits or, if you prefer, personality traits, secondly on personal experience, and thirdly on media influence. Finally, there is probably some interaction between people's risk assessments and media reporting, insofar as that the media exploit a topical nationwide interest even as they reinforce the same (18).

CAN COMMUNICATION BE USED TO HEIGHTEN SUBJECTIVE RISK PERCEPTION?

There are various ways to solve social problems in general and health problems in particular. Kurth (19) mentions the "three Es" for resolving social problems: Engineering, Enforcement, and Education. Engineering refers to modifying physical reality in order to remedy the problem at hand. In our case, that might entail limiting access and the opportunity to sunbathe, which may seem to be a problem that solves itself, at least in often sun-starved Scandinavia. The second way to solve a social problem is through enforcement, which involves building up a regulatory system using rewards and punishments and ensuring compliance with the rules. In our case, this could entail passing laws against being on the beach and banning artificial tanning methods like tanning salons. The third way to solve a social problem is through education: education and information are used in an attempt to persuade the public to adopt the correct behavior. The most common approach to social problems is to combine the three Es, but it should be mentioned in this context that while there are elements of communication in all three, the communication aspect is most distinct in the measure called education. Of these three instruments of social control, education is unfortunately the weakest means of rectifying a social problem, even as it is often the only instrument we have for various democratic, ethical, and moral reasons.

What I want to say with this argument is that it is considerably more efficient to legislate and restrict access in order to deal with a health problem than it is to try and influence public behavior by means of communication. However, the question is whether it is possible in practice to pursue legislation and accessibility issues towards preventing the occurrence of skin cancer? Are information and communication our only weapons in the battle against skin cancer? I will be addressing a few of those questions subsequently, that is, how one uses communicative measures to induce the public to adopt a behavior consistent with the actual health risk.

I SUPPOSE WE SHOULD RUN AN AD CAMPAIGN?

More than 40 years ago, Weibe asked "Why can't you sell brotherhood like you sell soap?" According to Solomon (20), that question was the birth of the theory of social marketing, that is, the theory that asked whether the same principles used to market products could also be used to market ideas, values, and so on. The difference between commercial and non-commercial marketing, however, is that the former often encourages people to do something, such as buy a product, whereas non-commercial marketing is often aimed at discouraging people from doing something, such as going out in the sun unprotected. Commercial and non-commercial marketing also differ in that with the former people are rewarded immediately, that is, they have the product in their hands, whereas the reward for changing their behavior in connection with a health-promotion campaign may not be noticeable until far into the future. Many researchers believe that the theory of social marketing has its limitations and consider it manipulative because it is associated with advertising and commercial products. Perhaps the most serious criticism is that the theory offers only simple solutions to complex health problems, such as "use condoms to stamp out AIDS" (20,21).

In this section, I will be discussing the characteristics of a communication campaign and the contexts in which a campaign may be considered justified in order to influence health behaviors in general and behaviors aimed at preventing skin cancer in particular.

Campaign is a word whose meaning is seldom defined and often taken for granted. "Campaign" in the context of communication says nothing more than that the sender's communication has a goal, that the recipients together form a collective, that the communication process has a particular duration, and that the process has a distinct beginning and end.

Rogers and Storey (22) define a campaign as follows:

1. A campaign has a purpose.
2. A campaign is aimed at a large recipient group.
3. A campaign has a clear time limit.
4. A campaign consists of a coordinated set of activities.

By this definition, relatively few communication activities in the health field would be classified as campaigns. The first criterion, that a campaign must have a purpose, may seem obvious but is not always met. The second criterion, that a campaign is aimed at a large recipient group, means that all interpersonal influence trials in small groups fall outside the limits of the campaign concept. The third criterion, that a campaign must have a clear time limit, means that certain continuously ongoing activities, such as pamphlets that are continually distributed, are not classified as campaigns. The last criterion, that a campaign consists of a coordinated set of activities, means for instance that a single advertisement or televised report does not suffice for the activity to be designated a campaign.

The ideal campaign that fits every situation does not exist. Every campaign must be tailored according to its unique conditions, goals, and target groups. In connection with health issues, the potential consequences of one behavior or another often do not become apparent until the future, that is, individuals cannot always clearly see the outcome of their own behavior.

Communication scholars generally agree that information campaigns are most effective when it comes to raising awareness of a particular problem. Campaigns may also fill a certain function with regard to stimulating interpersonal communication. Campaigns are considered less effective at achieving long-term changes in people's attitudes or behavior (23,24).

Campaigns can thus make people aware of a specific problem, such as that excessive sunbathing may cause skin cancer. Agenda-setting is a useful theory in this context. Rogers et al. (25) employ five phases to describe the agenda-setting process.

1. *The science agenda*: the issue/subject is discussed by experts in scientific journals and other professional publications.
2. *The media agenda*: the issue/subject is dealt with in the mass media.
3. *The public agenda*: the interpersonal agenda and the issue/subject are discussed in personal conversation among the target group.
4. *The polling agenda*: opinion polls start to be taken.
5. *The policy agenda*: policy decisions are discussed and made.

The most common order according to Rogers et al. (25) is that described above, but there are several situations/subjects in social debate wherein other combinations are conceivable. All issues/subjects, for instance, do not pass the interpersonal agenda on the way from the expert agenda to the policy agenda. Examples of this are the issue of alcohol's harmful effects on health and the fact that lying on the beach and exposing oneself to the sun may be hazardous to your health. Other issues/subjects may reach the interpersonal agenda before the media agenda, such as the issue of criminality among immigrants. An issue may also enjoy a high ranking on the media agenda without necessarily being particularly high on the interpersonal agenda.

Without exaggeration, one might say that the goal for health issues should be high placement on the interpersonal agenda, that is, to get people to start talking to their families, friends, and neighbors about what may be harmful versus less harmful to the health. Interpersonal communication is often more effective than mass communication at bringing about a behavioral change in the recipient (26). The position of a subject on the three first agendas—the science agenda, the media agenda, and the interpersonal agenda—may give us an indication of how far the subject has come in the individual information processing cycle. Health issues in general and the causes of cancer in particular that are discussed only on the science agenda are unlikely to be the subjects of discussion among ordinary people at the kitchen table or in the lunch room at work.

The preceding argument leads inevitably to the conclusion that the subjects suited for mass media campaigns are those that are not found on either the media agenda or the interpersonal agenda. Starting a large mass media campaign on the harmful effects of tobacco would at this juncture be rather meaningless. Tobacco as a danger to health is a clear example of a subject found on all five agendas. This reasoning in turn leads to the conclusion that mass media campaigns on, for instance, the danger of being in direct sunlight for too long may be effective from the perspective of opinion-shaping as well as to stimulate interpersonal communication. A campaign like that, however, is unlikely to have any direct effect on the behavior of the public.

Shaping of the Message

The question is how can the individual's subjective risk perception be heightened? First of all, we can state categorically that it is difficult if not impossible to elevate subjective risk perception by means of traditional mass media efforts, that is, with an advertising campaign. In order to bring about a change in behavior, the recipient group must genuinely feel that the behavior, such as excessive sunbathing, may be harmful and is a serious personal threat. Whether the message should contain threat sequences or not is of course debatable, but it is important that the message intrigues the target group and persuades them to believe that "this affects me." One common problem is that senders/ agencies wrap up the message in so much other information that it passes unnoticed. If one wishes to achieve effects other than getting the attention and increasing the interest of the target group, the message must be characterized by extensive adaptation to the target group and the situation. Although film and television, for instance, are suggestive media, so much time has elapsed between the communication of the message on television and the sunny day the person who saw the message decides to spend a long, lazy day on the beach that the impact of the message has worn off. Messages that have a chance of triggering the desired action are characterized by simple content and by delivery that is temporally and spatially as close to the action as possible, which is referred to as a point of action display. Initiatives of this type include stickers, posters, and so on in places where people sunbathe, such as beaches and resort towns. How a risk message should actually be formulated is a delicate task—perhaps the most difficult of all for the health information provider. Official agencies that are to inform the public about risks must first take into consideration the characteristics of various target groups, secondly, the available communication channels, and thirdly, the potential barriers for various target groups when it comes to interpreting a risk message.

How a health message should actually be formulated obviously depends on our purpose with the communication: do we want to introduce new facts, change attitudes, or change behavior? Regardless of our purpose, there are a number of factors that should be kept in mind when a message is formulated (27).

1. *Simplicity.* Simple messages contain as few technical, scientific, and bureaucratic terms as possible and exclude information that the public does not need to make personal decisions.
2. *Consistency.* Scientists often do not agree about what is dangerous and what is not nor about how individuals should actually behave to avoid poor health. Avoid this discussion in the message—it only creates confusion.
3. *The main point.* Make the main point clear in the message and do not hide it among less important information.
4. *The tone of the message.* The message may be presented in either a positive or a negative tone. The choice of presentation style may affect whether the public follows the advise and instructions given by the message.
5. *Credibility.* The source of the message—the sender—must be credible, consistent, and able to present the message clearly and persuasively.
6. *The needs of the target group.* For a message to be understood in the information noise that surrounds us, it is important that the message truly appeals to the recipients, that they realize that it affects them personally. The message must contain information about that which is most important to the recipient and not that which the sender and by extension government agencies think is the most important.

Unfortunately, we in the western world—in our endeavors towards achieving equality—have been careful to ensure that everybody gets the same information. What I finally wish to express in this context is that everybody does not seem to need the same information. Enlightenment and information initiatives thus need to be targeted and, first and foremost, adapted to the group of citizens who need them and of course combined with other supportive measures.

Media Selection

The choice of medium in connection with a communication activity is naturally dependent on which sender is used, the message, the target group, and the subject area to be addressed. Different media have different characteristics, whose importance varies depending on which communication activity is involved.

When selecting the medium, the first question should be the following: How do I come into contact with the target group? This may also be expressed as follows: even though my message seems to work, it is pointless to advertise it in the morning newspaper if the target group does not make a habit of reading it. As said, different media have different characteristics, and there is an entire array of media at our disposal in connection with health communication—everything from traditional mass media like newspapers and television to personal influence—each with its advantages and drawbacks. According to Lefebvre and Flora (28: 226), the following checklist may be useful in selecting a medium:

1. Capacity to transmit complex messages
2. Cost
3. Reach, frequency, and continuity
4. Number of intermediaries required
5. Potential for over-utilization, that is, whether saturation may occur so that the target group does not notice that you want to communicate with it
6. Options for coordination with other media
7. Degree of perceived authority and credibility.

Some of the opinions may need further explanation. The risk of over-utilization may arise, for instance, if you put out your message on billboards and posters in settings where there is already a lot of that—perhaps mainly commercial messages. The consequence may be that the target group, due to saturation, sees no messages at all. The fact that the credibility of various media differs among different target groups should also be considered when selecting a medium.

Several researchers emphasize how important it is for the health information provider to try and combine several different media if the goal is for a message to be noticed and bring about a change in behavior (27–29). Scholars also agree that mass media (such as radio, television, and newspapers) work mainly when the intent is to increase knowledge or spark interest in a subject among the target group (27,29). If the goal is to bring about behavioral change in the target group, people are often the best medium, that is, interpersonal influence.

CONSIDERATIONS FOR THE FUTURE

To succeed at health projects in general and in connection with skin cancer prevention in particular, different media strategies should be combined, that is, health information providers should use both mass communication and interpersonal communication.

Mass communication initiatives such as advertisements, posters, pamphlets, and so on may be used to arouse interest in the issue—the risks involved in sunbathing with respect to the target group—and to stimulate interpersonal communication and get co-workers, friends, and families talking about the issue. Research clearly shows that communication campaigns can fill those functions very well. Research also shows that interpersonal communication is considerably more effective in bringing about a change in the behavior of the recipients.

In the introduction, I mentioned that I would be taking an intermediate position between the social constructivist and the objectivist's perspectives. This intermediate position lies in the belief that we citizens have certain risk perceptions, be they adequate or not. The question is: Why do we have the risk perceptions we do in fact have? The media probably play a significant role here, in that they contribute by constructing and representing certain risks. The problem is that the risks the media report are not always those we citizens should actually perceive and be prepared for.

REFERENCES

1. Douglas M. Risk and Blame: Essay in Cultural Theory. London: Routledge, 1992.
2. Beck U. Risk Society. Towards a New Modernity. London: Sage, 1992.
3. Giddens A. Modernitetens följder. Lund: Studentlitteratur, 1996.
4. Cottle S. Ulrich Beck, "Risk Society" and the media. A catastrophic view? Eur J Commun 1998; 13(1):5–32.
5. Foucault M. Governmentality. In: Burchell G, Miller P, eds. The Foucaults Effect: Studies in Governmentality. London: Harvester Wheatsheaf, 1991.
6. Sjöberg L. Oro och riskuppfattning. In: Svensson LE, ed. Diffusa risker. Stockholm: Rikskollegiet, rapport 95:11, 1995.
7. Jarlbro G. Hälsokommunikation. En introduktion. 2nd ed. Lund: Studentlitteratur, 2004.
8. Höijer B. Från medborgarnas synvinkel. Vardagstänkande och massmediernas krisdiskurs. In: Lidskog R, Nohrstedt SA, Warg LE, eds. Risker, kommunikation och medier. En forskarantologi. Lund: Studentlitteratur, 2000.
9. Coleman CL. The influence of mass media and interpersonal communication on societal and personal risk judgments. Mag Commun Res 1993.
10. McCombs ME, Shaw DL. The agenda-setting function of the press. Public Opin Q 1972; 36:176–187.
11. Morton TA, Duck JM. Communication and health beliefs. Mass and interpersonal influences on perceptions of risk to self and others. Commun Res 2001; 28(5): 602–626.
12. Sjöberg L. Risk, Politik och näringsliv. Stockholm: Working paper series in Business Administration No 2002:6, 2002.
13. Storstads O, Haukenes A. Forbrukeroppfatninger om mat og risiko. Resultat fra en spörreundersögelse. Trondheim: Senter for Bygdeforskning, rapport 10/00, 2000.
14. Sjöberg L. Riskuppfattning hos experter inom området kost och hälsa. Uppsala: Livsmedelsverket, rapport nr 24, 1997.
15. Storstad O. Betydningen av forbrukertillit på det norske madvaremarkedet. Vol. 4. Norge: Sociologisk tidsskrift, 1999:285–304.

16. Wilkinson I. News media discourse and the state of public opinion on risk. Risk Manag Int J 1999; 21–31.

17. Tulloch J, Lupton D. Risk, the mass media and personal biography. Revisiting Beck's "knowledge, media and information society." Cult Stud 1999; 4(1):5–27.

18. Jarlbro G. Var det värre förr? Allmänhetens bedömningar av hälsorisker i ett sexårsperspektiv. In: Holmberg S, Weibull L, eds. Ljusnande framtid. SOM-undersökningen. Göteborg: SOM-institutet rapport nr.22, 1999.

19. Kurth T. Local campaigns and approaches by the forest community. In: Rice RE, Paisley WJ, eds. Public Communications Campaigns. Newbury Park: Sage, 1981.

20. Solomon DS. A social marketing perspective on communication campaigns. In: Rice RE, Atkin CK, eds. Public Communication Campaigns. Newbury Park: Sage, 1989.

21. Wallack L. Mass media and health promotion: promise, problem and challenge. In: Atkin C, Wallack L, eds. Mass Communication and Public Health. Newbury Park: Sage, 1990.

22. Rogers EM, Storey JD. Communication campaigns. In: Berger C, Chaffe SH, eds. Handbook of Communication Science. Newbury Park: Sage, 1989.

23. Alcalay R, Taplin S. Community health campaigns: from theory to action. In: Rice RE, Atkin CK, eds. Public Communication Campaigns. Newbury Park: Sage, 1989.

24. Thornton BC, Kreps GL. Perspectives on Health Communication. Illinois: Prospect Heights, 1993.

25. Rogers E et al. Aids in the 1980s. The agenda-setting process for a public issue. Journalism Monographs 1991; 126:1–47.

26. Jarlbro G. Forskning om miljö och massmedier. En forskningsöversikt. Lund University: Media and Communication Studies, Research report 2001:3.

27. Arkin EB. Translation of risk information for the public: message development. In: Covello VT, McCallum DB, Pavlova MT, eds. Effective Risk Communication. The Role and Responsibility of Government and Nongovernment Organizations. New York: Plenum Press, 1989.

28. Lefebvre RC, Flora JA. Social marketing and public health intervention. In: Thornton BC, Kreps GL, eds. Perspectives on Health Communication. Illinois: Prospect Heights, 1993.

29. Brown JD, Einsiedel EF. Public health campaigns: mass media strategies. In: Ray EB, Donohew L, eds. Communication and Health. Systems and Applications. Hillsdale: Lawrence Erlbaum Associates, Publishers, 1990.

20

Sun Protection at School

Cecilia Boldemann

Center for Public Health, Stockholm County Council, Stockholm, Sweden

Craig Sinclair

The Cancer Council Victoria, Carlton, Victoria, Australia

INTRODUCTION

Overexposure to ultraviolet radiation (UVR) causes approximately 60% of all melanomas and 80% to 90% of all non-melanocytic skin cancers in the world (1,2). Overexposure is most harmful during childhood, particularly in early childhood (3–5). Overexposure must be avoided in terms of sunburn and its contribution to the accumulation of UVR, as both the number of sunburns and the accumulation of UVR are positively related to the risk of skin cancer. Overexposure to UVR also causes damage to the eyes and the immune system (6,7). Targeting the behaviors and attitudes of pre- and primary school children and their peers is, therefore, valuable.

School policies can have a significant impact on children's exposure to the UVR, as the children spend a considerable proportion of the year and the vulnerable period of their lives at school where outdoor activities and break times mostly occur at peak UVR times (two hours either side of noon). Except during the winter months, at high latitudes (when outdoor sun exposure in the middle of the day is recommended), prolonged outdoor exposure in the sun can be harmful, irrespective of skin color or skin type. The variety of school systems, and cultures between and within groups, and environmental differences in terms of climate, geography, and UVR levels (Fig. 1) (8) put great demands on applying international or even national strategies so that they are suitable for

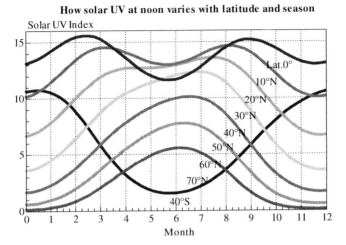

Figure 1   The need for sun protection is relevant all year round south of 40° north, and from April to September north of it. *Source*: Adapted from Ref. 8.

local intervention. Even though every school setting requires a uniquely tailored intervention for sun protection programs to be successfully implemented, they need to be a part of a socially and physically supportive environment, and of general health policies, as general good health is necessary for learning (9). Therefore, within the context of implementing sun protection programs, it is best that it is considered as part of a health-promoting schools' framework to enable the potential to coordinate efforts with other health programs, to contribute to a build-up of supportive environments for general health in a socioecological fashion, and to underpin the relevance of the message in relation to their special settings (9–11).

SUPPORTIVE ENVIRONMENT FOR SUN PROTECTION IN SCHOOL SETTINGS

Sun protection at school encompasses a broad age span of children and students from the earliest childhood (nursery school, pre-school) to adolescence and young adulthood (upper secondary school forms). However, supporting environments as being described in the Ottawa charter (build healthy public policy, create supportive environments, strengthen community action, develop personal skill, and reorient health services) are of benefit for all ages and all school systems. The creation of supportive environments can contribute to automate healthy behaviors. The school is not an isolated entity in society but is dependent on, exposed to, and communicating with other individuals, communities, and organizations. Having a strong supportive environment coming especially from parents and otherwise healthy social networks can under favorable conditions contribute significantly to the empowerment of schools to build healthy policies, to strengthen community action, and to develop personal skills in staffs and students, provided that political, economic, and social environments in the settings surrounding the schools are supportive. Environments supportive in all these aspects would also generate opportunities to promote other health behaviors.

A challenge is that the work situation among school leaders and teachers frequently creates a situation, in which they feel swamped with health programs and educational kits being added to their workload. Another challenge is that in countries with widely spread sunbed use, any efforts by schools to prevent the habit among their students may be warped when tanned skin is promoted by fashion and the tanning industry. Harmonizing efforts between authorities, professionals, and students are therefore necessary for the creation of an environment, which underpins any effort of sun protection at school and which feels supportive and relevant for all.

STRUCTURAL STRATEGIES FOR BEHAVIORAL MODIFICATION

Local authorities are in a position to take steps to control UVR exposure, as they are responsible to provide for a healthy, safe, and sustainable environment (12,13). It is sensible for UV protection to be a part of an overall official risk management strategy which includes minimizing the risk of overexposure to natural and artificial UVR in its population, particularly among pre-school and school children, as it would do to control other harmful Carcinogens, such as tobacco smoke.

A politically supportive environment may encompass comprehensive and sustainable sun protection policies, which require cooperation across local council departments. Providing healthy, safe, and sustainable environment will help the school environments and the whole of society to create consciousness about risks. Ratifying and effecting UV-protective policies (e.g., shade policies) in a "whole of organization" approach, involving councils and authorities across departmental boundaries (school, city architecture, parks and gardens, sports premises, etc.) are necessary for synergistic impact. Even though it is challenging to create supportive environments for a school, unintentional overexposure to UVR may be prevented, at least to some extent, by shade policies. Modifying the physical environment to be UV-protective is a major tool to reduce personal UV exposure. Combining well-planned and designed shade with favored play areas will attract children's playtime to places where risks associated with UVR are minimized and where there will be less reliance on the need to wear hats, clothing, and sunscreen (12,14). The consultation of school staff and other personnel working as local experts in the school environments is valuable for input in interdisciplinary boards with city architects and planners in charge of school playgrounds and school outdoor environments. Frequently, there are already existing policies that may relate to shade provision such as environment beauti-fication. It is then a matter of underpinning these activities by integrating them in the strategy.

For schools, natural shade from trees and shrubs is ideal for UV protection, in addition to scheduling outdoor education outside of the peak UVR hours. Outdoor education becomes increasingly popular in high-latitude countries, where it serves to strengthen health, and has been observed to have a positive impact on learning processes (15). In that context, rich vegetation is an invaluable asset. Vegetation yields low reflectance (1%) (16), gives rain and wind protec-tion, and offers good habitats for wildlife and many species. Other environmental benefits include fewer disposal problems, no or low expenditure of embodied energy, reduction of atmospheric carbon dioxide, and improvement of air quality. UV protection may be provided for by the integration of shade in the architectural design of new public places. In this way, costs associated with shade development are less when compared with developing shade structures at a later stage. Access can be given to green wedges for outdoor education or other outdoor activities, and trees can be planted in areas frequently used by school children and adolescents outside the school premises (e.g., public play-grounds, sports fields, swimming pools, skateboard ramps, play equipment, streetscape furniture, lunch areas, etc.). Trees with dense canopies provide open, safe areas with reduced UV exposure, whereas open canopied, deciduous trees yield benefits in providing winter sun without UV risks at high latitudes. Insect-pollinated, (for the prevention of allergies) resilient trees with non-inva-sive roots are practical, particularly in school environments and playgrounds. Shade structures may serve as valuable protection for lunch areas, for example, but require maintenance.

Successful UVR protective policies in supportive environments will decrease the likelihood of children under their care being at risk of sunburn. Schools may, for example, ensure that swimming or athletic sports days are held either side of the peak UV period. This may also yield the advantage of enjoying warm temperatures later in the day when UV levels are lower (Fig. 2) (17).

Creating Supportive Environments for Behavior Change

Good physical outdoor environments at schools may contribute to the develop-ment of sun-protective habits during childhood and, in extension, to more appro-priate sun behavior later in life. In young children attending pre- and primary school forms, any exposure to UVR from the sun is likely to be unintentional. In theory, unintentional exposure may be a consequence of sun-exposed physical environments in the daily school setting, unpurposeful scheduling of outdoor activities, and the dependence of younger children upon sun-seeking peers, for example, pre-school staff. Safe environments that fulfill architectural criteria relevant for children's self-triggered protective behavior (e.g., limited fraction

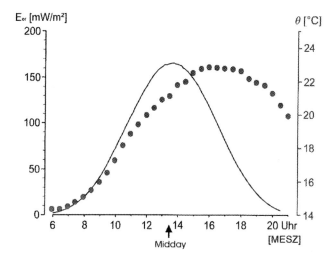

Figure 2 Solar peak and thermal peak. The thermal peak is in the late afternoon, when UV radiation is on the downward slope (Kiel, Germany). *Source*: Adapted from Ref. 17.

of free sky over the area, position of trees, etc.) (18,19) may work also to attract school staff and older students.

For young children, the access to healthy physical outdoor environments in everyday life is becoming increasingly important not only for sun protection, but also for the promotion of physical activity. Space and attractive opportunities for outdoor play with trees and shrubbery are vital not only for natural UV protection (provided there are enough trees and shrubs around) (14), but also for general health and academic performance (15,20–22). This also requires that the children have large surfaces in safe environments at their disposal (Photos 1–3). For very young pre-school children (ages one to four years), the dependency on sun-seeking peers may pose a problem, as children of these ages do not move around as freely as older children (20). Pre-school teachers must be made aware of the responsibility they carry for these children as role models. A recommendation to wear attractive, practical, and comfortable UV-protective clothing may, apart from education, be one route to encourage these employees to act as good role models.

In adolescents, the causes of overexposure to UVR are complex. In these age groups, sun-protection programs have been successful in increasing knowledge and, at the best, changing attitudes to some extent, but as yet there is little evidence of long-lasting behavioral change. The wish for a tan may increase the receptiveness for knowledge, but probably not for UV-protective behavior. It would be unrealistic to believe that outdoor intentional tanning or sunbed use (unless restrictive legislation concerning artificial tanning devices is strictly enforced) among secondary and upper secondary school students can be prevented outside of school hours. Restrictive legislation concerning sunbed use

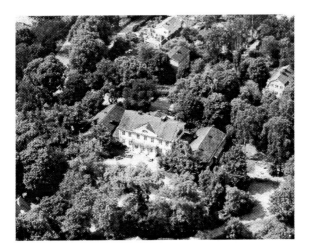

Photo 1 Attractive play constructions are placed under the canopies of tree crowns and invisible from above during the summer. *Note*: The sky view factors of these environments are small, that is, little visible sky is seen, and attractive play constructions are protected from direct UV radiation. *Source*: Adapted from Svenska Aero-Bilder AB.

would send a message to students of its harmfulness. Sunbed use is widespread among students in cold climates (23,24) and the habit is reported to increase at a disturbing pace among young people who live at lower latitudes (25) possibly due to a misconception of sunbeds being more "harmless" than the sun. In spite of efforts to prevent minors from using them, the opportunities to prevent sunbed use among adolescents are as yet limited, as school UV-protection programs have to compete with contradictory influences that come from the tanning and fashion industries. Education is required to ensure accurate information to all students via the school. For the time being, the role of the school is to deliver correct knowledge about the harmfulness of sunbed use and its contribution to the accumulation of UVR. Delivering a message of artificial UVR on the same terms as of natural UVR and other harmful environmental exposure may contribute to gain acceptance among the students for legal restrictions of sunbed use. Exposure to the natural sun during school hours may in the same way as for younger students be reduced by day planning of curricula and supportive political, social, and physical environments. Respectful guidance with straightforward rules and messages served by the school and the society around it will have a better chance to register, as supportive structural policies will influence interpersonal, social, and physical factors in the environment. Even though intentional risk behavior in adolescence is often difficult to prevent, research so far indicates that much is gained if adolescent students have had a childhood free of sunburn (even though intentional tanning and sunbed use in adolescence is always harmful). Any successful prevention of overexposure to UVR among children of pre- and primary school ages may therefore be regarded as a health gain not

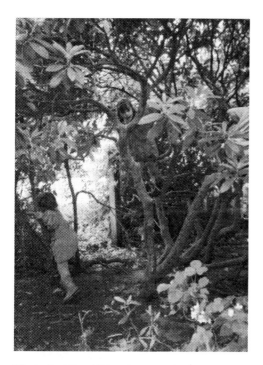

Photo 2 The children have ample space on broken ground with plenty of opportunities for dynamic play in an environment that is sun protective during the summer months. *Note*: The sky view factors of these environments are small, that is, little visible sky is seen, and attractive play constructions are protected from direct UV radiation. *Source*: Adapted from Maria Kylin.

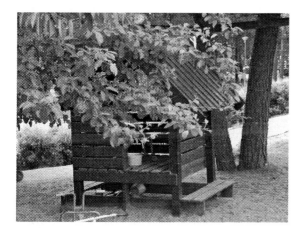

Photo 3 This play construction right outside a pre- and primary school building is placed among pine trees where UV radiation is low. *Note*: The sky view factors of these environments are small, that is, little visible sky is seen, and attractive play constructions are protected from direct UV radiation. *Source*: Adapted from Cecilia Boldemann.

only for these young children, but also for part of the adolescents they will become. Provided that one major route to prevent sunburn among young children is the access to shade in areas, which are attractive for play, the same may be applied for older students. Unintentional or even intentional sun protection could be triggered by creating attractive, shaded outdoor areas (trees or roofed over) inside and close to the school area, in the form of "welcoming" arbors or shaded areas by saving big, leafy trees for lunch breaks and outdoor reading. The same could be applied for other areas where young people gather in connection with lessons within and in the close surroundings of the school.

School Education and Information

For effective communication and acceptance, an education program must be relevant to its audience. The success also depends on the pedagogy and the teacher's ability to deliver the message, in which context the message is conveyed, and the supportiveness in the community in which the school is situated. The definition of successful communication and acceptance in terms of outcome must be behavioral change by consistent school policies resulting in increased sun-protective behavior. Long-lasting behavioral changes have been difficult to prove. In low-latitude areas, where the climate motivates large-scale UV protection approaches, it may be difficult to define to what extent a particular school intervention has contributed to modify children's behavior, as schools are often a part of broad campaigns and initial protection levels are high. However, multiunit presentations in classrooms (several presentations during several days) have proven successful for behavioral change among students aged 5 to 12. Five of these programs have been implemented in low-latitude areas (26–30) and two in a mid-latitude area (31,32). In high-latitude areas, sun-protection programs are otherwise more disparate and unsystematic, initial protection levels may be lower, as seems the motivation to adopt ambitious educational kits, possibly due to the climate during the winter months. Schools in these areas may also experience that the social environments, that is, other sectors in society, are less aware of UV risks which gives them less support than is the case in low-latitude areas. Yet, to support school-based strategies, the social environments need to integrate UV protection as an omnipresent element. If information about sun protection is being received by a multitude of sources, and the messages are easy to understand and comply to, any education or information on sun protection in school would be automatically underpinned. All provision of education/ information to teachers, caregivers, and others involved in delivering relevant information to children in school settings will be more likely to be successfully conveyed if supported by messages delivered by senders with broad coverage and impressiveness. Displaying information about the expected ultraviolet index (UVI), when relevant (e.g., reporting extreme UVI levels), in the weather forecast as an integral component of public information is one route to raise the awareness not only in school but also in rest of the society about UV exposure and its

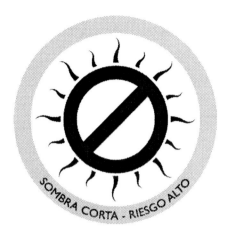

Figure 3 Pictogram saying "short shade—high risk." Example of nonverbal communication appealing to cognitive/affective sensations of danger. *Source*: Adapted from Ref. 33.

consequences. Visible symbols related to well-known road-signs crossing all culture and language barriers, a strategy which has proven successful on the South American continent would also serve this purpose (Fig. 3) (33). Communitywide interventions of the adult population, in conjunction with school-based policy, curriculum, and practice implementation with careful adaptation to geography, climate, and culture, would be the initial primary strategy (34–37).

Significance is also given to UV protection education by integrating it in pre-service education to teacher students in university curricula. For reinforcement, regular updates may be integrated into established systems of continued education for in-service school staff. In-service education may also apply to local agencies providing services for children, for example, family day-care programs and home-based child-care schemes. The provision of core messages may be the same to teachers, peers, parents or other proxies, local governments, politicians, city planners, administrative heads for health and environmental protection, pre- and primary school headmasters, and so on, as long as the recipients live in the same climate and same geography, and consequently share a motivation to receive the message.

However, frequently, it may be difficult to advocate for education in UV protection in schools and still less multiunit courses, due to competition between subjects on the curricula, particularly if, for various reasons ("climate" reasons and/or due to other health programs taking space), UV protection is not regarded as a high-priority issue. Apart from the climate, adversities such as social deprivation, mental ill health, drug abuse, and so on, among students may absorb resources. As good health in students is necessary for learning, health programs that are aimed at risk reduction in a long-term perspective (teaching sun protection, healthy food choices and physical exercise) normally require functioning of healthy schools' frameworks (besides supportive environments) with acute social and health problems being largely under control. Also, educational programs for normal-risk populations, (and young people in particular) which appeal to an individual's personal behavior versus concern for health frequently tend to fail if the risk of adverse effects lies too far ahead in the future instead of being an immediate threat. The prospect of skin cancer in a 20- to 30-year perspective is probably not perceived as "sufficiently" threatening to trigger behavioral change as a result of fear (especially not in a young person) and especially not if coupled with additional feelings of having to give up a pleasant habit ("enjoying the sun") (38). It is theorized that risks to personal health due to threats outside the range of own behavioral influence are perceived more risky and frightening than threats due to own risk behavior (39). For instance, pesticides in food may be regarded as more dangerous and threatening than a lack of fruits and vegetables in the own diet. In the same way, ozone depletion may be perceived as more threatening to one's health than own sun behavior, even though there is no evidence yet to suggest an impact on skin cancer rates due to ozone depletion. Yet, as adolescents are frequently concerned about issues of sustainable development, the link between global warming and ozone depletion may be mentioned in connection with sun exposure, as it could help to recognize the dangers of high UVR from more than one perspective.

In spite of ambitious educational schemes, personal trade-offs (i.e., gains and losses linked to compliance of the message) (38) may have an impact depending on the climate the addressee of sun-protection education lives in. In high latitudes, the desire for sunlight may be so strong that the message will either be filtered off or the dangers minimized at least by the older students (and their peers), unless a positive option to meet the requirements of sun protection is "served" at the same time (for instance, attractiveness of warm and low-irradiant late afternoon hours). On low latitudes, where the risk of inadvertent sunburn is much higher, and as sunburn is uncomfortable in a short-term perspective, the feeling of having abstained from pleasures due to sun protection is probably less likely. For effective communication to students and the key persons in their settings, it is therefore highly recommended to adapt messages to the climate (Table 1).

Short classroom presentations on one occasion have been assessed as unlikely to change sun-protection behavior in school students, an observation which seems to apply worldwide (40). However, one presentation in a classroom by a peer or agency representative from outside the school may result in a follow-up by the school staff. It is therefore important for the peer or agency delivering the presentation or lecture to serve as a "lifeline" and encouragement. At that stage, educational kits and teaching resources will enable the teachers to apply any pedagogic technique which will actively involve the students and test their knowledge and skills at the same time, as such techniques will serve as

Table 1 Sun Protection at School; Recommended Structural Action for Behavior Change

	Structural action for supportive environment		Education/information	
	Apply existing recommendations and teaching resources			
	Pre- and primary school forms	Secondary/upper secondary school forms	Pre- and primary school forms	Secondary/upper secondary school forms
Location/latitude				
Global	Provision of/use of spacious school outdoor environments with plenty of trees and shrubbery on broken ground. Provision of shade at sites used during mid-day hours.		Socio-cultural adaptation of information/messages, coordinated with messages of sustainable development. Provision of information/messages via channel with high acceptance and respected among students, peers, and key authorities ("a sender whose message everybody listens to"). Integration in curricula for relevant student education (teacher students, etc.) at universities, vocational study programs, etc. and regular in-service education of workforces and peers. Multiunit presentation and recurrent update.	

(Continued)

Table 1 Sun Protection at School; Recommended Structural Action for Behavior Change (*Continued*)

Location/latitude	Structural action for supportive environment		Education/information	
	Pre- and primary school forms	Secondary/upper secondary school forms	Pre- and primary school forms	Secondary/upper secondary school forms
		Legislation against sunbed use for minors. Mandate for law enforcement. Joint efforts by radiation-protection authorities, local authorities, and schools to prevent sunbed use. Education of providers of sunbeds.		Valid information of rules and regulations concerning sunbed use.
North of 40th latitude N Autumn, winter, early spring, and sea level/low elevation	Outdoor stay/activities whenever possible, especially during mid-day hours		Seasonal adaptation of sun protection education in students' schedules (multiunit presentations and information to parents (minors), considering climate and travel abroad.	
North of 40th latitude N Late spring, summer, and south of 40th latitude, and high elevation (UVI ≥ 3 October–March) year round	Outdoor lessons scheduled early morning and/or late afternoon, supply of protective clothing adapted to UVR (supplementary sunscreen SPF > 15 when required)		Integration of sun protection in school as permanent theme in curricula (multiunit presentations on a regular basis).	

Abbreviations: UVR, ultraviolet radiation; UVI, ultraviolet index.

memory cues as they build up the students' own knowledge and personal skills (35–37). Such a procedure would in turn form a multiunit intervention.

As multiunit presentations have proven most effective for behavioral change, it is recommended to work for an introduction of such schemes in low-latitude areas and/or in schools that run successful health policies, which would facilitate an integration of sun-protection education. In other areas or settings where multiunit presentations in classrooms are not prioritized due to immediate serious social health problems, the underlying causes have to be attended to, before a build-up of functioning healthy schools frameworks is possible. Schools are also encouraged to include a synergistic approach to UV protection, with culture and climate-specific adaptation, seasonally in high-latitude areas and on a more regular basis in the rest of the world.

SYNERGIES: GAINS FOR ENVIRONMENTAL PROTECTION AND HEALTH

In school settings, health programs increasingly compete for resources and attention. The target peers, headmasters and teachers, and the students themselves are exposed to massive input of information on a variety of health programs from a wide array of senders (media, authorities, NGOs, institutions, etc.) whose messages, though not conflicting, often seem disparate and unrelated. However, action for synergies may serve several purposes at the same time. Synergies become powerful if the health messages are experienced to be relevant to own life situations, across settings and age spans, and if two or more health messages overlap and interplay in one single recommendation for action.

For instance, the childhood obesity pandemic calls for any evidence-based action to increase the level of physical activity, preferably without increasing the risk of sunburn. Favorable physical outdoor environments trigger a variety of healthy behaviours that are crucial for general health, especially physical activity (Photos 1–3). Therefore, schoolyards with limited space and scanty vegetation should be investigated (Photos 4 and 5). Many children, at least the older ones, lack opportunity for unscheduled physical activity during school time, which makes it important to plan for outdoor environments disposing of extensive landscape with broken ground and plenty of vegetation. Combined with climate-specific scheduling of outdoor stay, and climate-specific recommendations regarding clothes and sunscreen, such environments yield sufficient sun protection. Frequent play among trees, shrubs, and broken ground promotes, in addition to physical activity, motor development, concentration abilities, and positive social interaction in free play, which in turn has implications for mental well-being (15,20–22,41). A recommendation to build or to give children daily access to outdoor environments and playgrounds which provide for space, broken ground, and plenty of trees and shrubbery would not only invite to sun-protective behavior, but also serve to promote children's health from several other aspects, besides serving the environment. Using the outdoor environment

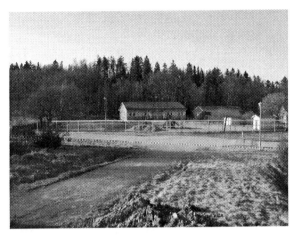

Photo 4   The children do not have access to the wood in the background, which would yield sun protection and also be a potential for play with much physical activity. *Note*: The fenced-in outdoor environments of these two preschools are fully exposed to the sun. *Source*: Adapted from Bertil Hjertell.

thus contributes to decrease the risks of skin cancer and diseases related to physical inactivity and to sustainable development.

In adolescence, risky life style cultures emerge, which frequently contain several risk elements. Concentrating on skin cancer prevention as an isolated subject may in this aspect be less effective than trying to elucidate the dynamics between UV-risk behavior and other risk behavior (e.g., behavior A increases the risk of behavior B, which increases the risk of behavior C). Smoking has been

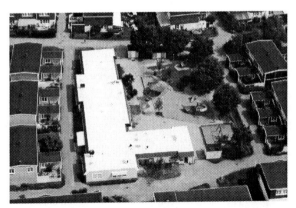

Photo 5   The area is cramped, and does not protect against the sun nor promote dynamic play. *Note*: The fenced-in outdoor environments of these two preschools are fully exposed to the sun. *Source*: Adapted from Svenska Aero-Bilder AB.

observed to be positively correlated with outdoor tanning and sunbed use among teenagers, especially in girls (24,42,43). Smoke-free adolescents also drink less alcohol than do the smokers (44), and even though there is as yet no evidence that freedom from smoking would have a restraining effect on outdoor and indoor intentional tanning, the top priority must always be to prevent children from starting to smoke. Freedom from smoking would in all likelihood, at least to some part, contribute to prevent an aggregation of risk behaviors.

Recognizing synergies that yield multiple health gains would help to simplify the implementation of health promotion in schools, provided that there are functioning intersectoral UV policies which are combined with other policies for health promotion and sustainable development (involving cooperation across departments on all governmental levels).

AUDITS, SURVEILLANCE, AND MONITORING OF POLICIES AND BEHAVIORS

As a part of UV-protection policies for supportive environments, shade may be added to the audits done by the school authorities, and the authorities for health and environmental protection, for instance, by using computerized tools to assess the proportion of free sky (sky view factor) to school playgrounds (19). A successful school policy would address all aspects of UVR protection, including shade, curriculum, and behaviour. Such policy would also enable inventories of the need of shade in these settings and shade as an element in planning and upgrading of these settings.

To identify where improvements can be obtained for UV radiation protection, the occurrence of UVR protection and UV-protective behavior may be assessed if questions related to UVR protection and exposure are added to national/regional instruments for public health surveys, which in many places are routinely used by national institutes and authorities for the surveillance of other health-related and environmental issues. Local surveys may include questions regarding the involvement of schools in the planning of interventions directed to them, frequency of sunburn before and after school time, impact of skill-based health education, use of shaded areas, use of protective clothing, and diffusion of information from students to parents. In surveys, questions may be combined in a way to give a clue whether intentions have been fulfilled or not (outcome evaluation) and why they have been fulfilled or not (process evaluation) which gives a tool for improvement and update.

CONCLUSION

The success of sun-protection implementation at school is dependent on the supportiveness of the social and physical environment, the adaptation of the message to socio-cultural and climatic conditions, the pedagogic methods by which the message is conveyed, and on functioning healthy school policies and healthy students.

The cooperation of authorities across departmental boundaries will serve to create supportive environments in order to make messages of sun protection understandable, relevant, and easy for students and peers to comply inside and outside school. An adaptation of the message to its special socio-cultural and climatic setting will increase the likelihood of the message as being perceived as relevant. For long-lasting behavioral change, multiunit education has so far been the only method with evidence of success and is therefore recommended, provided that education is adapted to its unique setting. Functioning school health policies may also be a tool to coordinate sun-protection education with other health programs and to maintain health and healthy (sun protective and other) habits among the students.

REFERENCES

1. World Health Organization. Protection against exposure to ultraviolet radiation. Geneva: WHO/EHC/UNEP, 1995.
2. Armstrong BK, Kricker A. How much melanoma is caused by sun exposure? Melanoma Res 1993; 3(6):395–401.
3. English DR, Armstrong BK, Kricker A. Case-control study of sun exposure and squamous cell carcinoma of the skin. Int J Cancer 1998; 77(3):347–353.
4. Kricker A, Armstrong BK, English DR, Heenan PJ. A dose-response curve for sun exposure and basal cell carcinoma. Int J Cancer 1995; 60(4):482–488.
5. English DR, Armstrong BK, Kricker A, Fleming C. Sunlight and cancer. (Review). Cancer Causes Control 1997; 8(3):271–283.
6. Sliney DH. Physical factors in caractogenesis: ambient ultraviolet radiation and temperature. Invest Ophtalmol Vis Sci 1986; 27(5):781–790.
7. Selgrade MK, Repacholi MH, Koren HS. Ultraviolet radiation-induced immune modulation: potential consequences for infectious, allergic, and autoimmune disease. Environ Health Perspect 1997; 105(3):332–334.
8. Wester U, Josefsson W. UV-Index and influence of action spectrum and surface inclination. In: Report of the WMO-WHO Meeting of Experts on Standardization of UV-indices and their Dissemination to the Public (Les Diablerets, Switzerland, 21–24 July 1997. World Meteorological Organization, Global Atmosphere Watch Report No. 127, 63–66).
9. www.gov.mb.ca/healthychild/healthyschools/healthy_schools_framework.pdf (June 14, 2005).
10. www.wahpsa.org.au/Content/healthpromotingschools.html# (June 14, 2005).
11. www.bced.gov.bc.ca/health/draft_frame.pdf (June 14, 2005).
12. Sinclair C, Hilditch A. UV radiation and Health, Local Authorities, Health and Environment briefing pamphlet series; 41. World Health Organization, 2003.
13. World Health Organization. Artificial Tanning Sunbeds: Risk And Guidance. World Health Organization, 2003.

14. Boldeman C, Dal H, Wester U. Swedish pre-school children's UV exposure—a comparison between two different outdoor environments. Photodermatol Photoimmunol Photomed 2004; 20(1):2–8.
15. Grahn P, Mårtensson F, Lindblad B, et al. How do children use the pre-school yard? The design of the pre-school yard as a function of play, motor development and concentration abilities (Swedish). Alnarp, Sweden: MOVIUM, Swedish University of Agricultural Sciences, 1997.
16. Diffey BL, Larkö O. Clinical climatology. Photodermatol 1984; 1(1):30–37.
17. Stick C. Pielke L. Ultraviolette Sonnenstrahlung und Sonnenbrandgefahr. Akt Dermatol 1997; 23:1–5.
18. Nezic B. Variations of erythemal UV-B irradiance load related to different human activities in the area of Gothenburg (in Swedish). Gothenburg: Department of Physical Geography, 1998. Report No. B110.
19. Grimmond CSB, Potter SK, Zutter HN, Souch C. Rapid methods to estimate sky view factors applied to urban areas. Int J Climatol 2001; 21:903–913.
20. Herrington S, Studtmann K. Landscape interventions: new directions for the design of children's outdoor play environments. Landscape Urban Plan 1998; 42:191–205.
21. Mårtensson F. The landscape in children's play. A study of outdoor play in preschools (Swedish). Alnarp: Swedish University of Agricultural Sciences, 2004.
22. Söderström M, Martensson F, Grahn P, Blennow M. The outdoor environment of day care centers. Its importance to play and development. Ugeskr Laeger 2004; 166(36):3089–3092.
23. Wichstroem L. Predictors of Norwegian adolescents' aunbathing and use of sunscreen. Health Psychol 1994; 13(5):412–420;1998.
24. Boldeman C, Jansson B, Nilsson B, Ullén H. Sunbed use in Swedish urban adolescents related to behavioral characteristics. Prev Med 1997; 26:114–119.
25. Marks R. The 10th World Congress on Cancers of the Skin, May 13–16, 2005 [personal communication].
26. Buller DB, Buller MK, Beach B, Ertl G. Sunny days, healthy ways: evaluation of a skin cancer prevention curriculum for elementary school-aged children. J Am Acad Dermatol 1996; 35(6):911–922.
27. Loescher LJ, Emerson J, Taylor A, et al. Educating preschoolers about sun safety. Am J Public Health 1995; 85(7):939–943.
28. Ramstack JL, White SE, Hazelkorn KS, Meyskens FL. Sunshine and skin cancer: a school-based skin cancer prevention project. J Cancer Educ 1986; 1(3):169–176.
29. Buller M, Loescher LJ, Buller DB. "Sunshine and skin health": a curriculum for skin cancer prevention education. J Cancer Educ 1994; 9(3):155–162.
30. Girgis A, Sanson-Fischer RW, Tripodi DA, Golding T. Evaluation of interventions to improve solar protection in primary schools. Health Educ Q 1993; 20(2):275–287.
31. Reding DJ, Krauska ML, Lappe KA, et al. Cancer education interventions for rural populations. Cancer Pract 1994; 2(5):353.
32. Reding DJ, Fischer V, Gunderson P, et al. Skin cancer prevention: a peer education model. Wis Med J 1995; 94(2):77–81.
33. Stengel F. Fundación Cáncer de Piel, Argentina 2005.
34. www.who.int/uv/intersunprogramme/en (June 17, 2005).
35. World Health Organization. Sun Protection. A Primary Teaching Resource. World Health Organization, 2003.

36. World Health Organization. Evaluating School Programmes To Promote Sun Protection. World Health Organization, 2003.
37. World Health Organization. Sun Protection and Schools. How to Make a Difference. World Health Organization, 2003.
38. Cooper J, Croyle RT. Attitudes and attitude change. Annu Rev Psychol 1984; 35:395–426.
39. Sjöberg L. The different dynamics of personal and general risk. Risk Manag: Int J 2003; 19–34.
40. Buller DB, Borland R. Skin cancer prevention for children: a critical review. (Review). Health Educ Behav 1999; 26(3):317–343.
41. Boldemann C, Blennow M, Dal H, et al. Impact of pre-school environment upon children's physical activity and sun exposure. Prev Med 2006; 42(4):301–308.
42. Feldman SR, Dempsey JR, Grummer S, et al. Implications of a utility model for ultraviolet exposure behavior. J Am Acad Dermatol 2001; 45(5):718–722.
43. Boldeman C, Jansson B, Dal H, et al. Sunbed use among Swedish adolescents in the 1990s: a decline with an unchanged relationship to health risk behaviors. Scand J Public Health 2003; 31(3):233–237.
44. Swedish Council for Information on Alcohol and Other Drugs. Swedish student's drug habits. Report No. 84, 2004.

21

The UV Index in Practice

Eva Rehfuess

Department of Public Health and Environment, World Health Organization, Geneva, Switzerland

Craig Sinclair

The Cancer Council Victoria, Carlton, Victoria, Australia

INTRODUCTION

Most fair-skinned populations worldwide have experienced a marked increase in the incidence of melanoma and nonmelanoma skin cancers since the early 1970s. Personal sun exposure habits, in particular, frequent travel to sunny destinations and the active seeking of a suntan as an expression of being healthy and beautiful, constitute the most important risk factor for UV radiation damage. Consequently, skin cancer is largely preventable when appropriate sun-protection measures are taken. As UV radiation cannot be seen or felt, it is important to visualize the level of danger and to alert people on a daily basis to take prompt, appropriate action to protect themselves.

Since the early 1980s, several countries, in particular Australia and New Zealand, pioneered the development of UV radiation scales and sun-protection programs. By 1994, at least six UV radiation scales were in use around the world, accompanied by different measurement approaches, forecast algorithms, and public health messages (1,2). To evaluate experience with existing UV indices and to facilitate the adoption of a single international standard for UV radiation scales and forecasting, the World Meteorological Organization (WMO), the World Health Organization (WHO), and the International Commission on Non-Ionizing Radiation Protection (ICNIRP) convened two expert meetings in 1994. On the basis of the recommendations of these meetings and the Canadian UV index scale (3–5), WHO, in partnership with WMO, the United Nations Environment Programme, and ICNIRP, issued the Global Solar UV Index as a tool to educate people about the dangers of UV radiation in 1995 (2).

Many countries have been using the UV index to promote sun protection, yet surveys suggested that a large percentage of the public, while aware of the existence of the UV index, did not understand its significance and failed to put recommendations into practice (6,7). Specific problems identified included confusion between the UV index and the sun-protection factor for sunscreens and the interpretation of reported "burn times" as an indication of "safe tanning times" (8).

This prompted WHO to spearhead the preparation of a comprehensive harmonized communications concept including the uniform graphical presentation of the UV index and clear and consistent sun-protection messages associated with different UV index values. In light of today's worldwide travel and tourism, the implementation of the harmonized approach, described in *The Global Solar UV Index: A Practical Guide* and published in 2002, is an important step forward in the fight against the skin cancer epidemic.

ALERTING PEOPLE ABOUT UV RADIATION

UV radiation levels are highly variable and depend on many geographical and climatic factors, such as sun elevation, latitude, cloud cover, altitude, levels of stratospheric ozone, pollution, and ground reflection (9). The Global Solar UV Index is a simple measure of the level of UV radiation at the Earth's surface. It has been designed to indicate the potential for adverse health effects to the skin: based on the reference action spectrum for UV-induced erythema (a reddening of the skin), one UV index unit is equivalent to $25 \text{ mW}/\text{m}^2$ of UV radiation reaching the Earth's surface (9).

The values of the index range from zero upward—maximum values range from 7 to 12 in mid-latitude countries but may reach 15 or more in tropical regions. The higher the index value, the greater the potential for damage to the skin and eye, and the less time it takes for harm to occur. UV radiation levels vary throughout the day, but reach their maximum around midday; in most countries, the UV index is presented as a forecast of the daily maximum UV radiation levels that are averaged over a 30-minute period. UV index reporting should take cloud cover into account; where this is not possible, forecasts should clearly state the UV index as "clear sky" or "cloud-free."

While addressing all populations, the basic UV index sun-protection scheme explicitly focuses on fair-skinned individuals and children as the most vulnerable groups. UV index values are grouped into five exposure categories, defined as low (0–2), moderate (3–5), high (6–7), very high (8–10), and extreme (11+), on a continuous colour scale that indicates the level of danger (Fig. 1).

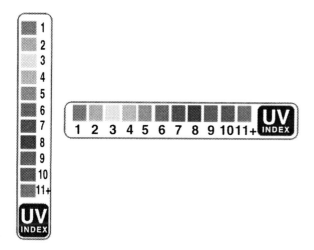

Figure 1 UV index values on a continuous color scale (shown here in gray scale). *Source*: Courtesy of the World Health Organization.

This sun-protection scheme takes a step back from the much practiced approach that increasing UV index values require successive use of sun-protection measures (9,10). Instead, it recommends that starting from a UV index of three, sun protection should include all protective means (Table 1). Even for very sensitive individuals, the risk of sunburn and long-term UV radiation damage below this threshold level is limited. At very high and extreme UV radiation levels of a UV index of eight and above, sun protection must be applied even more rigorously.

Sun protection is important in all settings, in particular, in relation to outdoor recreational activities. Simple precautions can prevent short-term and

Table 1 Basic Sun-Protection Messages

Limit exposure during midday hours.
Seek shade.
Wear protective clothing.
Wear a broad-brimmed hat to protect the eyes, face, and neck.
Protect the eyes with wrap-around-design sunglasses or sunglasses
  with side panels.
Use and re-apply broad-spectrum sunscreen of SPF 15 + liberally.
Avoid tanning beds.
Protect babies and young children: this is particularly important.

Abbreviation: SPF, sun-protection factor.

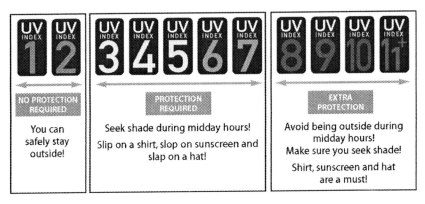

Figure 2 Recommended sun-protection scheme with simple "sound bite" messages. *Source*: Courtesy of the World Health Organization.

long-term UV damage to the skin and eyes while still making the time spent outdoors enjoyable. The WHO promotes a comprehensive sun-protection approach based on limiting exposure by ensuring people take particular care during midday hours and seeking shade, and wearing protective clothing, a hat, and sunglasses (Fig. 2). Sunscreen use is seen as a last line of defense on body parts that cannot be protected otherwise, such as the face and hands (11,12). Sunscreen should never be used to prolong the duration of sun exposure.

Children require special protection as they are at a higher risk of suffering damage from exposure to UV radiation than adults (13). In particular, a child's skin is more sensitive and even a short time outdoors in the midday sun can result in serious burns (14). Epidemiological studies indicate that frequent sun exposure and sunburn during childhood set the stage for a higher risk of melanoma later in life (15,16).

EXPERIENCES FROM AROUND THE WORLD

Today, the revised global solar UV index is in operation in Argentina, Australia, Canada, Germany, Hong Kong, Norway, Switzerland, the United Kingdom, and the United States of America. Plans for an introduction of this revised UV index are currently under way in parts of South America including Brazil, Ecuador, and Venezuela, and in several European countries. In each country, government authorities responsible for the delivery of meteorological services collect data on UV radiation levels and make the UV index accessible to the general public via a web-based presence and reports to the media.

The adoption of the global solar UV index by a country is usually accompanied by the development and dissemination of a range of information

---

Box 1   UV Index Media Success in Canada

In May 2004, Environment Canada updated their UV index program based on the recommendations provided in the *Global Solar UV Index: A Practical Guide*. The revised program drew upon UV index work that had started more than 12 years earlier.

An intersectoral working group, consisting of members from Environment Canada, Health Canada, the Canadian Cancer Society, the Canadian Dermatological Association, and the Canadian Association of Optometrists, developed sun-protection messages in relation to the new UV index categories. The Canadian activities were closely coordinated with the United States Environmental Protection Agency to ensure that consistent UV index information would be available on both sides of the border to minimize confusion, especially among travelers. As part of the launch of this revised UV index program, Environment Canada updated existing children's education programs and communication materials such as fact sheets and posters, and set up a new website on all facets of the UV index for the media and general public. A key partner in the launch was the Weather Network, a cable channel that provides 24-hour information on weather conditions.

A far-reaching public relations campaign targeted newspapers and magazines as well as national TV news programs. Spokespeople were coached for interviews and key media messages were developed to assist them. A scientific paper on the source and quality of UV index data for the United States and Canada was published prior to the launch date, and a presentation given at the annual congress of the Canadian Meteorological and Oceanographic Society. The launch was a remarkable success: more than 30 media outlets across Canada reported on the UV index launch, including 23 radio stations, 10 newspapers, and two television channels.

---

materials to help promote the index among the general population. These resources are often developed in collaboration with governmental and non-governmental agencies active in meteorology, environment, and health sectors. They include pamphlets for the general public, scientific articles or events for the medical and academic community as well as school-based curriculum materials. In addition, most countries conduct news conferences or other media events to engage print and electronic media (Box 1).

Despite meteorological agencies approaching the media, mainstream national-level newspapers, television, and radio stations often do not deliver UV index information on a regular and consistent basis. Argentina provides the exception as a national law obliges the government-run national radio and television stations to report the UV index on a daily basis. In Australia, training weather presenters has helped raise the awareness of those who have the potential to influence how weather forecasts are reported (Box 2). The well-established U.S.-based cable station The Weather Network regularly reports details of the UV index. Reporting of the UV index by the media is often confined to those times of the year when the UV index is rated moderate or above (≥ 3). This is in line with the recommendation by the WHO that sun protection is not required at a UV index of less than three.

Box 2   Overcoming UV Index Media Fatigue in Australia

Australia was one of the first countries in the world to adopt the revised UV index in 2002, in a collaborative project between Cancer Councils, the Bureau of Meteorology (BOM), and the Australian Radiation Protection and Nuclear Safety Agency (ARPANSA). Responsibility for delivering UV radiation information is largely in the hands of the BOM and the ARPANSA.

In the southern states ($>28°$ latitude), the UV index is reported to coincide with the introduction of daylight savings time (October–March); in the northern states ($<28°$ latitude), it is reported all-year-round. Particularly in the northern states, UV index levels can rise high into the teens for a large part of the year. This presents a major challenge as consistently high UV index values make it difficult to keep sun-protection messages newsworthy.

The development of resources to explain the UV index (17) and the training of weather reporters have been a joint effort between the Cancer Councils and the BOM (18). Unfortunately, most television outlets have developed their own graphical representation of the UV index, adding to confusion among the public.

In trying to overcome this problem, the state-based cancer councils have worked with BOM and ARPANSA to develop an effective way to communicate a more media-friendly UV index. The SunSmart UV Alert (Fig. 3) shows the times of day when UV levels are greater than 3. Following in-depth focus testing (19), it is published in every daily newspaper across Australia throughout the year.

DOES THE UV INDEX INFLUENCE BEHAVIOR?

Few studies to date have attempted to measure the impact of the UV index on people's knowledge, attitudes, and, in particular, sun-protection behavior. Notably, most of these studies were conducted following the launch of the 1995 UV index that focussed on the definition of the UV index as a physical measure. Few if any studies have been published since the launch of the 2002 UV index that complemented the original definition of the UV index with a comprehensive communications concept as well as clear and consistent sun-protection messages for each UV index value. Consequently, the overview of the research literature below provides an insight into the usefulness of the UV

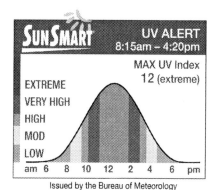

Issued by the Bureau of Meteorology

Figure 3 Highlighting dangerous hours. *Source*: Courtesy of the Australian Bureau of Meteorology.

index in general; it is not yet possible to assess the impact of the communications concept of the revised global solar UV index.

A 1997 Australian study by Alberink et al. (20) showed that out of 977 residents, the majority (92% of men and 86% of women) responded having seen or heard of the UV index forecast during the summer. A total of 28% of men and 46% of women reported that their outdoor behavior was influenced by knowledge of the UV index forecast.

Galler et al. (21), in a U.S. study of 700 white adults published in the same year, reported similar results (21). Nearly, 64% of the respondents had heard of the UV index; of these, 38% stated that they or their family had changed their sun-protection practices as a result. The study also showed that the majority of television weather forecasters and newspapers broadcast the UV index but noted that further evaluation was required to maximize the impact of the UV index on sun-protection practices.

Lovato et al. (22,23) conducted wide-ranging interviews with 4023 Canadians on their sun-protection attitudes and actions in the 1996 National Survey on Sun Exposure and Protective Behaviors. They found that 90% of Canadians had heard or seen the UV index during the previous summer. Of those, 56% indicated that they took extra precautions to protect themselves from the sun on days when the UV index was rated high.

In an innovative Australian study by Dixon et al. (24), 557 adults received a UV index reminder through their workplace email. Each of the participants was randomly allocated to receive one of three weather forecasts: a standard forecast (no UV index), a standard forecast plus UV index, a standard forecast plus UV index plus sun-protection message. Every Monday, they were e-mailed promptly to complete a Web-based questionnaire that asked about sun-related behaviors and any sunburn experienced during the previous weekend. The results indicate that the provision of UV index information as part of e-mail-based weather forecasts did not promote markedly enhanced personal sun-protection practices among the adults surveyed.

According to a series of surveys conducted in 1992, 1996, 2000, and 2004, 90% of the French population are aware of the existence of a UV radiation scale (25–29). The survey results also demonstrate that the UV index has made the population more aware of the concept of dangerous hours and the special vulnerability of children, and the consequent need to take precautions. In France, the possibility to quantify UV radiation levels in a simple way has also facilitated the education of children from the age of five years—whether in the context of a science curriculum or in the context of outdoor playtime.

In Switzerland, a representative population survey was conducted by computer-assisted telephone interview in 1998, 1999, 2002, and 2003 (30–33). Depending on the year, between 34% and 51% of the respondents claimed to be aware of the UV index. However, only about half of those who stated that they knew the UV index could also define it correctly. Between 17% and 26% of those respondents who defined the UV index correctly (approximately 5% of all respondents) reported that they had consulted the UV index during the last year.

In a Swedish randomized intervention trial, Branstorm et al. (34) investigated the impact of the UV index on sun-bathing practices and the frequency of sunburn. While overall knowledge of UV radiation was enhanced, there was no difference in behavior or frequency of sunburn between study participants that had received information about the UV index compared with study participants that had received more general written information about UV radiation.

As illustrated through the overview above, the limited research on the impact of the UV index shows mixed results. Although most studies report that the majority of people have seen or heard of the UV index, the forecast has not always had the desired effect. Thus, it is not yet possible to conclude that making the UV index widely available can motivate behavior change. The lack of knowledge on the usefulness and impact of the UV index has been a stumbling block for the widespread adoption and dissemination of the UV index among key players responsible for the delivery of the UV index in the United Kingdom. Significantly more research needs to be undertaken to ascertain the best method of delivering the information effectively and to determine what impact this has on behavior.

LESSONS LEARNED AND OPPORTUNITIES AHEAD

Problems encountered in relation to the UV index vary depending on geographic location and climate, awareness levels among the population regarding exposure to UV radiation and skin cancer, and the state of a country's UV index campaign. Nevertheless, a number of common problems emerge that, once identified, can be addressed through appropriate strategies.

Lack of variation in the UV index message: Several countries note problems with having to report the same category of UV radiation levels throughout the summer. For example, in Argentina, as much of the country is located in the tropical and subtropical regions, the use of the qualifying word "extreme" to cover all UV index values from 11 is considered too limiting, as the UV index reports and associated sun-protection messages stay the same for many months of the year. Furthermore, many Argentines have darker skin that has adapted over centuries to life in a high UV radiation tropical environment.

Limited media interest: A key challenge remains the unwillingness of the media to promote the daily UV index forecasts. Even focussed outreach strategies have shown limited success. In Switzerland, national TV stations and daily newspapers with a large-scale distribution do not find the UV index sufficiently attractive for inclusion in daily broadcasting. An additional difficulty is that most of the TV stations buy ready-made weather forecasts from private meteorological companies that have not shown a willingness to include the UV index in their programs. It emerges from the Australian experience that more needs to be done to engage the media as well as to encourage government agencies to promote the UV index in a more consistent fashion through standardized weather reports to the media.

Confused understanding of the UV index: Several countries launched UV index forecast programs from 1992 through 1996, yet a large fraction of the general public still do not understand its meaning. Even though the UV index is widely known in Canada, people do not have a clear idea how to apply it to their daily lives, despite continuing efforts to widely publicize the recommendations on appropriate sun-protective actions at various UV index levels. The Norwegian experience confirms the need for a comprehensive sun-protection message: it is simple to communicate a single number, yet it is essential to provide additional information based on which people can take action.

Restricted applicability to all skin types: While the values of the UV index represent a generally applicable physical measure of UV radiation levels, the sun-protection messages developed by WHO were specifically geared toward the most vulnerable segments of society: children and fair-skinned people. In countries, where much of the population has dark skin, there may be a need to adapt these messages or to develop specific messages for different population groups.

Without doubt, the most effective method to communicate the UV index to the general public is via the mass media and this route has not been fully exploited. More work needs to be undertaken to determine effective ways in which the UV index can be delivered to the media in a ready-to-use format. Television, in particular, provides an excellent medium to trigger changes in attitudes and behavior, and appealing TV or cinema spots could help provide emotive rather than intellectual access to the UV index. Opportunities also exist to draw the attention of weather presenters to the UV index, many of which have not been adequately trained as to its meaning and value as a public health tool.

Public outdoor venues represent another yet untapped opportunity (Box 3). UV index values could be displayed at outdoor sites, such as sporting clubs or national parks. Similarly, major outdoor events, such as tennis tournaments, swimming competitions, and local markets could serve as an entry-point to raise people's awareness about the need to protect themselves from the sun.

Box 3   Switzerland: The UV Index for Many Audiences and Settings

In Switzerland, a UV index service was first set up in 1998 and is accessible via telephone, fax, and the internet as well as print media, radio and, to some extent, television. Switzerland was also one of the first countries to adopt the revised global solar UV index. Since 2003, the Swiss Federal Office of Public Health, the Swiss Meteorological Office, and the Swiss Cancer League have joined forces in developing and launching a five-year UV index information campaign.

Realizing the need to address many different audiences if the UV index is to become well known and used, this campaign has been developing a variety of products. For example, a daily UV index display is distributed to medical surgeries, pharmacies, opticians, and tourism offices. School materials include an experimental kit about UV radiation and the weather as well as stories and lesson plans for different age groups of students. The academic and medical community are targeted through scientific articles, reports in print and electronic media, and presentations. And, given Switzerland's mountainous nature and attraction as a holiday destination, a poster campaign specifically addresses people walking, climbing, or skiing in the Alps.

The risks and benefits of UV radiation exposure vary for different population groups: while fair-skinned individuals and young children are very UV-sensitive, dark-skinned people living in northern latitudes and the elderly who tend to spend little time outdoors may lack sufficient exposure to UV radiation for vitamin D production. The UV index can be an important tool to provide more refined information as to when sun protection is not required to enable the body to generate sufficient vitamin D.

The inherently contradictive combination of a binary response (sun protection is required above a threshold UV index value of three) with a graded approach (extra protection is required at UV index values above seven) poses another challenge. Without losing the variation in the sun-protection message, this contradiction may be resolved by highlighting the times when sun protection is required. For example, at a UV index of six, sun protection may only be required for a period of four hours around midday, whereas at values of eight or above, sun protection may be required throughout the day. Australia has attempted to implement this scheme (Box 2), yet improvements in the graphical presentation and testing with the public and the media will be required to prove the usefulness of the dangerous hour scheme.

The UV index has the potential to become a very valuable public health tool to educate people about the importance of sun protection and, ultimately, to motivate changes in attitudes and behaviors. Therefore, the UV index must be promoted by health and environment agencies, weather bureaus, and media outlets at the country level. Different settings—schools, outdoor venues, pharmacies, medical surgeries—provide a range of entry-points for alerting people about UV radiation levels and sun protection. Yet, more needs to be done to evaluate the existing communication strategies and to learn from successes and failures to ensure that we maximize the existing uniform system of measuring and reporting UV radiation levels throughout the world.

ACKNOWLEDGMENTS

The authors would like to thank Ruben Piacentini (Argentina), Lilia Deschamps (Australia), Yvonne Bilan-Wallace, Kari Brintnell, Dave Broadhurst, Yvon Deslauriers, Angus Fergusson, Viteli Fioletov, Keith Keddy, Pascale Reinhardt, David Tarasick, David Wardle (Canada), Pierre Césarini (France), John YK Leung and WL Chang (Hong Kong), Terje Christensen (Norway), Beat Gerber (Switzerland), and Alastair McKinlay (United Kingdom) for their contribution of case studies and lessons learnt in countries around the world. A particular thanks goes to our Canadian colleagues for their detailed comments and insightful suggestions on an earlier draft of this chapter.

REFERENCES

1. Tena F, Martinex-Lozano JA, Utrillas MP, Martin MJ. UV monitoring and global solar UV index. International Non-Ionizing Radiation Workshop and Symposium, Seville, Spain, May 20–22, 2004.
2. World Health Organization, World Meteorological Organization, United Nations Environment Programme, International Commission on Non-Ionizing Radiation Protection. Global Solar UV Index. Neuherberg: International Commission on Non-Ionizing Radiation Protection, 1995.
3. Burrows W, Vallée M, Wardle D, Kerr J, Wilson L, Tarasick D. The Canadian operational procedure for forecasting total ozone and UV radiation. Meteorol Appl 1994; 1:247–265.
4. Kerr JB, McElroy CT, Tarasick DW, Wardle DI. Proceedings Quadrennial Ozone Symposium, The Canadian Ozone Watch and UV-B Advisory Programs, Charlottesville, VA, 1992.
5. World Meteorological Organization Global Atmosphere Watch. Report of the WMO meeting of experts on UV-B measurements, data quality and standardization of UV indices. Geneva: World Meteorological Organization, no. 95, 1994.
6. Geller AC, Hufford D, Miller DR, et al. Evaluation of the ultraviolet index: media reactions and public responses. J Am Acad Dermatol 1997; 37:935–941.

7. Morbidity and Mortality Weekly Report. Media dissemination of and public response to the ultraviolet index—United States, 1994–1995. Arch Dermatol 1997; 133: 907–908.

8. Repacholi MH. Global solar UV index. Radiat Prot Dosimetry 2000; 91:307–311.

9. World Health Organization, World Meteorological Organization, United Nations Environment Programme, International Commission on Non-Ionizing Radiation Protection. Global Solar UV Index: A Practical Guide. Geneva: World Health Organization, 2002.

10. Meves A, Repacholi MH, Rehfuess EA. Global solar UV index: a physician's tool for fighting the skin cancer epidemic. Int J Dermatol 2003; 42:846–849.

11. Meves A, Repacholi MH, Rehfuess EA. Promoting safe and effective sun protection strategies. J Am Acad Dermatol 2003; 49(6):1203–1204.

12. Vainio H, Bianchini F, eds. Sunscreens. IARC Handbooks of Cancer Prevention Vol. 5. Lyon: International Agency for Research on Cancer, 2001.

13. Rehfuess EA, von Ehrenstein OS. Ultraviolet radiation. In: Tamburlini G, von Ehrenstein OS, Bertollini R, eds. Children's Health and Environment: A Review of Evidence. Copenhagen: World Health Organization Regional Office for Europe and European Environment Agency, 2002:161–171.

14. World Health Organization. Protecting children from ultraviolet radiation. WHO Fact Sheet 261. Geneva: World Health Organization, 2001.

15. Westerdahl J, Olsson H, Ingvar C. At what age do sunburn episodes play a crucial role for the development of malignant melanoma? Rev Eur J Cancer 1994; 30A:1647–1654.

16. Whiteman DC, Whiteman CA, Green AC. Childhood sun exposure as a risk factor for melanoma: a systematic review of epidemiologic studies: review. CCC 2001; 12:69–82.

17. http://www.bom.gov.au/info/about_uvb.shtml.

18. Dixon H, Lemus-Deschamps L, Gies P. Meteorology meets public health: UV forecasts and reports for sun safety. Health Promot J Aust 2002; 13(3):252.

19. Centre for Behavioral Research in Cancer. Pre-Testing UV Index Graphics with Young Adult and Older Adult Focus Groups. Melbourne: AntiCancer Council of Victoria, 2000.

20. Alberink A, Russell P, Green A. Do forecasts of UV indexes influence people's outdoor behaviour? Aust N Z J Public Health 2000; 24:488–491.

21. Galler A, Hufford D, Miller D, Sun T, et al. Evaluation of the ultraviolet index: media reactions and public response. J Am Acad Dermatol 1997; 37:935–941.

22. Lovato C, Shoveller J, Rivers J. National Survey on Sun Exposure and Protective Behaviours: Final Report. Vancouver: Institute of Health Promotion Research, University of British Columbia, 1998.

23. Lovato C, Shoveller J, Peters L, Rivers J. Canadian National Survey on sun exposure and protective behaviours: parents' reports on children. Cancer Prev Control 1998; 2(3):123–128.

24. Dixon H, Hill D, Karoly D, Jolley D, Aden S. Solar UV forecasts: an evaluation of the impact on adults' sun protective behaviour. 53rd Annual Conference of the International Communication Association, San Diego, California, USA (MAz 2003), 2003.

25. IFOP. Sécurité Solaire. Sondage. 2000.

26. Institut National de Prévention et d'Education pour la santé, BVA—Institut de Marché et d'Opinion. Enquete INPES/BVA. 2004.
27. IPSOS, Sanofi. Sondage. 1992.
28. IPSOS, Sanofi. Sondage. 1996.
29. IPSOS, Sanofi. Sondage. 1997.
30. Institut érasm. Sondage sur la connaissance de l'index UV. Bern: Swiss Federal Office of Public Health, 1998.
31. Institut érasm. Sondage sur la connaissance de l'index UV. Bern: Swiss Federal Office of Public Health, 1999.
32. Krebs H. Sonnenexposition und Sonnenschutz 2002—Ergebnisse einer Repräsentativbefragung in der 15- bis 64-jährigen Bevölkerung. Bern: Swiss Cancer League, 2002.
33. Krebs H. Sonnenexposition und Sonnenschutz 2002—Ergebnisse einer Repräsentativbefragung in der 15- bis 64-jährigen Bevölkerung. Bern: Swiss Cancer League, 2003.
34. Branstorm R, Ullen H, Brandberg Y. A randomized population based intervention to examine the effects of the ultraviolet index on tanning behaviour. Eur J Cancer 2003; 39(7):968–974.

22

Prevention of Malignant Melanoma: Health Economics Aspects

Bengt Jönsson

Stockholm School of Economics, Center for Health Economics, Stockholm, Sweden

Ulf Staginnus

European Health Economics, Madrid, Spain

INTRODUCTION

Health economics is a science that deals with the economic aspects of health and healthcare. Individual and collected decisions that affect health are analyzed in terms of their costs and benefits (utility). Prevention involves using resources for avoiding the occurrence of events. Prevention can be seen as an investment, which involves costs up front and creates benefits in terms of disease and illness avoided in the future. Economic evaluation is a method aimed at assessing, in a systematic way, the costs and benefits of this investment. In an economic evaluation, resources used are valued according to their "opportunity cost," that is, their forgone value in the best alternative use. There may be an opportunity cost even if no money is paid out. For example, a visit to the physician for a check-up of an abnormality can have an opportunity cost even if it is free. The time used for the visit could have been used for other production or consumption. The identification, quantification, and valuation of resources used for prevention are an important part of an economic evaluation. But equally important is the assessment of the benefits gained by this investment. Those benefits may come much later in time and may only be arising with a certain probability, and will therefore be associated with a high uncertainty.

The most obvious benefit of a preventive program is a reduction in the number of future cases of the disease. However, to estimate the absolute risk reduction means having good estimates of both the absolute risk and the relative risk reduction from intervention. In addition, the number of cases avoided is only the first step toward a full economic evaluation. It is also necessary to estimate the effect of case reduction on survival and quality of life in order to come up with an estimate of the cost per quality-adjusted life-year gained from the intervention. Only this outcome measure allows a comparison with resource utilization from other interventions with the same purpose in order to improve health.

There are few health economic studies on the prevention of malignant melanoma. Hardly any references are found for the cost-effectiveness of primary prevention. The most common interventions aim at reducing the exposure to sunlight (UV radiation), either via direct avoidance or artificially through sun blockers. The benefits of those interventions are established, as exposure involves increased risk. However, the quantification of the risk is surrounded by uncertainty. Even more problematic is to assess the individual costs of complying with these measures. There are no published studies on how individuals perceive the risk and benefits, and whether these individual assessments can be regarded as rational. A cost can be easily assigned to information campaigns in terms of the resources used, but the benefits created can hardly be measured as such measures aim at changing individual behavior, which has unknown costs and benefits.

Early detection, through opportunistic screening (case finding) or formal screening program is a clear-cut candidate for economic evaluation. In fact, for economic evaluation in cancer, economic evaluation of prevention in general and screening in particular dominate the health economic references found in the literature. One reason for this is that treatments for cancer have been of limited effectiveness in most cases, which means that early detection can be a cost-effective alternative to ineffective treatment.

There are a number of criteria for screening programs to be an effective alternative. The most common are (1)

1. The performance of the screening method/diagnostic test (sensitivity/specificity)
2. Consideration of populations' covariate (general screening vs. high risk patients etc.)
3. Logistical and coverage issues (can the target population be reached effectively?), and, most importantly
4. Does a case detection ultimately lead to reduced morbidity and mortality?

Given the relatively high burden of disease due to melanoma in some countries, for example, in the United States the annual direct cost of treating newly diagnosed melanoma in 1997 was estimated to be $563 million (2).

A study of similar design from Sweden (3) assessed the annual direct and indirect costs of skin diseases caused by ultraviolet radiation. The researchers from the Karolinska Institute developed a model for cost-of-illness, whereby costs for hospital care, primary care, pharmaceuticals, mortality, and morbidity, for approximately 1.8 million inhabitants in Stockholm were evaluated. The total disease burden amounted to an annual discounted cost of 162 million SEK (approximately US $16 million in 2002). The indirect costs were the major cost driver (56% of total costs), mainly due to an estimated cost of mortality for cutaneous malignant melanoma of SEK84 million (US $8.4 million). The direct costs (approximately SEK71 million = US $7.1million) were predominated by hospital ambulatory care costs of about SEK33 million (US $3.3 million). Overall, direct cost amounted to only 0.4% of the overall healthcare costs for hospital care and primary health care in the Stockholm area. Areas with relatively low incidence of skin disease caused by ultraviolet radiation incur moderate economic losses in the community. Therefore, it may not be easy to make successful prevention of these diseases economically beneficial.

This may be entirely different in areas of high endemnicity such as Australia, southern Europe, or the southern states of the United States.

In these regions, it is suggested that aggressive primary prevention through sun protection and secondary prevention through intensive screening to enhance earlier detection could reduce the economic burden of melanoma care (4).

The available economic evidence of measures of primary and secondary prevention is further reviewed in this chapter opportunities for future research will be discussed.

PRIMARY PREVENTION

Primary prevention consists of limiting exposure to sunlight and using sunscreens. Light-skinned persons should be informed of the importance of limiting sun exposure and avoiding sunburns; this advice is particularly important for children and teenagers. This recommendation is based on risk reduction. However, considering the expected effects of sunscreen usage, a recent meta-analysis (5) found no association between this form of prevention and decreased incidence of melanoma. This finding may be explained due to the fact that sunscreens often provide a false sense of security and many times are used incorrectly, thereby leading to inadequate overall protection from exposure to ultraviolet light. On the other hand, studies from Spain and Australia arrive at the contrary conclusion (6). From an economic perspective, an Australian study (7) examined the potential cost-effectiveness of a national sun protection campaign using sunscreens (SunSmart). Model assumptions were made about the potential reduction of incidence and premature mortality due to the reduction of sun exposure. Cost-offsets in terms of lower management cost for skin cancer as compared to the cost of the campaign and cost per life-year gained were calculated. On the basis of the assumptions of the analysis (compared to a "do-nothing strategy") the annual net cost of the campaign (over a 20-year period) is estimated to be AUS $5 million and would result in 4300 premature death avoided with a cost of AUS $1.360 per life-year saved. The authors therefore conclude that a national campaign of this kind would be excellent value for money.

Evidence shows that some community-level campaigns effectively reduce sun exposure. For example, educational and policy approaches in elementary schools can change sun-protective behavior in children (8). Similar interventions in recreational and tourism settings can change sun-protective behavior in adults (9). However, it is still difficult to economically evaluate the individual behavior and the "memory effect" of information campaigns within the target population maybe rapidly declining, if not frequently repeated. Thus, a cost can be assigned to, for example, a TV advertisement, but the uncertainty around the compliance of the target audience and future benefits make a full economic evaluation difficult and require many assumptions that would need to be validated by longitudinal randomized or observational studies. Furthermore, there may be considerable external effects associated with primary prevention campaigns in the form of increased excision of benign skin lesions with significant associated cost that would need to be considered in such economic evaluations (10).

SECONDARY PREVENTION

Secondary prevention consists of routinely performing a total skin examination for a specific segment of the population or potential immunotherapy approaches.

In theory, routine screening for melanoma could save lives, because earlier detection of thinner tumors is associated with better survival rates. Screening can be performed on whole populations (population-based screening) or on high-risk subgroups of the population. Several organizations recommend routine screening solely for high-risk groups. Only the American Academy of Dermatology, the National Institutes of Health Consensus Conference on Early Melanoma and the American Cancer Society favor population-based screening in addition to screening for high-risk groups (11). However, there is no evidence to support population-based screening through randomized, controlled trials (12); however, first studies to answer that question are underway in Australia (13).

The health economic literature on the prevention of malignant melanoma is dominated by only a few and older studies of different formal screening programs or approaches to case finding. Some of the main publications are briefly reviewed hereunder.

Economics of Educational Campaigns and Screening

Melanoma is theoretically an ideal model for prevention campaigns to increase the avoidance of direct sun exposure. Various programs have been reported from different regions in the world. Any campaign, which can increase the notoriety of melanoma in the public, can probably improve early diagnosis and thereby potentially increase survival and reduce healthcare resources.

In an Italian study, Garattini et al. (14) researched the economic consequences of an educational campaign for early diagnosis of cutaneous melanoma as public educational campaigns for the early diagnosis of cutaneous increase the number of cases detected early and consequently lengthen patients' life expectancy. The researchers performed an economic evaluation of such a campaign in Bergamo, Italy, in order to quantify its costs and consequences. Cost-effectiveness analysis was used to compare the costs and effects of the public campaign with those of the do-nothing option. The analysis was performed from the perspective of the Italian National Health Service. Only direct costs related to publicly financed healthcare services were considered. Overall life-years gained were quantified by comparing the survival curves for four subgroups of patients with different lesional thicknesses at diagnosis. All costs were estimated in 1993 Italian lire (L). Overall undiscounted effectiveness amounted to 233.49 life-years gained; discounting with a 5% discount rate resulted in 171.3 life-years gained. The total cost of the educational campaign (i.e., the sum of the organizational and "induced" costs minus the costs saved) was estimated at L817 million (in 1993, US$ = 520 000), and L905 million (1993 US $575.000) after discounting at a rate of 5%. Thus, using discounted cost and effectiveness data, the cost of the educational campaign was estimated to be L5.28 million (US $3400) per life-year gained.

A similar approach has been published for France. The purpose of the study from Bonerandi et al. (15) conducted in the Provence-Alpes-Cote d'Azur-Corse region was to estimate the cost and effectiveness of a media campaign for the early screening of malignant melanoma at the national level. The campaign combined an effort to inform and heighten awareness in the medical community and the broadcast of an information movie for the general population on a regional TV channel. Following the broadcasting, the number of malignant melanoma diagnosed in a representative selection of pathology laboratories increased significantly compared with the same period of the previous year. This increase was mostly for malignant melanoma of low thickness, which has a good prognosis. Although the number of added cost generated by this campaign could not be precisely determined, the authors argued for a national prevention campaign based on the initial positive results and the lessons of this experience.

In the United States, Freeberg et al. (16) attempted to determine the effectiveness and costs of a visual screen to diagnose malignant melanoma in high-risk persons. They developed a decision analysis comparing no-skin-cancer screen with a single screen by a dermatologist. Clinical outcomes were malignant melanoma, nonmelanoma skin cancer, or no skin cancer. Subsequently, life expectancy and costs of care were calculated on the basis of the clinical results. They found that skin-cancer screening increased the average discounted life expectancy from 15.0963 years to 15.0975 years. On the basis of the prevalence of malignant melanoma, however, this translates into an increased discounted life expectancy of 0.9231 years for each person with diagnosed melanoma. Using a cost of $30 per screen, total skin cancer-related costs for a cohort of one million people increased from $826 million with no screen to $861 million with screening, with an increase of 1200 years of life. This resulted in an incremental cost-effectiveness ratio of $29,170 per life-year gained with screening. Sensitivity analysis showed that the cost-effectiveness ratio for screening remained below $50,000 per year of life saved if the prevalence of melanoma in the screened population was at least 0.0009, the probability that a melanoma detected in screening was at least 94.8%, or the cost of each screen was below $57. The key assumptions in the model, affecting the calculation of both effectiveness and cost, were that the proportion of late-stage melanomas would decrease from 6.1% without screening to 1.1% with screening. Similarly, the model assumed that invasive cancers would decrease from 20.1% to 12.6% of invasive melanomas. The researchers concluded that skin-cancer screening in high-risk patients is likely to be associated with only a small increase in discounted life expectancy and is reasonably cost-effective compared with other cancer screening strategies.

The country with the highest rate of skin cancer in the world is Australia. It is estimated that the incidence rate will be doubling every 10 years. Despite advances in the early detection and treatment of melanoma, about 800 people still die nationally of the disease each year (17). It is suggested by Girgis et al. (18) that a possible strategy for further reducing the mortality from melanoma is an organized program of population screening for unsuspected lesions in asymptomatic individuals. Up until now, arguments against introducing melanoma screening have been based on cost and the lack of reliable data on the efficacy of any screening tests. Few systematic economic assessments of the cost-effectiveness of melanoma screenings were available. The purpose of their research was to determine whether screening will be potentially cost-effective and, therefore, it warrants further investigation. A mathematical model was used to simulate the effects of a hypothetical melanoma-screening program that was in operation for 20 years, using cohorts of Australians aged 50 at the start of the program. On the basis of this calculation, cost-effectiveness estimates of melanoma screening were estimated. Under the baseline assumptions used in the model and setting the sensitivity of the screening test (visual inspection of the skin) at 60%, cost effectiveness ranged from AUS $6.853 per life-year gained for men, if screening was undertaken five-yearly, to $12.137, if screening was two-yearly. For women, cost-effectiveness ranged from $11.102 for five-yearly screening to $20,877 for two-yearly screening. The analysis suggests that a melanoma-screening program could be cost-effective, particularly if five yearly screening is implemented for men over the age of 50.

A more recent publication from McCarthy (19) outlines how primary and secondary prevention programs are now showing positive outcomes, especially in melanoma incidence and survival. In Australia, primary and secondary prevention initiatives are performed by a variety of nongovernment organizations such as the Australian Cancer Council, which is comprised of state anticancer groups, with some assistance from state and federal health agencies. Specific community groups at higher risk, noticeably teenagers and the older population, are the focus of current and future campaigns. The role of sun protection through creams and lotions as the primary preventative approach has been superseded by sunlight avoidance campaigns. McCarthy concludes that, when taking into account the increasing rate of early diagnosis, a low and falling morbidity of melanoma, improving general practitioner competence in skin cancer diagnosis and the growth of skin cancer clinics throughout Australia, it is not likely that the implementation of a skin-cancer screening program will be seen at the national level.

As demonstrated in the previous examples, campaigns to reduce delay in diagnosis by a combination of professional and public education have been reported from several centers around the world. The effects of these campaigns in reducing the depth distribution of cutaneous malignant melanoma have sometimes been encouraging, especially in combination with advertisements prior to screening programs (20), but in other instances have shown little effect (12,16).

Until there is clear evidence that early detection reduces mortality from melanoma, the opportunistic promotion of early detection may not be cost-effective and will fail to reach all sections of the community at risk, although some studies have demonstrated positive effects (21) and potential cost-effectiveness, for example, in high-risk populations. Therefore, at the present time, the emphasis should be on the primary prevention of skin cancer by emphasizing prospective personal responsibility for health (9,22,23).

Immunotherapy

Among the treatment options for malignant melanoma that have emerged in the past decades, cancer vaccine immunotherapy seems to present a promising and relatively safer approach as compared with chemotherapy and radiotherapy, according to Saleh et al. (24). The identification of different tumor antigens in the last 15 years, using a variety of techniques, allowed more refining of the cancer vaccines that are currently used in different clinical trials. In a subset of treated patients, some of these vaccines have resulted in partial or complete tumor regression, while they have increased the disease-free survival rate in others. These outcomes are more pronounced in patients suffering from melanoma (24).

Patients presenting with thick primary melanomas or those with regional nodal metastases have a high risk of recurrence after surgery alone (25). Chemotherapy has limited efficacy in the adjuvant setting, and whereas the use of high-dose interferon in the adjuvant setting has been reported to improve survival, treatment with interferon is not without significant cost and toxicity. There is mounting evidence that the immune system plays a prominent role in the natural history of melanoma and the clinical success of interferon highlights the potential for immunotherapy to prevent recurrence. Many researchers hope to use melanoma vaccines to reduce recurrence without significant toxicity and many different vaccine strategies are being investigated.

Notwithstanding the apparent and tremendous potential for vaccines in malignant melanoma, large prospective, randomized trial have to first demonstrate survival benefits to make them economically efficient for widespread adaptation. From a health economics perspective, vaccines have generally been a cost-effective option in many areas, for example, infectious diseases. However, it remains to be determined what the potential cost-effectiveness of future melanoma vaccines will look like. Important factors to be considered when conducting economic evaluation of vaccination programs for the prevention of skin cancer are: acquisition cost of the vaccine, the vaccine administration cost or logistics required to immunize target populations, costs of screening when necessary, costs of publicity and awareness campaigns, cost of side effects, and of course the efficacy of the vaccine program (26). Other important factors are the number of doses required (compliance issues) and the persistence (or waning) of the immune response.

Typical consequences of immunization programs are the number of new cases avoided, life-years saved, and quality-adjusted life-years gained. It can be expected that a relatively high efficacy will be required to make melanoma immunotherapy a cost-effective secondary prevention strategy.

ISSUES FOR FURTHER RESEARCH

Primary preventive measures do not lend themselves easy to evaluations in terms of costs and benefits. A more fruitful economics approach may be to use methods from behavior economics to improve the understanding of how individuals make decisions regarding activities that involve sun exposure and the risk of melanoma. A better understanding of the individual trade-offs, may give ideas for cost-effective interventions aimed at reducing risk.

Future research may also be directed to help the clinicians identify primary care patients at high risk for melanoma. Using such a risk-assessment technique would be the most promising strategy in addressing the excess burden of disease in the elderly and at the same time would improve cost-effectiveness as compared to the population-based screening initiatives.

As most economic evaluation of screening campaigns published in the health economics literature dates back to the early and mid 90s, re-evaluations and new cost-effectiveness studies of screening programs utilizing the latest evidence and new data seem indicated. Once randomized clinical trials of screening strategies become available, more comprehensive and economic models can be constructed in order to better inform decision-making on skin cancer prevention campaigns.

CONCLUSIONS

No randomized or case–control studies have been conducted that would demonstrate that routine screening for melanoma by primary care providers reduces morbidity or mortality. It is thus not possible to make a full economic evaluation of the cost-benefit and cost-utility of screening for malignant melanoma. Available studies indicate that screening, especially for high-risk patients, could be cost-effective; however, the ultimate evidence can only be provided after economic evaluations of the randomized controlled clinical trials can be performed. Immunotherapeutics may become a promising alternative in the future. However, only after the successful completion of the ongoing trials can their potential economic impact be evaluated. For the time being, primary prevention through direct sun avoidance seems to be the best approach. Measures that encourage personal responsibility are of increasing importance and behavioral economics might become an interesting field of research in the area of primary prevention of malignant melanoma.

REFERENCES

1. Sassi F, McKee M, Robers JA. Economic evaluation of diagnostic technology. Methodological challenges and viable solutions. Int J Technol Assess Health Care 1997; 3(4):613–650.
2. Tsao H, Rogers GS, Sober EJ. Reply. J Am Acad Dermatol 1999; 41(2 Pt 1):281–283.
3. Nilsson GH, Carlsson L, Dal H, et al. Skin diseases caused by ultraviolet radiation: the cost of illness. Int J Technol Assess Health Care 2003; 19(4):724–730.
4. Martin RH. Relationship between risk factors, knowledge and preventive behaviour relevant to skin cancer in general practice patients in south Australia. Br J Gen Pract 1995; 45:365–367.
5. Helfand M, Krages KP. Counseling to prevent skin cancer: a summary of the evidence for the U.S. Preventive Services Task Force. Rockville, Md.: Agency for Healthcare Research and Quality, 2003. Accessed November 31, 2005, at: http://www.ahrq.gov/clinic/3rduspstf/skcacoun/skcounsum.htm.
6. Darrell S, Rigel MD, Carucci JA. Malignant melanoma: prevention, early detection, and treatment in the 21st century. CA Cancer J Clin 2000; 50:215–236.
7. Carter R, Marks R, Hill D. Could a national skin cancer primary campaign in Australia be worthwhile?: an economic perspective. Health promotional international 1999; 14(1):73–83.
8. Hill D, Dixon H. Promoting sun protection in children: rationale and challenges. Health Educ Behav 1998; 26(3):409–417.
9. Austoker J. Melanoma: prevention and early diagnosis. Brit Med J 1994; 309(6948):168–174.
10. Del Mar CB, Green AC, Battistutta D. Do public media campaigns designed to increase skin cancer awareness result in increased skin excision rates? Aust NZ J Public Health 1997; 21(7):751–754.
11. Rager EL, Bridgeford ED, Ollila DW. Cutaneous melanoma: update on prevention, screening, diagnosis, and treatment. Am Fam Physician 2005; 72:269–276.

12. Helfand M, Mahon SM, Eden B, et al. Screening for skin cancer. Am J Prev Med 2001; 20(suppl 3):47–58.
13. Aitken JF, Elwood JM, Lowe JB, et al. A randomised trial of population screening for melanoma. J Med Screen 2002; 9:33–37.
14. Garattini L, Cainelli D, Tribbia G, et al. Economic evaluation of an educational campaign for early diagnosis of cutaneous melanoma. Pharmacoeconomics 1996; 9(2):146–155.
15. Bonerandi JJ, Grob JJ, Cnudde, N et al. Campaign of early detection of melanoma in the Provence-Alpes-Cote-d'Azur area 1989. lessons of an experience. Ann Dermatol Venereol 119(2):105–109.
16. Freedberg KA, Geller AC, Miller DR, et al. Screening for malignant melanoma: a cost-effectiveness analysis. J Am Acad Dermatol 1999; 41(5 Pt 1):738–745.
17. Katris P, Donovan RJ, Gray BN. Nurses screening for skin cancer: an observation study. Aust N Z J Public Health 1998; 22(suppl 3):381–383.
18. Girgis A, Clarke P, Burton RC, et al. Screening for melanoma by primary health care physicians: a cost-effectiveness analysis. J Med Screen 1996; 3(1):47–53.
19. McCarthy WH. The Australian experience in sun protection and screening for melanoma. J Surg Onc 2004; 86(4):236–245.
20. Katris P, Donovan RJ, Gray BN. The use of targeted and non-targeted advertising to enrich skin cancer screening samples. Br J Dermatol 1996; 135(2):268–274.
21. Brobeil A, Rapaport D, Wells K. Multiple primary melanomas: implications for screening and follow-up programs for melanoma. Ann Surg Oncol 1997; 4(1):19–23.
22. Marckmann G, Mohrle M, Blum A. Taking responsibility for one's own health: possibilities and limits using the example of malignant melanoma. Hautarzt 2004; 55(8):715–720.
23. Rhodes AR. Public education and cancer of the skin. What do people need to know about melanoma and nonmelanoma skin cancer? Cancer 1995; 75(suppl 2):613–636.
24. Saleh F, Renno W, Klepacek I, et al. Melanoma immunotherapy: past, present, and future. Curr Pharm Des 2005; 11(27):3461–3473.
25. Sabel MS, Sondak VK. Tumor vaccines: a role in preventing recurrence in melanoma? Am J Clin Dermatol 2002; 3(9):609–616.
26. Demicheli V, Jefferson T. Economics aspects of vaccination. Vaccine 1996; 14(10):941–943.

23

Screening for Melanoma

Frederick C. Beddingfield

*Department of Medicine, Division of Dermatology, David Geffen School
of Medicine at UCLA, Los Angeles, California, U.S.A.*

INTRODUCTION

Melanoma incidence and mortality have risen dramatically during this century in
almost all countries and, in particular, in fair-skinned populations (1,2). In the
United States, in 1935, one's estimated lifetime risk of disease was one in
1500 (3). In the year 2000, the lifetime risk of melanoma was estimated at 1 in
75 persons. In Australia, the lifetime risk has been estimated at 1 in 25 (3).
Some have questioned whether these statistics truly reveal an alarming increase
in disease or, in fact, are a sign of increased efforts at screening and diagnosing
the disease (4,5). Others do not hold this view (6). Some have suggested much of
the increase has been in a non-metastasizing biologically benign form of melanoma or simply in changes in the diagnostic criteria for melanoma by pathologists (4,5). The implications of this debate on public health initiatives are
substantial. In many countries, worldwide melanoma is of significant concern
and in these countries public interventions are being conducted to promote
earlier detection and treatment of the disease. Are these efforts worthwhile or
would resources be better spent elsewhere? The answer depends not only on
the interventions themselves, but also on the true nature of the epidemic. The
most recent data on melanoma incidence suggests that while melanoma is
being diagnosed earlier accounting for much of the increase in incidence, the
percent increase of localized tumors of all Breslow levels have increased since
the late 1980s (7–9). Moreover, mortality has been increasing at rates that

warrant concern (7), and higher mortality rates suggest that the increased incidence is not due to screening alone.

Is screening for melanoma worthwhile? The characteristics of a good cancer-screening program have been previously described (10).

1. Screening should be highly sensitive and specific.
2. The prevalence of the disease should be high enough to warrant screening.
3. Health implications should be high enough to warrant screening.
4. The disease should be slowly progressing and not immediately life-threatening.
5. The screening procedure should be simple, inexpensive, and acceptable to the population being screened.
6. The disease should be one for which early diagnosis results in improved prognosis.
7. Screening should lead to more effective treatment at an earlier stage. In addition to these criteria one might add the following.
8. The population to be screened should be identifiable and reachable so as to accurately target one's screening campaign.
9. The campaign's cost-effectiveness should be comparable to or better than other cancer screening campaigns.

Melanoma does appear to have many characteristics that might make it suitable to screening. It is identifiable at stages when treatment results in survival approaching 100%. The screening examination is sensitive and specific, non-invasive, inexpensive, generally acceptable, and does not pose a risk to patients. Furthermore, recent data have shown that screening for melanoma is relatively more cost-effective than many other types of screening for cancer that we currently perform (11–14).

INCIDENCE

The annual incidence of melanoma among Caucasians has risen rapidly between 3% and 7% over the last several decades (7–9). According to the most recent statistics in the United States, the incidence has not abated, though a recent Joinpoint analysis of Surveillance, Epidemiology, and End Results (SEER) (9) data showed the incidence rose less sharply in the most recent years (8). The incidence of melanoma in the United States, in 1997, was 14.3 per 100,000 (9). This is a sharp increase from 5.7 per 100,000 in 1973 (9). The incidence is not uniformly distributed over the population. Caucasians, the elderly, and men seem to have the highest rates (7,8). In the United States, men have higher rates than women (7–9), whereas in countries with lower incidence rates, women generally have higher rates than men (15). For men, the U.S. 1973 and 1997 incidence rates are 6.1 and 17.2 per 100,000, respectively (9). For women, the comparable 1973 and 1997 statistics are 5.4 and 12.0 per 100,000, respectively. Not only are elderly men at higher risk than elderly women, but the rate of increase in recent years among elderly men has also been higher than in elderly women (7). Caucasians are much more at risk with Hispanics, Asians, and African-Americans who had rates of 2.9, 1.1, and 0.8 per 100,000, respectively, from 1990 to 1997 (SEER) (9). In Australia, the incidence of melanoma is the highest in the world at more than 40 per 100,000 persons, whereas in certain Northern European countries the incidence is less than five per 100,000 persons (15). Persons with fairer skin types, who move closer to the equator, increase their risk of melanoma (15).

Birth cohort also influences one's risk of melanoma with later birth years being associated with higher age-specific incidence rates and with differences between successive birth cohorts increasing more rapidly over time (7). There has, however, been a leveling-off of the rate of rise in incidence in birth cohorts since the 1960s in Australia (16) and the United States (6). The causes of this slowdown in the rate of rise in the incidence for these latter cohorts are unknown but could relate to primary prevention effects.

Melanoma incidence is also dependent on age and gender (7–9). Incidence rises with age, especially in men. In the United States, women have a slightly higher risk of melanoma than men before age 40. After 40, men have a higher incidence and the difference becomes remarkably large with increasing age. By age 85, the incidence in men is approximately twice that in women (7,9).

Recent results suggest significant increases in early stage melanomas and in situ lesions (6,17). Some have questioned whether this increase is primarily due to early detection or to detection of clinically insignificant lesions (5,18), but further empirical analysis is needed. In a recent analysis of the SEER data, we found that melanomas of all stages increased from 1988 to 1997, but localized lesions and in situ lesions increased the most (8). However, among localized lesions, there was an increase in melanomas of all Breslow thickness levels. Breslow level is the best predictor of prognosis both independently and in multivariate analyses. In absolute numbers, thin lesions accounted for the majority of the increase. However, lesions of greater Breslow levels, though smaller in number, increased at comparable rates to thinner lesions. This strongly argues against the idea that the increase in incidence of melanoma is only due to early detection of thin lesions, at least during the time period studied, 1988–1997. If early detection of thin lesions alone were the case, one would expect for a time to see an increase in the incidence rates of thin melanomas followed by a decrease in the incidence rates of thin lesions. In that scenario, the apparent increase in incidence followed by a decline is attributable to the fact that first screenings detect the prevalent lesions and subsequent screenings detect only the cumulative incident cases since the last screening. However, in such a scenario, one would also expect a decrease in the incidence rate of thick lesions shortly after the increase in thin melanomas. This would happen because there would be less thin lesions to progress to thick lesions. These findings typical of early detection campaigns and screening were not detected in our analysis however, and this suggests increased screening is not the major factor responsible for the increase in melanoma incidence during the time period studied.

MORTALITY AND SURVIVAL

Two key factors are important regarding melanoma mortality rates. First, mortality rates have risen over the last three decades (9). Second, they have not been rising nearly as fast as incidence rates (9). Why are these two facts important? If the melanoma epidemic was due to biologically benign lesions *alone*, we would expect no increase in mortality, ceteris paribus. On the other hand, if one assumes that the treatment has not changed stage-specific mortality dramatically, the fact that mortality rates have not risen as fast as incidence rates suggests a change in the stage distribution of disease. This implies that relatively more of the increase in incidence is due to the detection of lesions, which are less lethal or less aggressive than is due to biologically aggressive lesions.

Mortality rates among fair-skinned people range from one to three per 100,000 people per year in the northern hemisphere (2,3). In Australia and New Zealand, the rates are even higher in the five to ten per 100,000 people range. Rates have not been changing equally among all strata of the population. While mortality rates in the United States have risen among older cohorts, younger cohorts have seen steady or declining mortality rates in recent years. Furthermore, on subgroup analysis from 1992 to 1998, the mortality rates among males increased, whereas the rate for females actually declined. The mortality rate in whites also increased more than in non-whites. Mortality rates, like incidence rates, also show age-specific trends. Older cohorts continue to show increased mortality in almost all countries, whereas younger cohorts show no increase or falling rates (15,16). These trends are not sufficiently explained by patterns of sun exposure alone.

While mortality rates have increased, survival for those diagnosed with melanoma has also increased in the United States, Europe, and Australia (15,17,19). For instance, the survival rates in Whites from 1960 to 1963 were estimated at 60%, the survival from 1974 to 1976 was 80%, and the survival from 1992 to 1997 was 89% (9). The reasons for this are not quite clear, though it likely has to do with earlier diagnosis at a more favorable stage rather than improved survival of late stage disease. These countries with improved survival also have made educational campaigns a priority though no clear causal link to improved survival from these plans has been documented.

DISTRIBUTION OF STAGES AT DIAGNOSIS

Most melanomas are localized and the trend is for the percentage of localized disease to continue rising (7,20,21). From 1992 to 1998, the stage distribution of U.S. melanoma cases in SEER was as follows: localized disease 82%, regional disease 9%, distant disease 4% (6% were unstaged). From 1988 to 1997, young patients and women had a higher incidence of melanomas of thinner Breslow levels when compared with older patients or men. Older patients and men had a higher incidence of melanomas of thicker Breslow levels compared with younger patients or women. For instance, in women under age 40, the incidence of melanomas less than or equal to 1 mm is nearly twice that of men. On the other hand, for men over age 60, the incidence of melanomas of greater than 4 mm is over twice that of women. From 1988 to 1997, the incidence of in situ lesions grew faster than localized disease, which increased faster than regional disease, which increased faster than distant disease (7). However, within localized disease, lesions of all Breslow levels increased at fairly comparable rates (7). Because of a shift in the stage distribution of melanomas toward thinner lesions with a disproportionate increase in incidence relative to mortality, some have questioned whether some of these thin lesions removed would have ever progressed (3,5,18,22). The idea these authors are suggesting is that some thin melanomas may be biologically benign and may never have become clinically relevant. The authors suggest these lesions are simply being detected now because of the increased propensity for physicians to biopsy pigmented lesions. While this may be true, there is no consensus that such biologically benign melanomas exist. Certainly, spontaneously regressing and slow growing, often benign-behaving, and sometimes remitting variants of other cancers are thought to exist, with actinic keratoses being one example. However, once a lesion is removed, one has lost the ability to follow its natural history. It is likely that the increases in incidence and changes in stage distribution do represent changes in biopsy patterns and diagnostic criteria to some degree. However, in the United States, increases in the incidence of lesions of higher Breslow levels are not consistent with this "epidemic" solely being due to biologically benign lesions.

ETIOLOGY AND RISK FACTORS

Studies trying to unravel the epidemiological causes of melanoma are difficult at best. Consistently though, studies point to a major role of ultraviolet light exposure as the most important risk factor for those with phenotypic susceptibility (23–25). The dramatic increases in melanomas seen over the last decades may be the result of changes in behavioral patterns relating to sun exposure and to a lesser extent ozone depletion (20,21,24). Studies suggest that a 1% reduction in ozone may lead to an increased incidence of malignant melanoma of 0.6% (24). The United Nations Environment Program estimated that in the event of 10% decrease in stratospheric ozone, an additional 300,000 cases of non-melanocytic and 4500 cases on melanoma could be expected worldwide on an annual basis. Studies show that in general melanoma prevalence increases with proximity to the equator controlling for other factors such as skin type.

As is almost always the case with cancer, environmental exposure affects people of different predispositions to melanoma differently. In the fair-skinned, red-haired, blue-eyed person who burns easily and rarely tans, the exposure to ultraviolet light appears to have an enormous real impact on melanoma risk. As an example, the risk of melanoma in whites in Australia is much higher than in Great Britain where it is also high, despite a common ancestry and phenotypic characteristics. The main reason for the different rate of melanomas appears to be predominantly the higher ultraviolet light exposure in Australia. An interesting study from Australia showed that immigration to Australia before the age of 10 increases one's risk of melanoma to that of a native Australian, while immigration after age 15 yields rates one-fourth native Australians (19).

It is thought that sunburns, especially in early life, are the most important risk factor for the development of melanoma. One or more severe sunburns in one's youth, roughly doubles the lifetime risk of melanoma (25). Case-control studies have shown with consistency that intermittent exposure, particularly if sufficient to cause sunburn, is an important factor for developing skin cancer (23–27). The male ear, which has a large amount of exposure to the sun, also has the highest incidence of melanoma of any body site per unit area (28). Also, patients with melanoma have increased solar elastosis, actinic keratoses, and nonmelanoma skin cancers, consistent with increased ultraviolet exposure (29). Ultraviolet exposure appears to result in melanoma after a long lag-time of years to decades. One of the strongest correlates of melanoma development is from those who recall many childhood burns before the age of 20. Of course, such studies are prone to recall bias, that is, the patient is more likely to remember he or she had severe sunburns only because they have developed a melanoma and thought about it sufficiently long. It may not be young age per se that is so important, as much as the behaviors associated with young age, namely sun exposure and sunburns. Superficial spreading melanoma appears to be the melanoma type most associated with intermittent sunburns. The evidence for total sun exposure as a risk factor is less clear. In fact, work-related exposure may be protective. Lentigo maligna is the skin cancer most associated with total sun exposure and unlike superficial spreading melanoma, is a disease almost exclusively of people older than 40, with a dramatic increase in incidence with age. It is also more common in men than women, and from age 45 to >85 the incidence increases approximately 15-fold (7).

From numerous studies, there appears to be a relationship between ultraviolet light exposure and the development of nevi, which are a key risk factor for the later development of melanoma (29,30–34). Complicating this is the fact that skin type is related to both tendency to develop melanoma and nevi. However, even when controlling for skin type, nevi are a central risk factor for the development of melanoma (34). Risk factors for melanoma include both clinically and/or histologically "atypical moles," increased numbers of acquired "normal" nevi, the dysplastic nevus (DN) syndrome, a family or personal history of melanoma, a personal history of nonmelanoma skin cancer, giant congenital nevi (more than 20 cm), and immunosuppression. The DN syndrome consists of people with at least one or two first- or second-degree relatives with melanoma and numerous nevi, some of which are atypical. People with this syndrome have a relative risk for melanoma from 33 to 1269, with a cumulative lifetime risk of almost 100% (31,35).

PUBLIC HEALTH INITIATIVES AND SCREENING

Efforts have been underway for years with varying amounts of vigor to fight the increased incidence and mortality from melanoma. Perhaps the mortality has not increased as much as incidence because of such efforts, but research has not yet determined this to be the case. Public health efforts aim at primary and secondary prevention strategies.

Primary prevention strategies attempt to prevent one from developing melanoma, mostly through avoiding exposure to the primary risk factor, ultraviolet light. There is particular emphasis on the avoidance of ultraviolet exposure in childhood and young adulthood when it appears the risk is greatest. When strict avoidance cannot be adhered to, sunscreens have been logically recommended. Interestingly, high-quality evidence to support the use of sunscreens has mostly been lacking. In fact, most reports have found no effect or an increased risk of melanoma with sunscreen use. As untenable as this seems, it deserves further evaluation, given the findings. It must be emphasized, however, that these studies showing increased risk are by and large non-randomized case series and/or retrospective analyses with inherent problems. The most obvious and foremost problem with such non-randomized studies is that people, who use more sunscreen, often do so because they are, or perceive themselves to be, at increased risk of melanoma due to behavior or constitutional risk. Furthermore, most of the older studies were performed when sunscreens were neither broad spectrum, nor of high SPF value. On the other hand, one recent randomized study (36) of sunscreen in school children found that children using a broad spectrum SPF 30 sunscreen developed fewer nevi than did those who were not randomized to use sunscreen (median counts, 24 vs. 28; $P = 0.048$). Sunscreen use was much more important for children with freckles than for children without and suggested that freckled children assigned to a broad-spectrum sunscreen intervention would develop 30–40% fewer new nevi than freckled children assigned to the control group (32). As nevi are considered to be the primary risk factor for melanoma, reducing the development of nevi may reduce melanoma risk. Though controversial among certain academicians, there appears to be little doubt among most clinicians and public health agencies on the value of sunscreens. Recently, however, public health campaigns and physicians have advocated sunscreens as part of an overall sun avoidance program and not as a substitute for directly avoiding the sun [information from American Academy of Dermatology (AAD) and American Cancer

Society]. Indeed, it has been hypothesized that one manner by which sunscreens could increase risk of melanoma may be by reducing the sunburn associated with UVB light, while allowing increased exposure time to ultraviolet light and especially harmful UVA light (36). UVA was not previously blocked effectively by less than broad-spectrum sunscreens and at times still may not be blocked effectively. Many current sunscreens are still not good UVA blockers. Sunscreens using physical sun-blocking products, such as zinc and titanium, provide excellent broad-spectrum coverage, but may be less cosmetically appealing and therefore a combination of physical and chemical sunscreens may be the most acceptable. Other research has shown that sunscreens are used incorrectly either in the amount recommended or in the re-application rate (37). Thus, many believe that primary prevention campaigns should focus more on sun avoidance and protective clothing, but still recommend sunscreens as part of an overall program.

Secondary prevention programs include early detection programs. As the outcome of melanoma is directly related to the stage at diagnosis, and as it is commonly held that melanomas take months to years to reach advanced stages, early detection has the potential to save lives. Thus, programs ranging from education of the public on self-screening and recognition of melanomas to physician screenings and screenings by other health professionals have been conducted. The effect of these programs on outcomes has not been extensively studied and there are almost no randomized trials, but there are reports of improvements in intermediate outcomes from some. Epstein et al. (38) in a retrospective study of patients presenting for treatment of melanoma found that just over one-half of the cancers were patient-detected (55%), but physicians were more likely to detect thinner melanomas (median thickness 0.23 mm vs. 0.9 mm; $P < 0.001$). Koh et al. (39) previously found that women are more likely to discover their own melanomas versus men and Epstein's study findings are in agreement with this. Studies such as these point to the fact that often a physician or someone other than the individual with a melanoma is needed to detect it and that this may be associated with earlier-stage melanomas.

The AAD has sponsored adult skin cancer screenings performed by dermatologists since 1985, resulting in more than one million screenings. Of those screened, approximately 50,000 possible nonmelanoma skin cancers and 10,000 possible melanomas have been discovered. Koh et al. (40) reviewed a 1986 and 1987 AAD-sponsored skin cancer-screening program in Massachusetts, which screened 2560 people. Of those screened, 787 (31%) were deemed to have a positive screen, which included suspected melanoma, squamous cell carcinoma, basal cell carcinoma, DN, and congenital nevus. They followed 22 of the 26 suspected melanomas and of these, nine (0.35%) were actually melanomas. Of these nine melanomas, four were in situ, three were superficial spreading melanomas, one was metastatic, and the other was of unknown stage. Of note, the stage distribution of melanoma patients whose lesions were discovered by screening was improved relative to SEER records of melanomas diagnosed in the general population.

Freedberg et al. (13) using similar updated data from AAD screenings in a decision analysis found screening for melanoma to be cost-effective, in the range of $30,000 per year of life saved. In a recent decision analysis, we calculated the cost-effectiveness of a one-time melanoma-screening program in moderately high-risk individuals at $51,000 per year of life saved (11,12). Cost of the screen and prevalence of melanoma in the target-screened group were key variables affecting cost-effectiveness. A recent analysis using a Markov simulation also determined that screening would result in a cost-effectiveness ratio <$50,000 per year of life saved (14). An assumption of these decision analysis studies is that the lesions detected are representative of routinely detected lesions of similar levels. Should a disproportionately large percentage of the lesions detected by screening indeed turn out to be nonaggressive and slow growing, then such decision analyses will suggest better cost-effectiveness ratios than would actually occur in a screening. There is no evidence for or against the assumption that screening may yield a higher proportion of less aggressive melanomas. In fact, the AAD screenings have detected melanomas of all localized Breslow levels as well as regional and metastatic disease, and this is not consistent with screening only detecting "biologically benign" melanomas. Importantly, these studies suggest that screening for melanoma is as cost-effective as many other cancer screening programs we currently perform. In fact, targeting the screenings to higher risk individuals such as those who are light-skinned and burn easily, or have a family history of melanoma, or even just those over age 50, results in a relative bargain in cost-effectiveness relative to other cancer screening programs (discussed subsequently).

Table 1   Cost-Effectiveness of Medical and Public Health Interventions

Intervention	Cost/YLS
Immunizations and fire detectors	Saves dollars and lives
β-Blockers post MI	$850–3000
Airbags + automatic lap belts	$17,000
BP medications for patients aged 40 (DBP 95–104)	$32,000
Lovastatin for men aged 45–54 with no heart disease and cholesterol >300	$34,000
Dialysis for ESRD	$51,000
Banning asbestos	$220,000
Cleaning up uranium toxic waste	Millions

Source: From Ref. 41.

Table 2   Cost-Effectiveness of Common Cancer-Screening Programs

	Cost/YLS	References
Prostate, PSA, one-time age 60	$158,000	(42)
Melanoma, all Caucasians, one-time	$108,000	(11,12)
Colon, FOB + Sigm, age 50–85 years	$93,000	(43)
Cervical, PAP years	$48,000	(44)
Melanoma, one-time all ages, self-selected	$48,000	(11,12)
Melanoma, one-time age >50	$17,000	(11,12)
Breast, mammography years, age 50–79	$17,000	(45)
Melanoma, one-time age >50, males only	$12,000	(11,12)

Education and self-examination are other means by which improved outcomes may be obtained. Berwick et al. (46) in a case-control study of skin self-examination found that melanoma patients who practiced self-examination had lesions that were thinner than those who did not. In a study from Scotland, educational campaigns resulted in a reduction of tumor thickness and a trend toward improved mortality among women (29). Self-examination strategies are a low-cost and seemingly viable way in which to improve outcomes among those who will do such exams. However, the proportion of individuals at risk for melanoma who can realistically be discovered and educated to do such exams prior to developing a melanoma remains unclear.

Currently only the AAD, the National Institutes of Health Consensus Conference on Early Melanoma, and the American Cancer Society recommend population-based screening. The U.S. Preventive Services Task Force, the International Union Against Cancer, and the Australian Cancer Society do not at this time recommend routine screening for melanoma. The reason for the variability in recommendation is the lack of hard evidence from quality studies such as randomized trials. In conclusion, over the last several decades, there have been increases in both melanoma incidence and mortality, but higher increases in incidence than mortality. Increases in incidence may be leveling off. This epidemic has arisen for a variety of reasons, including a true increase in melanomas of malignant behavior, a particularly high increase in localized and in situ lesions, and an increase in the number of biopsies performed that may have resulted in the increased detection of less aggressive lesions. The contribution of possible changes in the diagnostic criteria for melanoma to the increased incidence remains unknown. Ultraviolet light has been conclusively shown in a large number of epidemiological studies to be a factor in the increase in incidence. A variety of primary and secondary preventive strategies for controlling the problem have been attempted and may hold promise for the future. Screening of a targeted, relatively high-risk population for melanoma appears to be a relative bargain in the realm of cancer screening, but further evaluation of these programs is warranted.

REFERENCES

1. Armstrong BK, Kricker A. Cutaneous melanoma. Cancer Surveys 1994; 19:219–239.
2. Giles G, Thursfield V. Trends in skin cancer in Australia. Cancer Forum 1996; 20:188–191.
3. Burton RC, Armstrong BK. Non-metastasizing melanoma? J Surg Oncol 1998; 67(2):73–76.
4. Lamberg L. "Epidemic" of malignant melanoma: true increase or better detection? J Am Med Assc 2002; 287:2201.
5. Swerlick RA, Chen S. The melanoma epidemic. Is increased surveillance the solution or the problem? Arch Dermatol 1996; 132(8):881–884.
6. Dennis LK. Analysis of the melanoma epidemic, both apparent and real: data from the 1973 through 1994 surveillance, epidemiology, and end results program registry. Arch Dermatol 1999; 135(3):275–280.
7. Beddingfield FC III, Cinar P, Litwack S, Ziogas A, Taylor T, Anton-Culver H. An analysis of SEER and the California Cancer Registry data on gender and melanoma incidence. Presented at the Society for Investigative Dermatology, Oral and Poster Presentation, May 2000, Washington DC and at the Chao Family Comprehensive Cancer Center Conference on Carcinogenesis and Cancer Prevention: Non-Melanoma and Melanoma Skin Cancer. Oral presentation, Irvine, CA, June 2001 [abstr]. J Invest Dermatol 2002. In press.
8. Jemal A, Devesa S, Hartge P, Tucker M. Recent trends in cutaneous melanoma incidence among Whites in the United States. JNCI 2001; 93(9):678–683.
9. Surveillance, Epidemiology, and End Results (SEER) Program Public-Use Data (1973–1998), National Cancer Institute, DCCPS, Surveillance Research Program, Cancer Statistics Branch, released April 2001 based on the August 2000 submission.
10. McDonald CJ. Status of screening for cancer. Cancer 1993; 72(suppl):1066–1070.
11. Beddingfield FC III. Is screening for melanoma cost-effective? A decision analysis. Presented at the Society for Investigative Dermatology, Poster and Oral Presentation, Los Angeles, May 2002 [abstr]. J Invest Dermatol 2002. In press.
12. Beddingfield FC III. Melanoma: A Decision Analysis to Estimate the Effectiveness and Cost-Effectiveness of Screening and an Analysis of the Relevant Epidemiology of the Disease. RGSD-167; RGS dissertations, The RAND Corporation, 2003.
13. Freedberg KA, Geller AC, Miller DR, Lew RA, Koh HK. Screening for malignant melanoma: a cost effectiveness analysis. J Am Acad Dermatol 1999; 41:738–745.
14. Losina E, Walensky RP, Geller A, Gilchrest BA, Beddingfield FC III. Screening for malignant melanoma: clinical impact and cost-effectiveness analysis. Medical decision making. Arch Dermatol. In press.
15. Kricker A, Armstrong BK. International trends in skin cancer. Cancer Forum 1996; 20:192–195.
16. Giles GG, Armstrong BK, Burton RC, Staples MP, Thrisfield VJ. Has mortality from melanoma stopped rising in Australia? Analysis of trends between 1931 and 1994. Brit Med J 1996; 312(7039):1121–1125.
17. Lipsker DM, Hedelin G, Heid E, et al. Striking increase in thin melanomas contrasts with a stable incidence in thick melanomas. Arch Dermatol 1999; 135(12):1451–1456.
18. Swerlick RA, Chen S. The melanoma epidemic: more apparent than real? Mayo Clin Proc 1997; 72(6):559–564.

19. Holman CD, Armstrong BK, Heenan PJ, et al. The causes of malignant melanoma: results from the West Australian Lions Melanoma Research Project. Recent results. Cancer Res 1986; 102:18–37.
20. Hall HI, Miller DR, Rogers JD, et al. Update on the incidence and mortality from melanoma in the United States. J Am Acad Dermatol 1999; 40(1):35–42.
21. Wingo PA, Ries LA, Rosenberg HM, et al. Cancer incidence and mortality 1973–1995: a report card for the U.S. Cancer 1998; 82(6):1197–1207.
22. Burton RC, Armstrong BK. Recent incidence trends imply a nonmetastasizing form of invasive melanoma. Melanoma Res 1994; 4(2):107–113.
23. Elwood JM. Melanoma and sun exposure: contrasts between intermittent and chronic exposure. World J Surg 1992; 16:157–165.
24. Lee JAH. The relationship between malignant melanoma of skin and exposure to sunlight. Photochem Photobiol 1989; 50(4):493–496.
25. Wernstock M, Colditz G, Willett W, Stampfer M, Bronstien B, Mihm M, Speizer F. Nonfamilial cutaneous melanoma incidence in women associated with sun exposure before 20 years of age. Paediatrics 1996; 84:199–204.
26. Kok G, Green L. Research to support health promotion practice: a plea for increased co-operation. Health Promo Int 1990; 5(4):303–308.
27. Mackie RM, Marks R, Green A. The melanoma epidemic. Excess exposure to ultraviolet light is established as major risk factor. Brit Med J 1996; 312(7042):1362–1363.
28. Green A, Williams G. UV and skin cancer: epidemiological data from Australia and New Zealand. In: Young AR, Bjorn LO, Moan J, Nultsch W, eds. Environmental UV Photobiology. London: Plenum, 1993:233–254.
29. MacKie RM. The pathogenesis of cutaneous malignant melanoma. Brit Med J 1983; 287:1568–1569.
30. Greene MH, Clark WH, Tucker MA, Kraemer KH, Elder DE, Fraser MC. High risk of malignant melanoma in melanoma-prone families with dysplastic nevi. Ann Intern Med 1985; 102:458–465.
31. Holly EA, Kelly JW, Shpall SN, Chiu S-H. Number of melanocytic nevi as a major risk factor for malignant melanoma. J Am Acad Dermatol 1987; 17:459–468.
32. Slade J, Marghoob AA, Salopek TG, Rigel DS, Kopf AW, Bart RS. Atypical mole syndrome: risk factors for cutaneous malignant melanoma and implications for management. J Am Acad Dermatol 1995; 32:479–494.
33. Swerdlow AJ, English J, Mackie RM, et al. Benign melanocytic naevi as a risk factor for malignant melanoma. Brit Med J 1986; 292:1555–1559.
34. Tucker MA, Halpern A, Holly EA, Hartge P, Elder DE, Sagebiel RW, Guerry D IV, Clark WH Jr. Clinically recognized dysplastic nevi. A central risk factor for cutaneous melanoma. J Am Med Assoc 1997; 277(18):1439–1444.
35. Garbe C, Buettner PG, Weiss J, et al. Risk factors for developing cutaneous melanoma and criteria for identifying persons at risk: multicenter case–control study of the Central Malignant Melanoma Registry of the German Dermatological Society. J Invest Dermatol 1994; 102:695–699.
36. Gallagher RP, Rivers JK, Lee TK, Bajdik CD, McLean DI, Coldman AJ. Broadspectrum sunscreen use and the development of new nevi in white children: a randomized controlled trial. J Am Med Assoc 2000; 283(22):2955–2960.

37. Neale R, Williams G, Green A. Application patterns among participants randomized to daily sunscreen use in a skin cancer prevention trial. Arch Dermatol 2002; 138(10):1319–1325.
38. Epstein DS, Lange JR, Gruber SB, Mofid M, Koch SE. Is physician detection associated with thinner melanomas? J Am Med Assoc 1999; 281(7):640–643.
39. Koh H, Miller D, Geller AC, Clapp RW, Mercer MB, Lew RA. Who discovers melanoma? J Am Acad Dermatol 1992; 26:914–919.
40. Koh HK, Geller AC, Miller DR, Caruso A, Gage I, Lew RA. Who is being screened for melanoma/skin cancer? Characteristics of persons screened in Massachusetts. J Am Acad Dermatol 1991; 24(2 Pt 1):271–277.
41. Tengs TO, Adams ME, Pliskin JS, Safran DG, Siegel JE, Weinstein MC, Graham JD. Five-hundred life-saving interventions and their cost-effectiveness. Risk Anal 1995; 15(3):369–390.
42. Krahn MD, Mahoney JE, et al. Screening for prostate cancer: a decision analytic view. J Am Med Assoc 1994; 272:773–780.
43. Frazier AL, Colditz GA, Fuchs CS, Kuntz KM. Cost-effectiveness of screening for colorectal cancer in the general population. J Am Med Assoc 2000; 284:1954–1961.
44. Eddy DM. Screening for cervical cancer. Ann Int Med 1990; 113:214–226.
45. Lindfors KK, Rosenquist CJ. The cost-effectiveness of mammographic screening strategies. J Am Med Assoc 1995; 274(11):881–884.
46. Berwick M, Begg CB, Fine JA, Roush GC, Barnhill RL. Screening for cutaneous melanoma by skin self-examination. JNCI 1996; 88(1):17–23.
47. Burton RC, Coates MS, Hersey P, et al. An analysis of a melanoma epidemic. Int J Cancer 1993; 55:765–770.
48. MacKie RM, Hole D. Audit of a public education campaign to encourage early detection of malignant melanoma. Brit Med J 1992; 304:1012–1015.

Index